1873410

D1446612

Non-dopamine Lesions in Parkinson's Disease

Non-dopamine Lesions in Parkinson's Disease

Edited by:

Glenda M. Halliday, PhD
Neuroscience Research Australia
School of Medical Sciences
University of New South Wales
Sydney, Australia

Roger A. Barker, PhD
Department of Neurology
Cambridge Centre for Brain Repair
University of Cambridge
Cambridge, UK

Dominic B. Rowe, FRACP, PhD
Department of Neurology
Australian School of Advanced Medicine
Macquarie University
Sydney, Australia

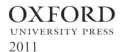

OXFORD
UNIVERSITY PRESS
2011

Oxford University Press, Inc., publishes works that further
Oxford University's objective of excellence
in research, scholarship, and education.

Oxford   New York
Auckland   Cape Town   Dar es Salaam   Hong Kong   Karachi
Kuala Lumpur   Madrid   Melbourne   Mexico City   Nairobi
New Delhi   Shanghai   Taipei   Toronto

With offices in
Argentina   Austria   Brazil   Chile   Czech Republic   France   Greece
Guatemala   Hungary   Italy   Japan   Poland   Portugal   Singapore
South Korea   Switzerland   Thailand   Turkey   Ukraine   Vietnam

Library of Congress Cataloging-in-Publication Data

Non-dopamine lesions in Parkinson's disease / edited by Glenda M. Halliday,
Roger A. Barker, Dominic B. Rowe.
    p. ; cm.
Includes bibliographical references and index.
ISBN 978-0-19-537108-6
1. Parkinson's disease—Pathophysiology.   I. Halliday, Glenda M.
II. Barker, Roger A., 1961–   III. Rowe, Dominic B.
[DNLM: 1. Parkinson Disease—physiopathology.   2. Brain—pathology.
3. Dopamine.   4. Parkinson Disease—complications. WL 359 N8128 2011]
RC382.N637 2011
616.8'33—dc22   2010006010

The science of medicine is a rapidly changing field. As new research and
clinical experience broaden our knowledge, changes in treatment and drug
therapy occur. The author and publisher of this work have checked with sources
believed to be reliable in their efforts to provide information that is accurate and complete,
and in accordance with the standards accepted at the time of publication. However,
in light of the possibility of human error or changes in the practice of medicine,
neither the author, nor the publisher, nor any other party who has been involved in the
preparation or publication of this work warrants that the information contained herein is in
every respect accurate or complete. Readers are encouraged to confirm the information
contained herein with other reliable sources, and are strongly advised to check the product
information sheet provided by the pharmaceutical company for each drug they plan to administer.

9 8 7 6 5 4 3 2 1

Printed in China
on acid-free paper

To the patients we have seen with Parkinson's disease and the colleagues who continue to challenge the way we view the disease.

Preface

We thank Craig Panner for asking us to think about organizing a book on non-dopamine lesions in Parkinson's disease, enthusing us about the idea and concept, and persisting with getting the book finished and published. We are grateful to Heiko Braak for stimulating so much interest in this topic with his landmark studies on the different pathological stages of Parkinson's disease. To be able to provide a comprehensive review of the non-dopamine lesions in Parkinson's disease, their pathophysiology and, where relevant, potential treatments, we are very grateful to our colleagues who said yes to contributing their expertise to this project, and particularly those we coerced to contribute at late stages. This book would really be nothing without their contributions, and it has been a pleasure and privilege to work with them. We also thank Heidi Cartwright who illustrated most of the chapters, making many of the more complex concepts in the book more understandable, as well as providing the main concept for the cover. The cell loss outside the dopamine system and the widespread neural inclusion formation and inflammatory response in the brains of patients with Parkinson's disease have too often been neglected in trying to understand the pathophysiology of their signs and symptoms. It is known that compensatory mechanisms, particularly in non-dopamine systems, must be substantial during the presymptomatic and early symptomatic phases as most patients do not seek medical attention during this time.

Unfortunately, over time the symptoms from these non-dopamine lesions become overwhelming. This book aims to provide a comprehensive assessment of how non-dopamine lesions contribute to both the diagnostic motor symptoms and the many additional symptoms that patients with Parkinson's disease have, including those that occur following symptomatic treatments. We hope that it will stimulate further advances in understanding the effects and progression of Parkinson's disease.

Glenda M. Halliday
Roger A. Barker
Dominic B. Rowe

Introduction

When James Parkinson first described the condition which now bears his name, he commented only on the motor features of the condition. This is not surprising, given the way in which neurological practice was undertaken and understood in the early part of the 19th century. Indeed, most of what Parkinson saw in his cases was in patients he observed walking along the streets of London rather than following detailed examinations in his consulting rooms[1].

Charcot, who gave Parkinson his due by naming the condition after him, was the first to show how the motor features of Parkinson's Disease (PD) may be helped by drugs—in particular anti-cholinergics[2]. Lewy then added his body to the story in the early part of the twentieth century when he described the pathology of PD, although why Lewy bodies form and what defines them is still a matter of debate[3]. Nevertheless, the discovery in the 1980s that they contain ubiquitin and in the 1990s, α-synuclein, has been important not only in allowing for them to be better detected immunohistochemically, but also in showing that they are intimately linked to the protein pathology of this condition.

Prior to these discoveries, in the 1960s it was shown that the central chemical deficit that defined PD was the loss of the then newly discovered neurotransmitter, dopamine[4]. The recognition that the loss of this specific transmitter lay at the heart of PD, led quickly to the development of dopaminergic drug therapies and the "awakening" of patients out of their akinetic disease state. This was then followed by the descriptions of a range of complications with L-dopa medications, including the development of dyskinesias and "on-off" phenomena[5]. Nevertheless, the powerful symptomatic benefits of L-dopa therapy were clear to see, and **Fahn and Halliday** in their chapter take us through the basis of this, both clinically and pathologically.

This ability to treat the motor features of PD with increasing success and sophistication[6], whilst undoubtedly true, has also revealed that not all the motor aspects of PD respond well to such therapeutic interventions—especially the gait disorder and tremor. This therefore raises the possibility that areas outside the nigrostriatal dopaminergic pathway may be involved in some of the motor manifestations of the disease process; a claim supported by the increasing evidence that PD has as many non-motor, as motor, features. This latter work concentrated on two main areas—namely the development of dementia in some patients with PD and cognitive deficits as a result of the dopaminergic dysfunction in PD [reviewed in[7]].

This realization that PD has non-motor features has grown over the last 40 years, as the ability to treat the motor problems continues to improve, allowing these other features to become more manifest and seen to be independent of dopaminergic systems. So for example, it has become clear that the depression of PD is not simply a reactive response to being given the diagnosis of PD, nor is it just a misdiagnosis of undertreated motor aspects of the disease, but a fundamental feature of the disorder. In this book, **Ehrt, Pedersen and Aarsland** discuss these aspects of PD, along with issues to do with apathy. This latter state is a difficult one to define, in so much as many features of depression can be construed as being apathetic, and vice versa. It is therefore useful to have this distinction dissected by these authors as they seek to describe the frequency of such features in PD, their basis, and how best they can be treated.

In a similar way, the sleep-related disorders of PD are now seen to be a central part of the disease rather than a reflection of poor nocturnal motor control and/or a side-effect of dopaminergic medication. Indeed, sleep problems may even precede the motor problems of the condition. That is not to say that inadequate motor control cannot contribute to sleep problems in PD, it is just not the only explanation. As **Hartmann and Halliday** discuss in their chapter on sensory abnormalities and pain in PD, these symptoms are not uncommon in PD, especially at night. Although this may be explained in terms of restless leg syndrome or early morning painful "off" dystonias, there is clear evidence that sensory processing can be abnormal and pain a feature of basal ganglia disorders[8].

This recognition that the non-motor features of PD exist is not only because we can now treat advanced motor PD with a whole range of novel therapies (e.g. DBS; Duodopa®), but because we now have more sophisticated ways to look for pathology.

PD can still only be diagnosed with certainty at death with the demonstration of α-synuclein positive Lewy body pathology in the substantia nigra. The development of immunohistochemistry in the 1970s and the identification of some of the key proteins involved in its pathogenesis, most notably α-synuclein in the 1990s, has led to a redefinition of the extent of pathology in this disease. So it is now possible to see that in all cases of PD, the α-synuclein pathology extends beyond the substantia nigra and involves a whole range of CNS (and even non-CNS) structures.

In this respect, Braak and colleagues have been instrumental in the evolution of this debate as they proposed a new pathological classification based on α-synuclein immunohistochemistry, in which involvement of the substantia nigra occurred at stage 3 of a 6 stage process[9]. The earliest pathology (namely stages 1 and 2) in their classification involves the lower brainstem, in areas linked to more "primitive" processes having to do with sleep, autonomic, and enteric functions. This redefinition of the pathological staging of PD has in turn had two major consequences to the field: (i) it has led many clinicians to search for the earliest non-motor clinical markers of PD[10] and (ii) it has led to new ideas on pathogenesis and in particular the extent to which PD may be a prion-like disease starting outside the CNS[11].

This search for the earliest features of PD, ahead of overt motor disease (the so-called prodromal stage of PD), has concentrated especially on sleep, as the development of a REM sleep behavioral disorder years ahead of the motor problems of PD now seems to be a common finding. This, though, is only one of the problems with sleep in PD, as **Unger, Oertel, Thannickal, Lai and Siegel** discuss in their chapter. It is now apparent that patients have a range of other abnormalities including daytime somnolence, which came to the fore following the problems with sudden sleep attacks and the use of newer dopamine agonists in the 1990s.

Other predictions from the Braak staging of pathology in PD would be early problems in olfaction, and this seems to be the case as discussed by **Doty, Hawkes and Berendse** in their chapter on lesions associated with olfactory dysfunction. The early loss of olfactory discrimination in PD has been proposed by some to be a useful marker by which to diagnose PD. However, it is clear that this sensory system is targeted by many neurodegenerative diseases, and thus is not a unique feature of PD. Nevertheless, it may be useful in establishing the diagnosis as some patients do report a loss of smell as part of their disease.

The extent to which there is autonomic and enteric nervous system involvement in PD is a controversial area, but there is no doubt that both systems are intimately wrapped up in the disease process. In the chapters by **Minguez-Castellanos and Rowe, and Post and Papapetropoulos**, this is fully explored and includes a discussion on when these problems first emerge in the course of the illness- and the extent to which they precede the motor features of PD—as Braak again would predict. This is a difficult area in clinical practice, as early prominent autonomic involvement would make one suspect the related synucleinopathy, multiple systems atrophy (MSA), as the diagnosis rather than PD.

In clinic, one of the useful questions to ask of patients referred with the possible diagnosis of PD is to do with their speech, more especially whether they have noticed their speech becoming quieter and/or difficulty with raising their voice. This can be misinterpreted as a hearing loss in the carer or partner, but is in fact part of the condition, and difficulties in this aspect of speech production can also evolve to problems with articulation, both of which tend to get worse as the disease progresses whilst language comprehension and generation is typically unaffected. In their chapter, **Bentivoglio, Quaranta, and Ho** explore all these features of PD both in terms of the pathological basis of the articulatory problems, as well as how they can best be treated at the different stages of disease—a discussion that is extended to other bulbar functions such as swallowing and sialorrhea by **Cersosimo and Benarroch**. These authors make the point that some of these symptoms are socially embarrassing, such as the sialorrhea, whilst others can be life threatening and need treatment by invasive procedures such as PEG feeding. Both can cause the patient great distress and may lead to social isolation as they refuse to go out given they are self conscious about these difficulties with eating and dribbling. Some of these features can be helped by medication, most notably the sialorrhea with anti-cholinergic medications, but this therapy runs the risk of worsening the cognitive deficits that many patients with PD develop.

The cognitive deficits of PD are becoming increasingly recognized as a major problem, especially in advancing disease where the development of visual hallucinations coupled to visuospatial difficulties and intermittent confusion typically heralds the dementia of PD. The basis of the hallucinations and psychoses of PD is not fully understood at the neurochemical or neuropathological level, but **Williams and Poewe** discuss this and generally support the idea that the hallucinations may have more of a cholinergic basis[12], whilst the psychosis is thought of more as a dopaminergic disorder[7]. In both cases though, the primary problem is Lewy body pathology in visual association areas.

In the chapter by **Evans, Revesz, and Barker**, they explore the range of cognitive deficits in PD, and their neurochemical and neuropathological basis and significance. They suggest that not all cognitive deficits in PD are a harbinger of PD dementia, and that there may be discrete, different cognitive syndromes in PD[13] and one of these has a basis in the frontostriatal dopaminergic network. This has implications as to how best to use dopaminergic treatments at different stages of disease.

Indeed, dopaminergic therapies are well known to exacerbate the cognitive deficits in PD in some cases, whilst in other individuals this type of drug can produce their own problems in terms of alterations in behavior especially with some of the newer types of dopamine agonists in younger patients. This treatment complication has only really been recognized in the last 10 years, and much of the work in this area has been done by **Andrew Evans,** whose chapter summarizes this field of work. One of the key questions in this area of dopamine dysregulation syndromes, is why do some patients develop this problem and others not? Why does it take different formats in different people? And more pragmatically, how can one treat it short of stopping their dopaminergic therapy with all the motor complications that will ensue from such a maneuver? Issues that are all discussed in this chapter.

Therefore, this book attempts to draw together all these strands of PD symptomatology and pathology to give a more complete picture of this disorder, with the hope that by better recognizing the range of deficits and their basis, the better we will become at treating them.

Roger A. Barker
Cambridge
October 2009

References

1. Williams DR (2007). James Parkinson's London. *Mov Disord.* 22:1857–9.
2. Elmer L (2005) Paralysis agitans- refining the diagnosis and treatment. In Ebadi M and Pfeiffer RF, eds. *Parkinson's Disease.* CRC Press. Pp11–19.
3. Harrower TP, Michell AW, Barker RA (2005). Lewy bodies in Parkinson's disease: protectors or perpetrators? *Exp Neurol.* 195:1–6.
4. Hornykiewicz O (2007). Dopamine, levodopa and Parkinson's disease. *ACNR.* 6:14.
5. Poewe W (2009) Treatments for Parkinson disease–past achievements and current clinical needs. *Neurology.* 72(7 Suppl):S65–73.
6. Lewis SJG, Caldwell MA, Barker RA (2003). Modern therapeutic approaches in Parkinson's disease. *Exp Review in Molecular Med.* 5:1–20.

7. Williams-Gray C, Lewis SJG, Barker RA (2006). Cognitive deficits in Parkinson's disease: A review of the pathophysiology and therapeutic options. *CNS* Drugs 20: 477–505.

8. Barker RA (1988). The basal ganglia and pain. *Int J Neurosci.* 41:29–34.

9. Braak H, Bohl JR, Müller CM, Rüb U, de Vos RA, Del Tredici K (2006). Stanley Fahn Lecture 2005: The staging procedure for the inclusion body pathology associated with sporadic Parkinson's disease reconsidered. *Mov Disord.* 21:2042–51.

10. Hawkes CH (2008). The prodromal phase of sporadic Parkinson's disease: does it exist and if so how long is it? *Mov Disord.* 23:1799–807.

11. Brundin P, Li JY, Holton JL, Lindvall O, Revesz T (2008). Research in motion: the enigma of Parkinson's disease pathology spread. *Nat Rev Neurosci.* 9:741–5.

12. Manganelli F, Vitale C, Santangelo G, et al. (2009). Functional involvement of central cholinergic circuits and visual hallucinations in Parkinson's disease. *Brain.* 132:2350–5.

13. Williams-Gray CH, Evans J, Goris A, et al. (2009). The distinct cognitive syndromes of Parkinson's disease: 5 year follow-up of the CamPaIGN cohort. *Brain* 132:2958–69.

Contents

Contributors

Dag Aarsland, MD, PhD
Section of Geriatric Psychiatry
Division of Psychiatric
Stavanger University Hospital,
Stavanger, Norway

Roger A. Barker, PhD
Department of Neurology
Cambridge Centre for Brain Repair
University of Cambridge
Cambridge, UK

Eduardo E. Benarroch, MD
Department of Neurology
Mayo Clinic
Rochester, MN

Anna Rita Bentivoglio, MD, PhD
Institute of Neurology
Department of Neuroscience
Catholic University
Rome, Italy

Henk W. Berendse, MD, PhD
Neuroscience Campus Amsterdam
Department of Neurology
VU University Medical Center
Amsterdam, The Netherlands

Maria G. Cersosimo, MD
Parkinson's Disease and Movement Disorder Unit
Hospital de Clínicas
University of Buenos Aires
Buenos Aires, Argentina

Richard L. Doty, PhD
Smell and Taste Center
Department of Otorhinolaryngology: Head and Neck Surgery
University of Pennsylvania School of Medicine
Philadelphia, PA

Uwe Ehrt, MD
Section of Geriatric Psychiatry
Division of Psychiatric
Stavanger University Hospital,
Stavanger, Norway

Andrew H. Evans, FRACP
Department of Neurology
The Royal Melbourne Hospital
Melbourne Neuropsychiatry Centre; and
Department of Medicine
University of Melbourne
Parkville, Australia

Jonathan R. Evans, MD, MRCP
Department of Neurology
Cambridge Centre for Brain Repair
University of Cambridge
Cambridge, UK

Stanley Fahn, MD
Division of Movement Disorders
Department of Neurology
Columbia University
New York, NY

Glenda M. Halliday, PhD
Neuroscience Research Australia
School of Medical Sciences
University of New South Wales
Sydney, Australia

Andreas Hartmann, MD, PhD
Centre d'Investigation Clinique
Hôpital de la Pitié-Salpêtrière
Paris, France

Christopher H. Hawkes, MD, FRCP
Neuroscience Centre
Institute of Cell and Molecular Science
Barts and The London School of Medicine and Dentistry
4 Newark Street
London E1 2AT

Aileen K. Ho, PhD
Department of Psychology
School of Psychology and Clinical Language Sciences
University of Reading
Reading, UK

Yuan-Yang Lai, PhD
Departments of Psychiatry and Biobehavioral Sciences
University of California at Los Angeles
Los Angeles, CA

Andrew W. Michell, MRCP, PhD
Consultant in Clinical Neurophysiology,
Department of Clinical Neurosciences,
Addenbrooke's Hospital,
Cambridge, UK

Adolfo Mínguez-Castellanos, MD, PhD
Servicio de Neurología
Hospital Universitario Virgen de las Nieves
Universidad de Granada
Granada, Spain

Wolfgang H. Oertel, MD
Department of Neurology
Philipps-University Marburg
Marburg, Germany

Spyridon Papapetropoulos, MD, PhD
Department of Neurology
Division of Movement Disorders
University of Miami, Miller School of Medicine
Miami, Fl

Kenn F. Pedersen, PhD
Norwegian Centre for Movement Disorders
Stavanger University Hospital
Stavanger, Norway

Werner Poewe, MD
Department of Neurology
Medical University of Innsbruck
Innsbruck, Austria

Kathryn K. Post, MD
Department of Neurology
Division of Movement Disorders
University of Miami, Miller School of Medicine
Miami, Fl

Davide Quaranta, MD
Neuropsychology and Neurorehabilitation Unit
Institute of Neurology
Department of Neuroscience
Catholic University
Rome, Italy

Tamas Revesz, MD, FRCPath
Division of Neuropathology
Institute of Neurology
University College London
London, UK

Dominic B. Rowe, FRACP, PhD
Department of Neurology
Australian School of Advanced Medicine
Macquarie University
Sydney, Australia

Jerome M. Siegel, PhD
Departments of Psychiatry and Biobehavioral Sciences
University of California at Los Angeles
Los Angeles, CA

Thomas C. Thannickal, PhD
Departments of Psychiatry and Biobehavioral Sciences
University of California at Los Angeles
Los Angeles, CA

Marcus M. Unger, MD
Department of Neurology
Philipps-University Marburg
Marburg, Germany

David R. Williams PhD, FRACP
Van Cleef Roet Centre for Nervous Diseases
Monash University
Melbourne, Australia

Non-dopamine Lesions in
Parkinson's Disease

Chapter 1

Lesions Associated with the Classic Triad of Parkinsonian Motor Features

Stanley Fahn and Glenda M. Halliday

Parkinson's disease (PD) is clinically defined by its movement disorder, which was first described by James Parkinson in 1817.[1] His account included "involuntary tremulous motion… in parts not in action… with a propensity to bend the trunk forward, and to pass from a walking to a running pace, the senses and intellect being uninjured." Thus, he described tremor-at-rest, flexed posture and festinating gait due to the person's center of gravity being in front of his feet. As the disease progresses, movements "are accomplished with considerable difficulty, the hand failing to answer with exactness the dictates of the will." In this sentence, Parkinson is referring to what is now called bradykinesia and hypokinesia (slowness and decreased amplitude of voluntary movement). These classic features are still considered the core symptoms of PD that are largely initially responsive to levodopa therapy in cases with typical disease.

Classic Parkinsonian Motor Features

The classic clinical triad of parkinsonian motor features is bradykinesia, rigidity and rest tremor. However, there is considerable clinical heterogeneity in the dominance of these features and only two of these features are necessary for a clinical diagnosis of PD in association with levodopa responsiveness.[2] A flexed posture, as noted in Parkinson's description, develops later in the disease. A loss of normal postural control can also be a motor feature of PD, although this feature is not common early and is often more dominant in other forms of parkinsonism. A sixth motor feature that can appear, also occurring late, has been called the "freezing phenomenon," in which the person's feet get transiently "glued to the ground." Both loss of postural stability and the freezing phenomenon can lead to falls, and these are a major source of disability in advanced PD. Flexed posture, postural instability and the freezing phenomenon are largely unresponsive to levodopa therapy and will not be discussed or considered with the more typical clinical triad in this chapter.

Bradykinesia/hypokinesia or poverty of movement—Within the triad of early motor features of PD, poverty of movement is the main problem in causing disability of activities of daily living for most patients. Features of cranial bradykinesia are loss of facial expression, decreased frequency of blinking, reduced amplitude of voice with loss of inflection, and reduced frequency of spontaneous swallowing resulting in accumulation and drooling of saliva. Features of limb bradykinesia are a smaller and slower handwriting, and difficulty shaving, brushing teeth, and putting on make-up. Walking becomes slow, with shortened stride length, decreased arm swing, and with a tendency to shuffle feet. Difficulty arising from a deep chair, getting out of automobiles, and turning in bed are symptoms of truncal bradykinesia.

From clinical observation, the actual composition of movement is preserved, and when a slow movement is all that is required PD patients have little difficulty, even if the movement requires fine control and accurate sensory feedback. This suggests limited qualitative problems with the motor programs that determine the actual structure and control of movement. The specific PD deficit is in the speed of movement. Rapid movements normally consist of a triphasic pattern of agonist burst, antagonist burst and second agonist burst.[3] The antagonist burst functions to brake the initial pulse of movement, while the second agonist burst dampens down the unstable oscillations that might otherwise result.[3] As perhaps expected, the basic motor program of the triphasic pattern is preserved in PD. However, instead of a single triphasic pattern, there is a whole series of smaller triphasic bursts as the motor system "underestimates" and then corrects for the effort required.[3] In this way PD patients adopt a strategy usually reserved for large movements in normal subjects, where movement amplitude is scaled by varying movement duration rather than movement speed.[3] This movement deficit therefore suggests a quantitative problem, with poor scaling of agonist bursts rather than a limit on size, and a relative tardiness in development of maximal force.[3]

While bradykinesia is one of the main movement problems in typical PD, there is considerable clinical heterogeneity in the severity of this feature and its progression over time. Individual variability in the annual rate of progression can be from 0.5% to 8.9% of the maximum motor score possible.[4,5] However, it should be noted that on average there is a consistent, significant decline in the bradykinesia sub-scores throughout the course of the disease in patients with PD.[6]

Rigidity or increased muscle tone in the resting state when not actively engaged in voluntary activity—This rigidity in PD appears to be due to increased activity of the main descending drive from the CNS to the muscles, that is an increase in tonic reflex mechanisms.[3] This notion is supported by the fact that steady-state reflexes, polysynaptic reflexes mediated by skin afferents, long latency (possibly transcortical) reflexes to maintain stretch, and the tonic vibration reflex all tend to be increased in PD, but the H-reflex remains normal.[3] In other words, rigidity in PD reflects the fact that patients' muscles are never at rest, but subject instead to a continuous descending activation which at the same time activates the more complex steady-state reflexes.[3]

Like bradykinesia, there is also considerable clinical heterogeneity in the severity of rigidity in PD and its progression over time. Similar individual variability in the annual rate of progression of rigidity can be observed.[4,5] However, in contrast to bradykinesia, there is a slowing in the rate of decline in measures of rigidity as the disease progresses,[5] particularly with follow-up over 4 years and with significantly more advanced disease.[4,6]

Resting tremor—The characteristic PD tremor is a 4–6 Hz distal resting tremor, although patients may have a resting tremor, an action tremor, or both. It is most commonly unilateral in onset, lost during sleep and inhibited during movement, but may reoccur with the same frequency when adopting a posture.[7] It is worsened by excitement, anxiety, or apprehension. Unlike the other typical motor features of PD, resting tremor does not show any significant progression over time.[5,6]

The classic triad of motor features is initially responsive to dopamine replacement therapies in patients considered to have typical PD, with levodopa the most effective agent.[8] However, these drugs do not have an immediate antiparkinsonian effect, and it may take several days to weeks of high dosage therapy to achieve the desired degree of benefit. This is due to a priming effect, and because the treatment response is not equivalent for all PD features. Bradykinesia and rigidity have the most benefit from dopamine replacement therapies over time, whereas the therapeutic response for tremor is much more variable as it is sometimes quite resistant to dopamine replacement therapies.[9] While oral dopamine replacement therapies have been a revolutionary breakthrough for the treatment of PD, the progression of the disease and ongoing compensatory mechanisms cause motor fluctuations and dyskinesias often after 5 years of treatment.[10] Over time, the clinical severity becomes similar to the level prior to therapy and additional, more disabling, clinical features become evident.[10]

Clinical Heterogeneity of Classic Parkinson's Disease

It has been known for some time that clinical cohorts of patients with PD are heterogeneous, even excluding those who are not responsive to dopamine replacement therapies. Clinical phenotypes include those with different symptoms (resting tremor versus akinesia and rigidity and/or postural instability and gait disorder), with differing rates of progression (rapid versus slow) and with different ages of onset (early versus late), often with overlap between these phenotypes.[11] Even the responsiveness to levodopa, such as those who develop motor fluctuations and those who do not, represents differences between patients with pathologically proven PD.[12] A recent study using exploratory factor analysis in a data-driven approach identified bradykinesia and rigidity as strongly related clinical features, whereas rest tremor was separate and unrelated to these cardinal motor features in PD.[13] It is therefore not surprising that the classic motor triad is found in only a minority of PD cases at onset, with around 25% of cases never having rest tremor and only approximately 50% having rest tremor as a dominant feature.[14,15] It is more difficult to determine the true prevalence of the other two cardinal motor features, as they are more likely to be discussed together in the literature. However, of these two motor features, bradykinesia is considered more prevalent and is a core feature for the clinical diagnosis of PD in the UK Brain Bank criteria.[2] As stated above, this motor feature worsens over time and appears to become the dominant motor feature in many PD patients, progressing to marked slowness and immobility.

In three independent cohort studies using cluster analysis, two to four clinical subtypes have been consistently identified depending on when in the disease course the patients have been assessed.[16–18] After ten years only two subtypes are seen, whereas at five years there are three subtypes, and a fourth rapidly progressive and under-reported subtype is found only very early in the disease process (this subtype has a rapid progression to dementia).[16–18] The three main subtypes are (1) those with a younger onset (around the age of 50 years), (2) those with tremor dominant PD (with both of these subtypes having a longer benign disease course), and

(3) a non-tremor dominant subtype of later onset with a shorter disease course and with cognitive deficits occurring only a few years into the course of the disease. Cognitive deficits, however, appear to be related to the age of patient and not solely to the phenotype of PD.[12] These studies confirm the wide variability in the type and progression of PD observed in individual patients.

Diagnostic Pathology

There are two pathological features required for a diagnosis of PD—substantial loss of the dopaminergic pigmented neurons in the substantia nigra, and the finding of Lewy body inclusions in remaining brainstem pigmented neurons (Fig. 1-1). Both features characterize PD but are not found only in PD, although when these features occur in the absence of other degenerative pathologies there is a high likelihood that the patient had at least some of the cardinal motor features of PD. Significant loss of the dopaminergic pigmented neurons in the substantia nigra is also a feature of other parkinsonian conditions (multiple system atrophy, progressive supranuclear palsy, corticobasal degeneration) and Lewy body inclusions in brainstem pigmented neurons are also a feature of dementia with Lewy bodies.[19] In some cases of dementia with Lewy bodies, significant loss of the dopaminergic pigmented neurons in the substantia nigra also occurs [19] and α-synuclein-positive Lewy bodies can also be a feature of many cases with Alzheimer's disease, although their distribution varies.[20,21] The main difference between such cases and those with motor PD is the co-occurrence of other age-related neurodegenerative pathologies in addition to the pathologies of PD.

Both PD-related pathologies progress over time, with greater degeneration of the dopaminergic pigmented cells within the nigra with longer disease durations [22–25] as well as more Lewy body infiltration in the brain with longer disease durations.[26,27] At the onset of motor symptoms, a proportion of the pigmented cell population in the brainstem already have abnormal inclusions in their cytoplasm, and as the disease progresses, inclusion pathology infiltrates higher centers in the forebrain in a stereotypic fashion.[26,27] This infiltration of Lewy body inclusions is extremely slow, taking 13 years on average for 50% of PD patients to have Lewy bodies in limbic regions of the forebrain and 18 years for all PD patients to have such pathology.[27] At present there is only speculation concerning the pathophysiology behind the continued progression of these neuronal inclusions from one cell population to another.

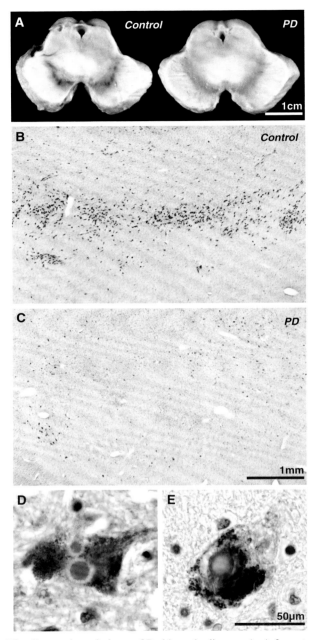

Figure 1-1. The diagnostic pathology of Parkinson's disease. A. A 3mm transverse midbrain slice at the level of the decussation of the superior cerebellar peduncle showing a well-pigmented control substantia nigra pars compacta (at left) and a de-pigmented substantia nigra pars compacta in a patient with Parkinson's disease (PD, at right). B. A cresyl violet-stained 50μm transverse tissue section through the substantia nigra, showing the normal

Cell Loss and α-Synuclein Deposition Within Systems Regulating Movement

Volitional movements are achieved by descending neural drive from so-called 'motor cortical' centers generating corticospinal and corticobulbar outputs, with the pyramidal tract containing the bulk of direct corticofugal outputs destined to recruit spinal motoneurons.[28] There is no cell loss and limited α-synuclein deposition in these descending pathways in PD,[29] and patients with PD are capable of normal movement, supporting an absence of significant pathology within these descending corticospinal and corticobulbar pathways.

Two subcortical systems are crucial for adequate volitional movement: cortical interactions with the motor thalamus and the integration of information through the basal ganglia.[30] The basal ganglia comprise a large number of integrated regions, which, when lesioned, impact the motor system at the level of the thalamus and brainstem. Depending on the location of lesions or stimulation, there can be extreme poverty of all movements, abnormal postures, and/or uncontrollable rhythmic motor outputs.[31] Basal ganglia regions include the caudate nucleus, putamen, internal and external segments of the globus pallidus, subthalamic nucleus and substantia nigra, while thalamic regions participating in motor control include specific ventral, posterior and intralaminar nuclei.[32] These regions have complex anatomical interconnections. Cortical drive to initiate movement is received by the primary motor cortex from a number of specialized nearby cortical regions (the ventral and dorsal premotor areas, supplementary motor areas, and cingulate motor areas) that provide strong excitatory drive to the large layer V pyramidal output neurons, as well as reinforce the thalamic input to these neurons.[33] The thalamus is the main facilitator of information transfer from one cortical region to another through a feedforward mechanism.[34] In particular, the ventral anterior thalamus feeds forward executive information to premotor cortices (under basal ganglia influence), the ventrolateral anterior thalamus feeds forward premotor

---

Figure 1-1. (continued)
distribution of darkly pigmented dopaminergic neurons. Scale equivalent to that in C. C. A cresyl violet-stained 50μm transverse tissue section through the substantia nigra of a patient with Parkinson's disease (PD) showing a severe loss of the pigmented dopaminergic neurons. D. High magnification hematoxylin and eosin-stained 10μm midbrain tissue section showing 2 round haloed eosinophilic Lewy bodies within a pigmented nigral neuron from a patient with Parkinson's disease. Scale equivalent to E. E. High magnification 10μm midbrain tissue section immunohistochemically stained for α-synuclein and counterstained with cresyl violet, showing a positive round haloed Lewy body within a pigmented nigral neuron from a patient with Parkinson's disease.

information to the primary motor cortex (under basal ganglia and cerebellar influence), and the ventrolateral posterior thalamus provides feedback from the primary motor cortex (under cerebellar influence). These reciprocal and non-reciprocal cortico-thalamo-cortical connections form cohesive integrated circuits for the overall control of movement.[34]

As required for diagnosis, there is substantial degeneration of the dopaminergic pigmented neurons in the substantia nigra that project to the caudate nucleus and putamen, with the innervation of the posterior putamen affected first and most severely, and α-synuclein deposition found within a proportion of remaining nigral neurons. In addition to the loss of dopaminergic regulation in PD, there is also a substantial loss of the glutamatergic projection from the caudal intralaminar nuclei of the thalamus to the caudate nucleus and putamen in PD, again with the putamen innervation bearing the brunt of the degeneration.[35] However, there is no deposition of α-synuclein in the remaining caudal intralaminar neurons.[35,36] This substantial denervation of the putamen and caudate nucleus results in a significant remodelling of the GABAergic projection neurons in these regions to lose their spines and significantly change their dynamic regulation.[37,38] However, there is no further substantial cell loss or α-synuclein deposition in these neurons or neurons in other regions of the basal ganglia or motor thalamus in PD. There is, however, a selective loss of glutamatergic projection neurons in the presupplementary motor area in PD, again without significant α-synuclein deposition.[29] These cortical neurons are active before the onset of movement and innervate the premotor cortices to assist with the selection of and preparation for the specific movements required. As stated above, there is no further loss of cortical neurons in PD.[29]

Overall cell loss in the motor system in PD is not restricted to the loss of the dopaminergic innervation of the putamen (and over time the caudate nucleus), but also involves a loss of the glutamatergic innervation from the thalamus to the same basal ganglia regions and a remodelling of the inhibitory projection neurons in these regions. In addition, there is a substantial loss of the glutamatergic projection neurons from the presupplementary motor cortex to the premotor cortices in PD, and for the most part these changes are not accompanied by a significant deposition of α-synuclein. The pathologies within these regions directly regulating movement are schematically depicted in Figure 1-2.

Pathophysiology Relating to Motor Symptoms

Dopamine release within the putamen improves rigidity and bradykinesia, but not resting tremor in PD.[39] This supports the dogma that different brain

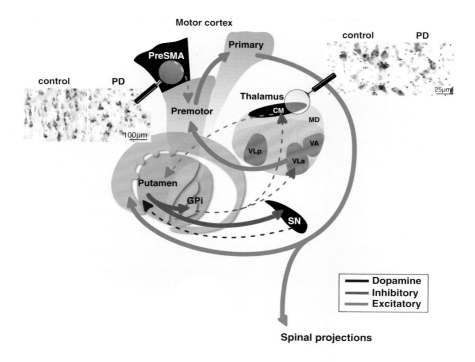

Figure 1-2. Diagram of the main motor pathways affected in Parkinson's disease (PD). Two major inputs to the putamen degenerate in PD, the dopaminergic SN and the glutaminergic CM. This causes significant remodeling of the projection neurons in the putamen and an increase in their inhibitory activity on the GPi and SN. Disinhibition of the input from the GPi to the VLa increases the excitatory drive to the premotor and motor cortices, increasing descending tone in the spinal motor pathways in patients with PD. In addition to these changes within the basal ganglia circuit, there is a loss of the initiating motor input from the pyramidal neurons in the preSMA to the premotor cortex in PD, leaving modulation by the basal ganglia circuit as the dominant influence on motor output. Photomicrographs at left show the loss of pyramidal neurons in the preSMA in PD. Further specific staining techniques have revealed that the population of neurons lost are the short corticocortical projection neurons.[29] Photomicrographs at right show the loss of projection neurons in the CM in PD. Further specific staining techniques have revealed that the population of neurons lost are those projecting to the putamen.[29] CM=centromedial nucleus of the caudal intralaminar thalamus, GPi=internal segment of the globus pallidus, MD=mediodorsal thalamus, preSMA=presupplementary motor cortex, SN=substantia nigra, VA=ventral anterior thalamus, VLa=ventrolateral anterior thalamus, VLp=ventrolateral posterior thalamus.

circuits mediate these different motor features, with even potential differences in the brain circuits mediating rigidity and bradykinesia.

There are considerable similarities in the progression of dopaminergic cell loss in the substantia nigra,[22–25] the progression of dopamine terminal depletion in the putamen,[40–42] and the progression of the severity of rigidity (see above), to link these features in PD. In all cases there appears to be a faster progression in the early versus the later phases of PD. The severity of rigidity has been correlated with the degree of dopamine terminal depletion in many but not all studies (eg.[43–45]) and, as stated above, dopamine release within the putamen improves rigidity.[39] The severity of motor deficits directly correlates with the severity of degeneration of the dopaminergic substantia nigra,[25] and the severity of α-synuclein deposition in the degenerating substantia nigra inversely correlates with the amount of remaining dopamine terminals in the putamen.[46] These correlations suggest that a reduction in putaminal dopamine due to the degeneration of nigrostriatal neurons increases descending drive in the corticospinal tract, a finding consistent with increased metabolic activity in the primary motor cortex in patients with PD.[42]

Bradykinesia is also responsive to dopamine replacement therapies, but as discussed previously, has a different progression to that observed for rigidity and the loss of the nigrostriatal dopaminergic projection. The different dynamics may indicate involvement of the presupplementary motor cortex degeneration in the development of this clinical feature. The selective loss of the corticocortical innervation from the presupplementary cortex to the supplementary motor and premotor areas in PD overlaps with the thalamocortical innervation of the supplementary motor and premotor areas that are most influenced by the basal ganglia, and therefore by any dopamine replacement therapy in PD patients. This places the impact of these two deficits on the same premotor cortical regions (particularly the supplementary motor area) with perhaps the initial response to dopamine replacement therapy able to overcome both deficits. Of interest is the substantial innervation of the putamen by the supplementary motor area with activation of the circuit from the supplementary motor cortex through the putamen, globus pallidus, and thalamus, to the primary motor cortex directly related to the rate of self-generated fine-finger movement.[47] Of even greater interest is the increased metabolism in exactly this circuit in patients with PD, a change that is largely unaffected by dopamine replacement therapies.[42] If these PD-related changes were generated by the loss of the non-dopaminergic presupplementary motor neurons, the changes in the metabolic circuits noted in PD patients[42] would be predicted.

From direct recordings, the resting tremor of PD appears to arise from spontaneous oscillatory activity in the ventrolateral anterior thalamus.[48]

This part of the thalamus provides the feed-forward regulation of premotor information to the primary motor cortex and is under both basal ganglia and cerebellar regulation.[34] Changes in the dynamic regulation of this thalamic region by the cerebellum versus the basal ganglia appear to play a role in the generation of resting tremor. Lesions or high frequency stimulation of this region of the thalamus permanently improves PD resting tremor in 80% of cases.[49] Depending on the role of either basal ganglia disruption or changes in cerebellar regulation of this region of the thalamus, dopamine replacement therapies may or may not significantly influence the resting tremor in patients with PD.

In addition to the generation of the classic clinical motor triad by the degenerative changes in the motor system found in patients with PD, additional motor complications occur over time in association with levodopa replacement therapies. The initial long duration benefit most patients have with levodopa wanes, resulting in clinically detectable fluctuations in the rapidity of onset and duration of benefit of a medication dose.[50,51] In some patients there can be a sudden loss of movement unrelated to the timing of medication dose,[52] there may be significantly worsening of motor features at the onset or end of a dose, or there can be a complete dose failure. Dose failures are often due to gastrointestinal factors relating to absorption.[51,53] Patients also often experience levodopa-induced involuntary movements called dyskinesias in association with medication fluctuations.[51,54] The exact mechanisms for these motor fluctuations remain unclear, but ongoing dopaminergic and non-dopaminergic degeneration in the critical motor system regions outlined, in concert with the neuronal remodeling that occurs in the putamen and caudate nucleus in response to the massive denervation of these structures (see above), are likely to play a significant role. Further research on the timing and progression of degeneration and compensatory changes in the non-dopaminergic motor regions in association with the onset and progression of medication-induced motor fluctuations is needed.

Conclusion

While degeneration of the dopaminergic nigrostriatal pathway is important for the classic motor triad of PD, it is only one of three main regions in the motor system that degenerates to a similar degree in PD (Fig. 1-2). The other two regions are glutamatergic and influence either the same basal ganglia region (caudal intralaminar thalamus projection to the putamen and caudate nucleus) as the nigrostriatal pathway or the same premotor cortical regions (presupplementary motor cortex projection to the supplementary and premotor cortices) as influenced by the basal ganglia output to thalamocortical relays. In this way both dopamine and non-dopamine lesions contribute to the cardinal motor features of PD. In addition to these regions of substantial degeneration, over time there is considerable remodeling of the projection neurons in the putamen and caudate nucleus due to their substantial denervation. This remodeling, in association with ongoing degenerative changes, drives additional poorly characterized abnormal cellular responses to dopamine replacement therapies. Understanding the non-dopaminergic changes in these motor systems is necessary to determine optimal therapies for the classic and adaptive motor features that characterize patients with PD.

References

1. Parkinson J. *Essay on the Shaking Palsy*. London: Sherwood, Neely and Jones; 1817.
2. Hughes AJ, Ben-Shlomo Y, Daniel SE, Lees AJ. What features improve the accuracy of clinical diagnosis in Parkinson's disease: a clinicopathologic study. *Neurology*. 1992;42:1142–1146.
3. McAuley JH. The physiological basis of clinical deficits in Parkinson disease. *Prog Neurobiol*. Jan 2003;69(1):27–48.
4. Schrag A, Dodel R, Spottke A, Bornschein B, Siebert U, Quinn NP. Rate of clinical progression in Parkinson's disease. A prospective study. *Mov Disord*. May 15 2007;22(7):938–945.
5. Post B, Merkus MP, de Haan RJ, Speelman JD. Prognostic factors for the progression of Parkinson's disease: a systematic review. *Mov Disord*. Oct 15 2007;22(13):1839–1851; quiz 1988.
6. Goetz CG, Stebbins GT, Blasucci LM. Differential progression of motor impairment in levodopa-treated Parkinson's disease. *Mov Disord*. May 2000;15(3):479–484.
7. Sethi KD. Tremor. *Curr Opin Neurol*. Aug 2003;16(4):481–485.
8. Riederer P, Gerlach M, Muller T, Reichmann H. Relating mode of action to clinical practice: dopaminergic agents in Parkinson's disease. *Parkinsonism Relat Disord*. Dec 2007;13(8):466–479.
9. Visser M, Marinus J, Stiggelbout AM, van Hilten JJ. Responsiveness of impairments and disabilities in Parkinson's disease. *Parkinsonism Relat Disord*. Jun 2006;12(5):314–318.
10. Katzenschlager R, Lees AJ. Treatment of Parkinson's disease: levodopa as the first choice. *J Neurol*. Sep 2002;249 Suppl 2:II19–24.
11. Jankovic J, McDermott M, Carter J, et al. Variable expression of Parkinson's disease: a base-line analysis of the DATATOP cohort. The Parkinson Study Group. *Neurology*. Oct 1990;40(10):1529–1534.
12. Kempster PA, Williams DR, Selikhova M, Holton J, Revesz T, Lees AJ. Patterns of levodopa response in Parkinson's disease: a clinico-pathological study. *Brain*. 2007 Aug;130(Pt 8):2123–2128.

13. van Rooden SM, Visser M, Verbaan D, Marinus J, van Hilten JJ. Motor patterns in Parkinson's disease: a data-driven approach. *Mov Disord*. May 15 2009;24(7): 1042–1047.

14. Hughes AJ, Daniel SE, Blankson S, Lees AJ. A clinicopathologic study of 100 cases of Parkinson's disease. *Arch Neurol*. 1993;50:140–148.

15. Alves G, Forsaa EB, Pedersen KF, Dreetz Gjerstad M, Larsen JP. Epidemiology of Parkinson's disease. *J Neurol*. Sep 2008;255 Suppl 5:18–32.

16. Graham JM, Sagar HJ. A data-driven approach to the study of heterogeneity in idiopathic Parkinson's disease: identification of three distinct subtypes. *Mov Disord*. Jan 1999;14(1):10–20.

17. Lewis SJ, Foltynie T, Blackwell AD, Robbins TW, Owen AM, Barker RA. Heterogeneity of Parkinson's disease in the early clinical stages using a data driven approach. *J Neurol Neurosurg Psychiatry*. Mar 2005;76(3):343–348.

18. Post B, Speelman JD, de Haan RJ. Clinical heterogeneity in newly diagnosed Parkinson's disease. *J Neurol*. May 2008;255(5):716–722.

19. McKeith IG, Dickson DW, Lowe J, et al. Diagnosis and management of dementia with Lewy bodies: third report of the DLB Consortium. *Neurology*. Dec 27 2005;65(12):1863–1872.

20. Hamilton RL. Lewy bodies in Alzheimer's disease: a neuropathological review of 145 cases using alpha-synuclein immunohistochemistry. *Brain Pathol*. Jul 2000;10(3): 378–384.

21. Leverenz JB, Hamilton R, Tsuang DW, et al. Empiric refinement of the pathologic assessment of Lewy-related pathology in the dementia patient. *Brain Pathol*. Apr 2008;18(2):220–224.

22. Fearnley JM, Lees AJ. Ageing and Parkinson's disease: substantia nigra regional selectivity. *Brain*. 1991;114:2283–2301.

23. Halliday GM, McRitchie DA, Cartwright HR, Pamphlett RS, Hely MA, Morris JGL. Midbrain neuropathology in idiopathic Parkinson's disease and diffuse Lewy body disease. *J Clin Neurosci*. 1996;3:52–60.

24. Clarke G, Collins RA, Leavitt BR, et al. A one-hit model of cell death in inherited neuronal degenerations. *Nature*. 2000;406:195–199.

25. Greffard S, Verny M, Bonnet AM, et al. Motor score of the Unified Parkinson Disease Rating Scale as a good predictor of Lewy body-associated neuronal loss in the substantia nigra. *Arch Neurol*. Apr 2006;63(4):584–588.

26. Braak H, Del Tredici K, Rüb U, de Vos RAI, Jansen Steur ENH, Braak E. Staging of brain pathology related to sporadic Parkinson's disease. *Neurobiol Aging*. 2003;24:197–211.

27. Halliday G, Hely M, Reid W, Morris J. The progression of pathology in longitudinally followed patients with Parkinson's disease. *Acta Neuropathol*. Apr 2008;115(4): 409–415.

28. Dum RP, Strick PL. Motor areas in the frontal lobe of the primate. *Physiol Behav*. Dec 2002;77(4–5):677–682.

29. Halliday GM, Macdonald V, Henderson JM. A comparison of degeneration in motor thalamus and cortex between progressive supranuclear palsy and Parkinson's disease. *Brain*. Oct 2005;128(Pt 10):2272–2280.

30. Sherman SM, Guillery RW. On the actions that one nerve cell can have on another: distinguishing "drivers" from "modulators." *Proc Natl Acad Sci U S A*. Jun 9 1998;95(12):7121–7126.
31. Vilensky JA, Gilman S. Integrating the work of D. Denny-Brown and some of his contemporaries into current studies of the primate motor cortex. *J Neurol Sci*. Jan 1 2001;182(2):83–87.
32. Darian-Smith C, Darian-Smith I. Thalamic projections to areas 3a, 3b, and 4 in the sensorimotor cortex of the mature and infant macaque monkey. *J Comp Neurol*. Sep 8 1993;335(2):173–199.
33. Matelli M, Luppino G, Geyer S, Zilles K. Motor cortex. In: Paxinos G, ed. *The Human Nervous System*. 2nd ed. New York: Academic Press; 2004:973–996.
34. Haber SN, McFarland NR. The place of the thalamus in frontal cortical-basal ganglia circuits. *Neuroscientist*. 2001;7:315–324.
35. Henderson JM, Carpenter K, Cartwright H, Halliday GM. Degeneration of the thalamic caudal intralaminar nuclei in Parkinson's disease. *Ann. Neurol*. 2000;47:345–352.
36. Henderson JM, Carpenter K, Cartwright H, Halliday GM. Loss of thalamic intralaminar nuclei in progressive supranuclear palsy and Parkinson's disease: clinical and therapeutic implications. *Brain*. 2000;123:1410–1421.
37. Zaja-Milatovic S, Milatovic D, Schantz AM, et al. Dendritic degeneration in neostriatal medium spiny neurons in Parkinson disease. *Neurology*. Feb 8 2005;64(3):545–547.
38. Smith Y, Villalba R. Striatal and extrastriatal dopamine in the basal ganglia: an overview of its anatomical organization in normal and Parkinsonian brains. *Mov Disord*. 2008;23 Suppl 3:S534–547.
39. Pavese N, Evans AH, Tai YF, et al. Clinical correlates of levodopa-induced dopamine release in Parkinson disease: a PET study. *Neurology*. Nov 14 2006;67(9):1612–1617.
40. Heiss WD, Hilker R. The sensitivity of 18-fluorodopa positron emission tomography and magnetic resonance imaging in Parkinson's disease. *Eur J Neurol*. Jan 2004;11(1):5–12.
41. Schwarz J, Storch A, Koch W, Pogarell O, Radau PE, Tatsch K. Loss of dopamine transporter binding in Parkinson's disease follows a single exponential rather than linear decline. *J Nucl Med*. Oct 2004;45(10):1694–1697.
42. Huang C, Tang C, Feigin A, et al. Changes in network activity with the progression of Parkinson's disease. *Brain*. Jul 2007;130(Pt 7):1834–1846.
43. Tissingh G, Bergmans P, Booij J, et al. Drug-naive patients with Parkinson's disease in Hoehn and Yahr stages I and II show a bilateral decrease in striatal dopamine transporters as revealed by [123I]beta-CIT SPECT. *J Neurol*. Jan 1998;245(1):14–20.
44. Haapaniemi TH, Ahonen A, Torniainen P, Sotaniemi KA, Myllyla VV. [123I]beta-CIT SPECT demonstrates decreased brain dopamine and serotonin transporter levels in untreated parkinsonian patients. *Mov Disord*. Jan 2001;16(1):124–130.
45. Spiegel J, Hellwig D, Samnick S, et al. Striatal FP-CIT uptake differs in the subtypes of early Parkinson's disease. *J Neural Transm*. Mar 2007;114(3):331–335.

46. Kovacs GG, Milenkovic IJ, Preusser M, Budka H. Nigral burden of alpha-synuclein correlates with striatal dopamine deficit. *Mov Disord.* Aug 15 2008;23(11):1608–1612.

47. Taniwaki T, Okayama A, Yoshiura T, et al. Reappraisal of the motor role of basal ganglia: a functional magnetic resonance image study. *J Neurosci.* Apr 15 2003;23(8):3432–3438.

48. McAuley JH, Marsden CD. Physiological and pathological tremors and rhythmic central motor control. *Brain.* Aug 2000;123 (Pt 8):1545–1567.

49. Speelman JD, Schuurman R, de Bie RM, Esselink RA, Bosch DA. Stereotactic neurosurgery for tremor. *Mov Disord.* 2002;17 Suppl 3:S84–88.

50. Muenter MD, Tyce GM. L-dopa therapy of Parkinson's disease: Plasma L-dopa concentration, therapeutic response, and side effects. *Mayo Clin Proc.* 1971;46:231–239.

51. Fox SH, Lang AE. Levodopa-related motor complications–phenomenology. *Mov Disord.* 2008;23 Suppl 3:S509–514.

52. Fahn S. "On-off" phenomenon with levodopa therapy in parkinsonism: Clinical and pharmacologic correlations and the effect of intramuscular pyridoxine. *Neurology.* 1974;24:431–441.

53. Melamed E, Bitton V, Zelig O. Episodic unresponsiveness to single doses of L-Dopa in parkinsonian fluctuators. *Neurology.* 1986;36:100–103.

54. Fahn S. The spectrum of levodopa-induced dyskinesias. *Ann Neurol.* 2000;47 (Suppl 1):S2–S11.

Chapter 2

Lesions Associated with Motor Speech

Anna Rita Bentivoglio, Davide Quaranta, and Aileen K. Ho

Introduction

Motor speech impairment is very common during the course of Parkinson's Disease (PD), affecting up to 70% of subjects.[1] From an observational point of view, it is mainly characterized by monotony of pitch and loudness; reduced stress and prosody; variable changes in speech rate (ranging from slowness to festination); short rushes of speech; and imprecise pronunciation of consonants.[2,3] Dysarthria may emerge at any stage of the disease, with a definite worsening in later stages, leading to impaired communication, social isolation, and severe psychosocial sequelae.

In the last decade, the interest in this aspect of PD has increased. In a recent review, Yorkston[4] reported that 110 papers concerning PD dysarthria were published from 1996 to 2007, covering as much as 70% of the literature about "degenerative dysarthria." Although motor speech disorders in PD are commonly referred to as "dysarthria," it must be noted that dysfunction includes two main categories: dysarthria and apraxia of speech.

Neuroanatomic and Neurophysiologic Substrates of Motor Speech Control

Speech production requires multiple and complex performances of motor control mechanisms, requiring fast and accurate execution of oro-facial-lingual movements, finely adjusted timing, and coordination of laryngeal and respiratory activities. First observations about speech motor control were based on clinical descriptions of patients with identified central nervous system (CNS) lesions and dysarthria. The direct consequence of this clinical approach was a "phenomenological" classification of dysarthria corresponding to specific sites of lesion. This classification has been successively implemented by refined studies about the perceptual characteristics of speech disturbances in patients affected by neurological diseases. This approach provided insight to the different role played by cerebral structures in the planning and execution of movement leading to vocal emission.

The final common pathway of speech production consists of 3 fundamental muscular groups: **voluntary expiratory muscles** which maintain a constant pressure below the glottis; **vocal cords**, which are adducted and vibrate the air during production of voiced speech sounds or are abducted and free of vibration during production of unvoiced speech sounds; and the **articulators** (soft palate, tongue, jaw, and lips), which modify the passage of expired air (Figure 2-1). The muscular activation is controlled by 2 neural pathways: a direct one, consisting of the corticobulbar and corticospinal tracts, which control skilled speech movements; and an indirect one, also originating from the cerebral cortex, with synapses in the brainstem, committed in the control of posture and tone necessary to maintain an appropriate framework while refined speech movements are carried out.[5] The muscular groups involved in speech are disproportionately allocated in the motor cortex, thus reflecting the refined representation of movement programs concerning speech. Bilateral lesions affecting motor cortex, corticospinal and corticobulbar tracts, and the indirect pathway lead to *spastic dysarthria*, characterized by slowed speech tempo, hypernasality due to insufficient velar elevation, tongue retraction, increased constriction of the pharynx, and hyperadduction of the shortened vocal folds.[6]

Control of the speech sounds produced and the rapidity of transitions between them relies on a highly integrated system involving basal ganglia, cerebellum, and different cortical structures (Figure 2-2).[5,7–10] Basal ganglia play a crucial role in regulating and maintaining normal posture and static muscle contraction upon which skilled movement can be performed. They regulate amplitude, velocity, and the initiation of movement; furthermore, they may play a role in movement selection and learning. The basal ganglia circuitry is important in generating components of motor programs for speech, particularly those which help in maintaining a sustained muscular contraction that makes possible the execution of discrete movements.[5] Functional neuroimaging studies have confirmed that specific regions of basal ganglia are involved in speech production, but different

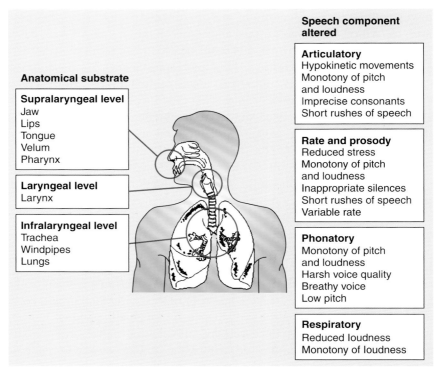

Figure 2-1. Anatomical substrate of speech components and parkinsonian dysarthria characteristics. PD speech has been defined as a hypokinetic dysarthria, and can be associated with specific changes to 3 of the main components of speech production: respiration, phonation, and articulation. The prosodic component can also be taken into account because several speech components are involved in the dysfunction. (Reprinted with permission from Pinto et al.[3])

studies have produced conflicting data on the role played in different speech tasks. Wise et al[11] reported a focal activation of left posterior pallidum during repetition of single words. Wildgruber and colleagues[7] reported that activation of the left putamen (as well as cerebellum, supplementary motor area, and motor cortex) changed during syllable repetition tasks, depending on the repetition rate. An elegant fMRI study by Bohland and Guenther[9] observed that during tasks of overt production of syllables, putamen and pallidum are activated bilaterally; interestingly, they reported that besides the functioning of a "minimal network" controlling speech production, additional areas are recruited when syllables and sequence complexity increases.

Dysfunction of the basal ganglia has been categorized in two different kinds of speech disturbance, reflecting a "classical" approach to the

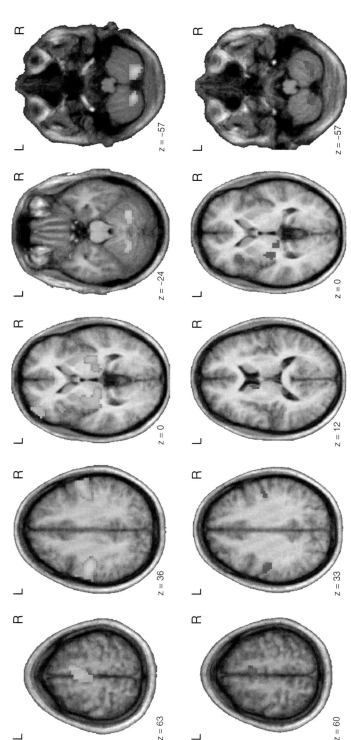

Figure 2-2. Hemodynamic changes during syllable repetitions. (Top) Main effects calculated across all 6 frequency conditions and subjects (yellow/orange spots). (Bottom) Rate/response functions characterized by a positive linear (red spots) or a negative linear relationship (blue spots) displayed on transverse sections of the averaged anatomic reference images. (z=distance to the intercommisural plane; L=left hemisphere; R=right hemisphere) (Reprinted with permission from Riecker et al.[10])

semiology of movement disorders, which divides movement disorders into hypokinesias and hyperkinesias. Consequently, hypokinetic dysarthria is associated with parkinsonism and other hypokinetic movement disorders: it is characterized by lowered voice volume (hypophonia) concomitant with normal or accelerated speech tempo; imprecise consonant pronunciation; "prosodic insufficiency," regarded as monotony of pitch and loudness, and reduced stress[5,12–14]; *vide infra* for more details. Core features of the so-called hyperkinetic dysarthria are variable in respect to the underlying pathological condition (e.g., chorea, dystonia, athetosis, tics, etc.) and will not be discussed.

The cerebellum participates in motor speech control through reciprocal connections with cerebral cortex and brainstem structures involved in the above-mentioned indirect pathway; auditory and proprioceptive input from speech muscles, tendons and joints; and cooperation with the basal ganglia.[5] Two cortical-cerebellar pathways appear to be critical for speech. The first, originating in the primary motor and premotor cortices, reaches the cerebellar hemispheres via pontine nuclei; the return pathway reaches the same cortical regions, via cerebellar deep nuclei and ventral thalamus. This loop is considered important in planning and programming learned movement. A second pathway from the corticospinal tract is directed to the intermediate regions of the cerebellar hemispheres, with a return pathway to the primary motor cortex through deep cerebellar nuclei and ventral thalamus. This circuit provides an "on-line" control of skilled movements using cortical output information. The intermediate regions of the cerebellar hemispheres also project to brainstem and spinal motor centers. Functional studies on normal subjects reported an activation of cerebellar structures during phonation; in particular, Wise et al[11] reported increased activity during speech production in the rostral paravermal cerebellum. Wildbruger et al[7] signaled activation in Larsell's H VI region (where tongue and lip muscles are represented[15]). Furthermore, they reported cerebellar activation to be absent for syllable production rate inferior to 2.5 Hz, whereas it was constant at higher frequency. This result suggests that cerebellar function might be important in speech production under time-critical conditions. Patients with cerebellar dysarthria exhibit slowed speaking rates with predominant lengthening of unstressed syllables, sometimes associated with voice tremor or irregular pitch shifts.[14,16]

The highest level of neural organization participating in motor speech is at the interface between the conceptual organization of language and the sequence of coordinated neural activities leading to phonation and articulation. The organization of this "high level" system is complex and several theoretical models about it have been proposed.

1 The first steps of speech production are "linguistic" in nature and consist of the activation of lexical representations of concepts stored as semantic representations.

2 Afterwards, motor commands for the production of phonetic segments must be retrieved and activated. This process passes through two steps: planning, i.e. the formulation or recall of a general representation ("engram") of speech units; and programming, i.e. the correct and coordinated activation of different learned motor sequences (subprograms) which provide specific parameters for muscular groups.

Premotor and the supplementary motor area (SMA) of the language-dominant hemisphere are involved in planning functions. The former contributes relays through the corticospinal and corticobulbar tracts, mainly indirectly influencing the primary motor cortex through a loop involving the basal ganglia and thalamus. The premotor cortex is mainly involved in the choice among competing alternative programs. In non-human primates, lesions in the premotor cortex have been associated with uncoordination of lip, tongue and jaw movements.[17] Levelt and coworkers[18,19] proposed that overlearned syllable-sized programs (i.e., motor programs for high frequency syllables) might form a "mental syllabary" housed within the premotor cortex. The SMA projects to primary motor and premotor cortices, parietal lobe and cingulate gyrus, and receives afferent fibers from the basal ganglia and primary motor and premotor cortices. It s also connected with limbic structures. SMA is considered to play a crucial role in the preparation of internally driven movements and in initiation of spontaneous speech, control of rhythm, phonation, and articulation.[20] Accordingly, functional inactivation of SMA through repetitive magnetic stimulation induces slowing of speech or arrest of vocalization[21]; moreover, surgical lesion of the left SMA results in mutism or reduced spontaneous speech.[22]

In recent years the role of insular cortex has been studied,[23,24] but its function in motor speech is still poorly understood. Lesions of the intrasylvian region lead to speech disturbances characterized by effortful and groping articulatory movements, dysprosody, inconsistent distortions of speech sounds (''phonetic variability''), and compromised initiation of verbal utterances, while motor execution in terms of force development is unimpaired. This condition is known as *apraxia of speech* (AOS) and it is considered as the manifestation of "inefficiencies in the translation of a well-formed and filled phonological frame to previously learned kinematic parameters.''[25] Dronkers[26] found the anterior insula to represent the area of maximum overlap of lesion sites responsible of AOS, while the posterior aspects of the intrasylvian cortex seem to be less engaged in speech motor control.[27] Ackermann and Riecker[24] and Bohland and Guenther[9] reported that left anterior insula was activated during overt speech and "silent" during covert speech, thus suggesting that the insula may support the coordination of the activity of muscles engaged in speech production. On the other hand, Broca's area, which is essential for linguistic functions, does not seem to participate in strictly motor aspects of speech, according to neuroimaging studies.[7,9,11,24]

In speech production, emotionally driven output reaches its more important expression. The emotive status of the speaker, more than through word content, is expressed by the modulation of speech features, such as variation in pitch, loudness, and duration (for example, sentences produced in a happy tone exhibit larger pitch fluctuations and higher amplitudes than utterances produced in a sad mood[24]). In this sense, it is conceivable that limbic structures, together with the right hemisphere, might play a key role.

Pathophysiology of Motor Speech Disorders in Parkinson's Disease

Progressive disruption of the nigrostriatal pathway is the key pathogenetic process in PD leading to basal ganglia motor loop dysfunction. Akinesia, rigidity, and tremor are the core symptoms of PD, and all may contribute to hypokinetic dysarthria, influencing the muscular parameters (strength, stiffness, velocity of contraction) of the effectors. Dysarthria may be attributed mainly to the dysfunction of basal ganglia circuitry, and to the impairment of the dopamine pathway, as shown by several studies on the levodopa-induced improvement of speech parameters.[28-30] On the other hand, it is well known that non-dopamine lesions precede the onset[31,32] of motor symptoms and become prominent in the late stages of PD, when even dysarthria worsens.[3,33]

Scanty functional studies have provided initial insight on the involvement of structures other than the basal ganglia in the pathogenesis of PD dysarthria. Pinto et al[34] reported a lack of activation of the right orofacial M1 cortex and the cerebellum, and enhanced activation of the SMA, dorsolateral prefrontal cortex, the right superior premotor cortex and the left insula, during speech production and articulation in PD. The authors concluded that PD dysarthria is associated with an altered recruitment of the motor cerebral regions and a compensatory recruitment of premotor and prefrontal cortices (bilateral dorsolateral prefrontal cortex, SMA, superior premotor cortex) (Figure 2-3). Liotti et al[35] obtained partially overlapping results: abnormalities of cerebral activation were essentially represented

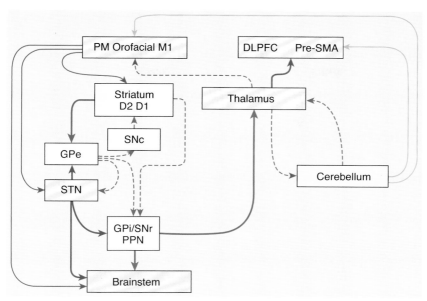

Figure 2-3. Cerebral activation abnormalities during speech in PD. The 3 main kinds of cerebrocortical dysfunction during PD speech are: an overactivation of the rostral part of the pre-supplementary area (pre-SMA) and the bilateral dorsolateral prefrontal cortex (DLPFC); an underactivation of the orofacial motor cortex M1; and an underactivation of the cerebellum. These results reinforce the fact that 2 parallel neural pathways are implicated in motor control of speech production: the basal ganglia are involved in the first and the cerebellum in the second. In PD, dysfunction of the first pathway seems to affect the second. (D1, D2=D1 and D2 striatal dopamine receptors; GPe=external globus pallidus; GPi=internal globus pallidus; PM=premotor cortex; PPN=pedunculopontine nucleus; SNc=substantia nigra pars compacta; SNr=substantia nigra pars reticulata; STN=subthalamic nucleus; red lines=excitatory glutaminergic projections; blue lines=inhibitory GABAergic projections; dotted lines=underactivity of the projection, and thickness of the continued lines represent the range from supposed normal (thin) and hyperactive (thick) activities; yellow lines=corticocerebellar connections).(Reprinted with permission from Pinto et al.[3])

by an overactivation of the orofacial primary motor cortex, inferior lateral premotor cortex, and SMA. In an fMRI study, Rektorova et al[36] reported an increased BOLD response in the right primary sensorimotor cortex. Data from functional studies led to the hypothesis that the hyperactivation of cortical regions may reflect compensatory mechanisms. These findings were confirmed by Dias et al,[37] who studied the neurophysiological effects of repetitive transcranial magnetic stimulation (rTMS) on voice and speech in 30 individuals with PD. Repetitive TMS modulation of the M1-mouth region of the cortex resulted in a significant improvement of fundamental voice frequency and intensity. The role of basal ganglia in speech production has been confirmed in the results of brain surgery in PD (see the effects of therapy below).

Clinical Features of Dysarthria in Parkinson's Disease

The principal speech disorder in PD is hypokinetic dysarthria, with the principal complaints of patients being an excessive rate of speech and "indistinct" word production; also the negative effects of fatigue on speech are often subjectively reported. On the other hand, patients often deny or minimize changes in voice loudness.[5]

Several alterations in the functioning of oral structures responsible for speech production (articulators) are found on clinical examination. Tremor of the jaw, lips, and tongue may be present at rest or during sustained posture (mouth opening or lip retraction). Furthermore, PD patients display a reduced rate of swallowing, which can lead to saliva accumulation. When segmental strength of oro-facial muscles is examined, it is generally normal. Non-speech alternating movements of oral muscles may be impaired because of akinesia (difficult in starting movement). They are often rapid and restricted in range; on the other hand, simple movement can be normal in range or greater than the ones observed during speech. Speech movements and their timing are generally accurate. Individual movements are slowed in PD, whereas repetitive movements are commonly characterized by a tendency to progressive acceleration, particularly for limited range of movement. In both individual and repetitive movements the range and force of movement are reduced in PD. The presence of excessive muscular tone (rigidity) can contribute to decreased range of movement.

The characterization of dysarthria can follow two principal methods of speech therapy investigations, *perceptual characterization* and *instrumental investigation.* From the perceptual point of view, the features of PD dysarthria have been well characterized by the classic works of Logemann et al[13] and Darley et al.[2] Logemann et al[13] reported that about 90% of patients complained of voice alterations, characterized by hoarseness, *tremulousness,* and *breathiness*, whereas about a half of subjects had articulatory problems. Darley et al[2] proposed that PD dysarthria could be labeled as *prosodic insufficiency.* It is characterized by:

- monotony of pitch: a reduction in the normal pitch and inflectional changes;
- monoloudness: the voice lacks normal changes of loudness;

- reduced stress;
- short phrases;
- variable rate: frequently appears accelerated while the subject is performing rapidly alternating movements; this alteration may appear more evidently as *short rushes of speech* which are characterized by the production of several words together, separated from other parts of an utterance by inappropriate pause; other subjects may show an increased speech rate within segments. These features can be referred to as festination (the tendency to speed up when performing repetitive movements);
- imprecise consonants: Logemann and Fischer[38] described in detail the abnormalities in consonant production and reported that they principally affect stops, fricatives, and affricates. Stops were often perceived as fricatives, probably because of incomplete articulatory contact and continual air emission during the stop period; the same pattern was detected as for affricates. Fricatives, on the other hand, were perceived as reduced in sharpness, probably because of an insufficient constriction of the articulators.

These features together give rise to the "flat" quality of PD speech.

Other features commonly observed in PD dysarthria are inappropriate silence that may reflect difficulties in starting movement (akinesia) or a more cognitive-mediated reduced initiation of spontaneous behavior; and a tendency to repeat phonemes, especially at the beginning of the utterances or after pauses (somehow resembling the freezing phenomenon). Palilalia, that is the repetition of syllables, words or even phrases, with increasing rate and reducing loudness, is less common.[5] Re-emergence of childhood stuttering is also well described, but very uncommon, as a manifestation of PD.[39] Also, a true voice tremor is quite uncommon as it more likely reflects head tremor.

The motor speech alterations are studied by speech therapists at different levels of function. The fundamental mechanical phenomena that underlie the correct emission of sounds are:

- respiration, which is responsible for the correct coordination of voluntary air emission with upstream structures;
- phonation, which depends upon the vibration of vocal folds and produces *voiced sounds*; the vibrating vocal folds produce a periodic excitation, termed the glottal flow; the spectra of sounds produced under normal conditions are characterized by a harmonic comb structure, i.e., distribution of energy at the fundamental frequency (F0, ranging from 100 Hz in males up to 400 Hz in infants) and its harmonic integer multiples ($2 \cdot$ F0, $3 \cdot$ F0, etc.)[40]; the F0 and its harmonics are the primary acoustical cues underlying pitch perception[41];

- resonance, a process through which sounds produced by the phonatory activity are amplified and modified by the vocal tract resonators (mouth cavity, velopharyngeal structures, nasal cavities); the vocal tract weights the comb structure by other resonances, termed the formants (F1, F2, F3, etc.), that determine the vowel category. The different vowel sounds are determined by different shape and width of the resonance cavity, which are dependant upon lip and tongue position;
- articulation, the modification of sounds that lead to the production of recognizable words, through the complex coordination of the vocal tract articulators (the tongue, soft palate, and lips); at this level, primary sounds produced by phonation are transformed into consonants; this phenomenon happens through the "forcing" of occlusion and passage through the narrowing of the articulatory system (lip, tongue, palate).

Several studies have addressed the physiological features of PD dysarthria in relation to these functions.

Respiratory alterations conceivably contribute to some characteristics of PD dysarthria, especially through the modification of the posture and tone of the chest wall. Solomon and Hixon[42] reported reduced rib cage volumes and large abdominal volumes at the initiation of speech in PD subjects producing fewer words and speaking for less time per breath group. Murdoch et al[43] reported that approximately half of the PD subjects exhibited irregularities in their chest wall movements while performing vowel prolongation and syllable repetition tasks. Some subjects display increased latency before exhalation, after inhalation, and before phonation during exhalation, as well as difficulty in altering automatic respiratory rhythms for speech.[5] These alterations, together with a reduction of vital capacity and the execution of short breath cycles, may account for some of the PD dysarthria features, such as reduced loudness, short rushes of speech, and inappropriate pauses.

Several studies have addressed the phonation abnormalities in PD dysarthria. Variations of the F0 have been variously reported. Some studies reported increased F0 values during speaking tasks[44]; however it is not clear if this feature is specific to PD, as compared to age-matched controls the increase is not always significant.[45] The analysis of F0 variability in PD revealed patterns of variability changes which are task-specific. Long-term measures, such as syllables and sentences, have revealed a decrease in F0 variability, in support of the perceptual characteristics of monopitch and monoloudness.[5] On the other hand, increased variability of F0 has been documented for sustained vowel tasks.[44,46,47] An influence of gender has been also reported, even if data are conflicting: Hertrich et al[46] reported an increase of F0 instability in female subjects, while Midi et al[47] reported the same in male patients. Studies investigating intensity are more consistent, as reduced vocal intensity in speech, vowel prolongation, and Alternate Motion Rates AMR tasks have been widely documented.

Voice tremor is not a prominent feature of PD dysarthria; nevertheless, some videostroboscopy studies[29,48,49] documented laryngeal and/or arytenoid tremor in about a half of the examined subjects. Holmes et al[50] reported that voice tremor was associated with later stages of the disease. Abnormalities in acoustic perturbation measures, such as jitter (varying pitch in the voice) and shimmer (change in amplitude of the voice), may be present in PD, possibly reflecting an impaired control of laryngeal abductory and adductory mechanism. Abnormal shimmer values have been correlated to perceptual measures of breathiness, probably related to vocal fold bowing which causes increased airflow turbulence and intensity variations.[51] Several acoustic studies suggest reduced laryngeal control. Some patients are slow to initiate phonation (events correlated to inappropriate silences).[51] Incoordination of voicing has been regarded as responsible of perceived omission of final consonants, and voiceless vowels-consonants transitions within syllables.

Laryngoscopy has documented different visible abnormalities. In most patients a vocal fold bowing (related to laryngeal muscle rigidity) during phonation, causing glottal gap, was correlated with perceived breathiness and reduced intensity. Electromyography studies provided further evidence that limited vocal fold motion may reflect a loss of appropriate reciprocal activity between agonist and antagonist muscles, rather than weakness.[29] Aerodynamic studies documented subglottic pressure, and laryngeal resistance is abnormally increased during speech in some hypokinetic speakers. These findings suggest the presence of increased glottal or supraglottic muscle tension during phonation, caused by phonation with a smaller glottal aperture or a greater resistance to deformation of the folds with decreased pulsing of airflow;[28] this is related to an abnormally effortful speech.

Resonance abnormalities usually are not perceptually prominent in hypokinetic dysarthria. However, a few studies have demonstrated that nasal airflow can be increased,[52] that nasalization may spread across several consecutive syllables, and that the degree and the velocity of velar movements during speech tasks can be reduced. It has been hypothesized that the perception of resonance abnormalities may be masked by phonatory abnormalities.[52] Velopharyngeal dysfunction seems to be a consequence of slow movement, rigidity, and reduced range of movement. These can lead to the perception of hypernasality and weak intraoral pressure during consonant production.

Acoustic and physiologic studies of articulatory dynamics of patients with hypophonic dysarthria support imprecise articulation and rate abnormalities, and reduction in the range of articulatory movements. Articulatory "under-shoot," or failure to sustain contacts for sufficient duration, impairs precision. *Spirantization* (correlated to articulatory under-shooting) is characterized by the replacement of a stop-gap by low intensity frication. As a consequence, acoustic contrast and detail is reduced.[38] Range of movement is reduced; moreover, articulator movements have abnormal speed due to muscle rigidity. Several studies documented lip muscle stiffness, and reduced amplitude and velocity of lip and jaw movements. Abnormal reciprocal adjustment of antagonist muscles, or a loss of reciprocal suppression between functionally antagonist muscle pairs, also accounts for reduced range of movement of articulatory muscles.

Numerous studies have examined speech rate and the results have been inconsistent as the variability in rate across subjects ranges from abnormally slow to abnormally fast. It is interesting to outline some considerations: 1) first, the variability is not simply a function of severity, thus suggesting the possibility of subtypes of the disorder; 2) hypokinetic dysarthria is the only type of dysarthria in which the speed is perceived as rapid or accelerated. However, Kent and Rosenbek[53] suggest that articulatory imprecision and continuous voicing reduce discrete acoustic contrast and may lead to a perception of increased rate even when rate may not actually be rapid. Hirose[54] compared abnormally fast speech rate to festination and speculated that this may reflect a disturbance of CNS inhibitory function, such as a release of automatic oscillators. Moreau et al[55] reported that oral festination is strongly associated with gait festination but not with the severity of freezing of gait or dysarthria overall, concluding that oral festination may share the same pathophysiology as gait disorders. Finally, some PD patients have difficulty in altering rate when requested, suggesting that a major problem for these subjects is in controlling alterations in rate even if the temporal organization of speech may be adequate.[51] Weakness and reduced endurance have been found in the upper lip, velum and tongue which in some studies have been correlated to articulatory precision and speech impairment. Pathological tremor in the jaw, lip, and tongue during sustained postures and active and passive movements may also interfere with maintaining muscle contraction (e.g. tongue elevation) thus contributing to the impairment of articulation.

Besides the above-mentioned characteristics which underlie PD dysarthria, other features influence the perception of prosodic insufficiency, such as pauses during speech. Illes et al[56] found that hypokinetic speakers exhibited fewer interjections during narrative speech. It has been speculated that hypokinetic speakers display silent pauses instead of fillers, and this loss may be an akinetic sign such as hypomimia or reduction of arm swing during gait. Furthermore, there is some degree of relationship between dysarthria and cognitive impairment in PD.[57]

Impaired Speech Performance in Parkinson's Disease

Problems with speech are not commonly the initial symptom (3.8%) in PD,[58] but they are often encountered over the course of the illness. While there is some suggestion that speech problems increase with advancing disease severity,[59] this relationship is not always found[60,61] and findings are often mixed.[50,62] This unequivocal picture, and the mixed findings on the impact of levodopa medication on speech performance, invites further speculation regarding the role of non-dopamine influences on speech and how this may interact with dopamine influences.[63] Just how widespread the occurrence of speech disorder is in any given PD population depends less on who may be providing the answer than the level at which speech performance is evaluated. When PD patients themselves were asked if they had any difficulty with speech,[64] or considered their speech impaired,[1] or that their voice had changed,[61] responses were 65%, 70% and 76% respectively. When patients' speech was rated by listeners for functional communication[65] or intelligibility,[61,66] again similar figures were obtained (74%, 65% and 70% respectively).

These figures across raters, studies, and over time, are remarkably consistent, pointing to just under three quarters (65–75%) of patients with PD experiencing a significant interference to speech performance which impacts their daily experience of life. However, if a more detailed technical definition of speech impairment is adopted, i.e. clarity of articulation,[13] then a higher figure of 89% emerges. This highlights the importance of the issue of different levels of speech assessment in this population, and has implications in terms of the widely adopted World Health Organization International Classification of Functioning, Disability and Health (ICF) conceptual framework. For example, there may be discrete acoustic changes in the way a PD patient speaks due to neuropathophysiological and/or orolaryngeal changes at the level of impairment to body structure and function, but this may or may not result in activity limitation, depending on whether overall speaking performance or communication is significantly impaired. Different means would be appropriate to tap into the various concepts of changes in body structure and function, and activity limitation, and yet again different measures to gauge participation restriction. This concept is important as it aims to contextualise the actual distal impact of any disease-related changes, but is also most challenging because multiple extraneous factors may affect participation restriction, and it may not be readily inferred from the other limitations. For example, severity of speech dysarthria per se does not necessarily predict communicative difficulties.[67]

Assessment of Speech Performance

In a clinic setting, speech language therapists typically interview patients and care givers, and will form a clinical impression of patients' speech from hearing the perceptual qualities of speech output,[68,69] largely based on the Mayo Clinic speech and voice dimensions.[70,71] Another commonly used clinician-based voice assessment is the GRBAS Scale,[72] an acronym which stands for grade (i.e. overall severity of dysphonia), roughness, breathiness, asthenia and strain. These five voice parameters are graded by the clinician on 4-point or visual analog scales based on any variety of speech samples produced during the interview, such as spontaneous speech, specific vowel sounds, and the production of phonetically balanced samples of various lengths. Perceptual assessment has been and will remain the backbone of clinical evaluation, despite its limitations[69] due to the pragmatic time and resource constraints of a clinic setting. More formal assessment using auditory perceptual assessment may be conducted in order to gather information to form an initial assessment of speaking adequacy, and/or to provide a comprehensive picture of a patient's overall speech profile. Three of the most widely used PD dysarthria assessments are described below.

1. Frenchay Dysarthria Assessment[73]
This assessment consists of using a 5-point rating scale (based on appearance, activity and function) to examine a series of tasks performed by the patient on command, after an initial demonstration. The anchors (e.g. for time allocation to complete task) on the rating scale are derived from information from a normal healthy population. Areas covered are reflexes (cough, swallow, noted or reported drooling), respiration (deep breath let out as audibly and slowly as possible, counting to 20 on one breath), lips (repeat /p/, oo-ee 10 times), jaw (observation during speech and rest), palate (observe velar elevation during a series of /a/'s, note nasal resonance and emission during /may pay/ and /nay bay/), vocal cords (maximum phonation time, singing a scale, counting to 5 increasing volume for each number, quality of connected speech), tongue (protrude and retract tongue 10 times, point tongue towards nose and then chin 5 times, move tongue from side to side 5 times) and intelligibility (single words selected

from an array-blind, sentences selected from an array-blind, conversation, rate i.e. words/min). In PD patients it is most commonly used during initial assessment to check that there are no other speech disturbances than classical hypokinetic dysarthria,[60] or as an overall indication of speech performance (intelligibility).[74]

2. Robertson Dysarthria Profile[75]
A 5-point rating scale (normal to unable to perform) surveys performance on respiration (sustain, crescendo, diminuendo /s/, repeat series of /s/), phonation (maximum phonation time for /a/, loud /a/, crescendo, diminuendo /a/, repeat series of /a/), facial musculature for articulation (purse/stretch lips, maintain lip closure, protrude/retract tongue, lateral tongue movement), diadochokinesis (oo-ee, pa-pa, la-la, ka-la, p-t-k, rapidly), articulation (vowels, consonants, consonant clusters, polysyllabic words), and intelligibility (passage reading, spontaneous speech, maintenance of rate, intonation, rhythm). Ideally, ratings are performed by several parties, e.g. speech and language therapist, relative or close friend, and a stranger. This provides a useful assessment of the patient's strengths and weaknesses, and has been used to examine the effect of therapy.[76]

3. Assessment of Intelligibility of Dysarthric Speech[77]
This index of intelligibility is based on the premise that a rater should not have prior knowledge of what the speaker is trying to say, therefore it involves the procedure of audiotaping randomly selecting words or sentences from large sets of such items, which can then be rated by the clinician. For the single-word task, 2 response formats may be used to arrive at the percentage of words correctly produced. First, a multiple choice format where the rater selects the target word from a list of 12 alternatives, and second the rater simply writes down what they heard and compares it with the target word. In the sentence task, sentences of 5 to 15 words long are transcribed verbatim to determine percentage correct. Other measures are speaking rate (words per minute), rate of intelligible speech (number of intelligible words per minute), and communication efficiency ratio (rate of intelligibility of the patient relative to that of healthy normal speakers). This assessment has been used as an index of intelligibility to compare baseline and treatment or experimental conditions in PD.[60,78–80]

It should be borne in mind that the concept of intelligibility depends both on the listener as well as the rater, and that listener familiarization exerts a significant impact on improving intelligibility scores across successive trials.[81] Furthermore, the type of material spoken is yet another important factor in PD, as this affects performance. For example, more complex scenarios involving a high cognitive load are more susceptible to performance decrements[82,83]; and intelligibility of spontaneous speech is most impaired compared to other speech conditions, repetition, reading, repeated singing, and spontaneous singing.[84]

Assessment of the Impact of Dysarthria

With the increasing acceptance of the ICF conceptual framework, the focus on measuring the real-life consequences of a speech impairment has been heightened. The concept of participation is important because it represents the final consequences or impact of upstream changes and is therefore central to the person's experience. While it may be argued that existing instruments do not yet fully tap the construct of communicative participation (for review see Eadie et al[85]), the most commonly used patient-based scales which seek to ascertain the impact of impaired speech on the individual are detailed below.

1. Voice Handicap Index[86]
This scale comprises three 10-item subscales (functional, emotional, and physical) with scores from 0 to 40 points, with the total score the sum of the 3 subscales (range 0 to 120). Subjects read each of the 30 items (e.g., I speak with friends, neighbors and relatives less often because of my voice) and rate their response on a 5-point scale as "never," "almost never," "sometimes," "almost always," and "always" to indicate how frequently they have the experience. Functional, emotional, and physical subscales are calculated as the sum of the responses to the 10 items in each scale. Total Voice Handicap Index is the sum of the scores on the 3 subscales. Recently, this index has been used in intervention studies in PD patients in order to assess impact of voice changes.[87]

2. Voice-related Quality of Life Index[88]
This 10-item scale asks how much of a problem certain situations cause respondents (e.g., I have trouble using the telephone because of my voice), where 1 = Not a problem, 2 = A small amount, 3 = A moderate amount, 4 = Frequently and 5 = Problem is as "bad as it can be." This scale has recently been used as on outcome measure to determine the efficacy of experimental intervention.[37]

These scales are increasingly included in research studies of PD. They are likely to become more important due to the increasing recognition of the importance on functional communication and psychosocial aspects of communicative participation. In most previous PD research, the trend has been to focus on the limb movement impairments, cognitive and mood-related changes, and also increasingly on non-motor symptoms.[89,90] While an item on speech and communication may appear on clinical rating scales like the Unified PD Rating Scale, or specific quality of life instruments such as the PDQ-39[91] or PDQL,[92] these items tend to be rather general, and even so are seldom examined in their own right. Nevertheless, the significant impact of speech-related difficulties in PD has been suggested by some studies using generic health-related quality of life measures. For example, a recent study using the 15D instrument showed speech to be among the 4 most affected areas of life.[93] Another study adopting a different methodological approach showed that for 38% of patients speech change was among their top 4 PD concerns.[61] The full extent of difficulties stemming from compromised speech function and communication will be better documented as future studies provide more comprehensive information.

Effect of Parkinsonian Therapies on Speech

Drug therapies

Dopamine replacement therapies are the first treatment line for PD subjects. Patients usually display a favorable response to the administration of dopamine replacement drugs in the first phases of the disease. However, as the disease worsens the response to pharmacological treatment decreases. Several studies have investigated the effect of dopamine replacement and non-dopamine treatments on dysarthria. However, to date the small number of subjects enrolled in these studies and the heterogeneity of clinical outcome measures and assessments have lead to contradictory results.

A trend towards levodopa improvement of both spontaneous speech and oral reading was reported in the 1970s.[94] Similarly, an increase of speech volume after levodopa improves speech intelligibility in PD[95] with coupled acoustic and glottographic measurements showing an increase in sound pressure level but no change for other phonatory factors.[28] An acoustic analysis showed a significant increase of fundamental frequency after levodopa administration, which seems directly related to the decrease of laryngeal hypokinesia and rigidity.[30] Similar results have been reported by electromyographic studies of laryngeal muscles.[29] Pitch variation improves with levodopa therapy, although the speech rate was unchanged.[96] Dysfluency changes have been noted in some patients, supporting the hypothesis that speech dysfluencies may be related to an increase or decrease in the concentration of dopamine in the brain.[97] A recent acoustic analysis showed a significant reduction of intensity variation and the frequency tremor intensity index following levodopa therapy.[30]

Levodopa restores orofacial muscle activity assessed with electromyography,[98] leading to a decrease of tonic hyperactivity of labial muscles[99] and the restoration of labial motor control involved in speech.[100] This beneficial effect results in the reduction of reaction and movement times measured during lip kinematical analysis,[101] and the improvement of lip contractions.[102] Pergolide, with or without levodopa, did not achieve significant improvement for dysarthria[103] but perceptual assessment of dysarthria showed a trend towards improvement during co-administration of bromocriptine and levodopa.[104,105]

However, in some patients dopamine replacement does not affect speech quality;[106] some studies showed no change in phonatory factors after levodopa administration.[107] Hence, the effect of dopamine replacement therapy seems to be limited and variable. Ho et al[108] found that although speech stimuli showed a consistent tendency for increased loudness and faster rate during the "on" state, this was accompanied by a greater extent of intensity decay, while pitch and articulation remained unchanged. Levodopa effectively upscaled the overall gain setting of vocal amplitude and tempo, similar to its well-known effect on limb movement. However, unlike limb movement, this effect on the final acoustic product of speech may or may not be advantageous, depending on the existing speech profile of individual patients.

Brumlik and colleagues[109] observed a tendency towards improvement in maximum intensity speech range and speaking rate in patients taking trihexyphenidyl compared with those taking placebo. Little improvement in articulation after administration of other anticholinergic drugs has been described.[110] Furthermore, the motor complications of the long duration syndrome, i.e. orofacial or respiratory dyskinesias, oromandibular dystonias,[111] and "peakdose dysphonia,"[112] may affect the therapy-induced improvement of voice in PD.

Surgical therapies

Before the introduction of dopamine replacement therapies, functional neurosurgical procedures (mainly thalamotomy and pallidotomy) were used to treat PD symptoms. In more recent years, a better understanding of basal ganglia circuitry, advances in neuroimaging and neurosurgical techniques, and positive reports of clinical studies, led to a renaissance in the neurosurgical treatment of movement disorders associated with PD. Some significant improvement after surgical treatment has been observed for motor impairment of limbs. As for dysarthria, the effect of ablative neurosurgery is more commonly deleterious.[3] Deep cerebral stimulation (DBS) of basal ganglia has more recently become the first line treatment for severe PD patients. Variable effects on speech have been described as a consequence of stimulating different targets.

Pallidotomy was introduced with the purpose of alleviating PD signs and reducing controlateral dyskinesias—lesions involved the posteroventral portion of the internal part of the globus pallidus (GPi). In most cases a worsening of dysarthria was observed,[113] along with facial weakness, swallowing problems, and alteration of verbal fluency.[114] Barlow et al[115] reported that half of the patients involved in a study of labial force production and stability experienced improvement on this motor component of speech after bilateral posteroventral pallidotomy; they reported significant reduction in laryngeal airway resistance, increased mean vocalic airflows, more consistent syllable production rates, reduced voice onset variability, and improved force control of the perioral apparatus. Positive changes in phonatory and articulatory measures in patients with PD who underwent unilateral pallidotomy have also been reported. Acoustic analysis of speech and voice parameters in 6 patients with PD following unilateral pallidotomy identified considerable variability amongst the subjects; in 4 of 6 patients a positive effect after pallidotomy was reported either on phonatory or both phonatory and articulatory measures, consisting of greater intensity, more syllables per second, and longer extended vowel duration after surgery.[49] Speech impairment was observed also in subjects who had underwent GPi stimulation,[116,117] and Hariz et al[118] reported this adverse event in 5% of patients with GPi-DBS after a long term follow up; however, it has been reported that dysarthria can be improved by adjusting the stimulation parameters.[119]

Subthalamic lesioning in PD patients seems to exert a negative effect on speech,[120] while subthalamic DBS has been reported to induce both speech impairment and improvement[121] with dysarthria one of the most reported side-effects.[122] From a neurophysiological point of view, Pinto et al[34] reported that STN stimulation was able to revert the cortical activation abnormalities observed on PET during speech production and articulation (see above). Lateralized effects of STN stimulation have also been reported. However, in a recent paper on long term adverse DBS events, after 4 years, 9 out of 49 patients (18%) who underwent the surgery reported speech impairment.[118] Wang et al[123] reported that, while a mild improvement was observed in all subjects in the stimulation-on condition, 3 subjects who received left-STN stimulation showed a significant decline in vocal intensity and vowel duration from their baseline. In a subsequent study, the same group[124] reported that the speaking rate was generally slower for the left STN DBS group in comparison to the right STN DBS group; furthermore, they measured diadochokinetic syllable rate and found that active stimulation decreased the syllable rate in the left STN group while it increased the rate of syllables in the right STN group. Santens et al[125] found selective left-sided stimulation to have a negative effect on prosody and articulation, whereas right-sided stimulation did not display this kind of effect. Because no significant difference in speech characteristics was found between bilateral stimulation on and off, the authors suggested that a balanced tuning of bilateral basal ganglia networks is necessary for speech, and that the left circuit is probably dominant. Pinto et al[126] investigated oral force control in PD subjects treated with bilateral STN stimulation; the forces of the upper lip, lower lip and tongue were measured: an improvement in a series of indices was observed (maximal voluntary force—an index of hypokinesia; reaction time—an index of akinesia; movement time—an index of bradykinesia; imprecision of the peak force; hold phase). Similar results were obtained by Gentil et al.[127] Dromey et al[128] reported small increases in sound pressure level and fundamental frequency variability in response to STN stimulation. D'Alatri et al[129] reported that stimulation of the STN improved motor performances and vocal tremor and provided a major stability to glottal vibration.

Thalamic stimulation does not significantly improve speech; moreover, dysarthria has been reported as a side effect of the surgery.[130] Stimulation of the thalamus has been reported to produce silencing and slowing of speech.[131] More recent reports suggest that bilateral thalamic stimulation more frequently causes dysarthria than unilateral procedures.[132,133] Thalamotomy was mainly used to improve parkinsonian tremor and the lesion was generally made in the ventrolateral and the ventral intermediate nuclei of the thalamus. Unilateral thalamotomy worsens several aspects of speech (initiation and maintenance of speech) when the lesion is in either the dominant or the non-dominant hemispheres[134]; patients with PD who underwent unilateral or bilateral thalamotomy were more dysarthric after surgery.[106] Bilateral thalamotomy has been associated with word blocking, slow speech and hypophonia, and a persistent worsening of dysarthria.[135,136] The negative effect on speech has been the main reason for abandoning bilateral thalamotomy in favor of other techniques.

In conclusion, the effects of levodopa, dopamine agonists, and other drugs on dysarthria in PD are variable. The available data have been obtained in small and diverse groups of patients, leading to a low level of evidence and reliability. Albeit the available information is insufficient for clinical practice to allow any viable prediction regarding speech response to levodopa, as a general rule it is common to observe that, at least in the early stages of the disease, the dopamine drugs improve speech, whereas in later stages this is not common. On the other hand, from a clinical point of view, DBS appears to not affect speech at all, or worsen it, even though some reports on selected voice parameters pointed out some degree of improvement.

Speech Therapy in Parkinson's Disease

Despite the implications of speech changes on the lives of people with PD, only a minority have any form of speech therapy. In the UK, this figure was 3%–4.4% approximately 30 years ago.[64,137] This appears to have increased 4 to 5 fold to 15%–20% in a span of about 20 years,[138,139] and plateaued at this level as reported recently.[140] This pattern of speech therapy engagement over time is likely to resonate with that in other countries with similar traditions of speech therapy provision, due to the change in perception and progress in the field.

The most prevailing early view expressed for the most part of the last century was that PD, as a progressive neurological condition, was irreversible, therefore not suitable for therapy in general. In terms of speech therapy, speech impairments in PD only started attracting some interest from speech and language therapists in publications from the 1950s and 1960s. The author of a study[141] describing a 15-year speech-training program with over 300 patients concluded that in PD patients there is no permanent improvement, that 'therapeutic efforts are probably of greatest benefit to the patient's psyche rather than to his ability to speak', therefore reinforcing the view that the degenerative pathophysiology of PD 'does not yield to therapeutic incursion' (p274). This reinforced the pessimistic view that effective therapy for this population of patients was not realistic, with not enough real gains to be made per unit of time. The program of treatment generally involved average treatment for 2hrs per week for 6 months. A wide range of different techniques were used, mainly prosodic exercises (targeting maintenance and control of intensity level; increased facial mobility; increased mobility, speed, accuracy of lip, tongue, and jaw movement; and improved articulation) with visual (mirror) and auditory playback of patients' speech, and auditory cueing (metronome) for individuals and groups. Although there was no positive outcome documented, some interesting points were made regarding the importance of awareness and motivation in patients. A smattering of other subsequent, small anecdotal studies[142,143] reported inconsistent or lack of success, reinforcing the commonly held view and leading to a further general lack of interest in the area. However, it must be borne in mind that this was also the era of pharmacological prominence in treatment and management of PD with the advent of levodopa therapy in the late 1960s.

Twenty years on, with the keen realization of the limits of levodopa medication and the impetus around physiotherapy for patients with PD, there was a renewed interest in what speech therapy might offer. Therefore, the 1980s saw an increase in the number and quality of studies, with more participants and better experimental design such as random assignation and clearer outcome measures. Most studies investigated the utility of prosodic multi-focused therapy emphasizing benefit to the rate of speech, articulation, loudness and pitch, by using breathing[144] and prosodic exercises, sometimes with the provision of visual feedback on performance.[76,145–148]

Scott and Caird[149] conducted a study with 9 PD patients comprising 10 one-hour sessions over 2 weeks at home. Two treatments were used in a random order: 1) prosodic or intonational exercises on pitch, volume, duration in production, and recognition, with visual feedback for monitoring and reinforcement (vocalite –voice-operated light source); and 2) proprioceptive neuromuscular facilitation focusing on intensive multisensory input for speech movement exercises with proprioceptive feedback. Perceptual ratings were made for breathing pattern, initiation of speech, ability to vary volume, and prosodic abnormality, with high numbers poorer. Intonational exercises were found to improve ability to vary volume and prosodic abnormality; proprioceptive abnormality improved only prosody. Eight patients were retested 6 months later and only the prosodic abnormality was significantly better than baseline, although it was poorer than immediately post treatment. The study recommended that intonational exercises were more practical, but suggested that 'therapist rather than the treatment method may be responsible' (p1088), echoing earlier studies' commenting about the importance of motivation. A similar larger follow-up study of 26 PD patients found there was an improvement on prosody and intelligibility which was maintained for 3 months, and that there was limited benefit from using a visual reinforcement device compared to just conducting the multi-focused prosodic exercises alone.[146] A similar but more intensive focused prosodic approach was taken in another study.[76] Here, 12 randomly selected patients received 3.5–4 hrs of therapy daily in a group setting, with individual sessions as required, resulting in a total of 35–40 therapy hours at the end of 2 weeks. The remaining 10 patients formed a no-therapy control group. Treatment focused on respiration, pitch variation and loudness of voice, articulatory movement range, strength and speed, rate of speech control, variation of intonation, and stress pattern, similar to a previous study conducted in a residential setting.[150] Types of activities included reading out dialogues and monologues, with role play and video feedback and discussion. The results showed that the treatment group improved all aspects of the dysarthria profile immediately after treatment and this was maintained over 3 months.

The 1990s saw a streamlining of the multi-focused traditional prosodic treatment plans of the 1980s to emphasize the key impairment in the hypokinetic dysarthria of PD, that is, vocal speech intensity, or loudness. The novelty of only having a single common treatment focus across all specific presentations of PD speech was an approach that reduced the cognitive components of therapy and has been the most effective therapy to date, as documented in a series of studies with rigorous controls.[151,152] Other key elements to its effectiveness include the intensive nature of the program (4 times per week, for 4 weeks, with daily homework exercises), and the highly motivational one-on-one therapist-client relationship. The combined use of behavioral strategies such as cueing target behavior through means of a mental prompt and cognitive retraining in terms of learning to over-ride down-scaled sensory perception of speech output. The efficacy of this single-focused treatment program has been shown to impact other aspects of speech such as intelligibility as well as facial movement, and current research is exploring ways of increasing its accessibility to PD patients, e.g. via Internet and webcam technology.[153]

As effective speech therapy and new ways of delivering treatment become more available to patients with PD, it is hoped that the availability and uptake of speech therapy will continue to increase over time in order to lessen the burden of PD on patients and their care givers.

References

1. Hartelius L, Svensson P. Speech and swallowing symptoms associated with Parkinson's disease and multiple sclerosis: a survey. *Folia Phoniatr Logop*. 1994;46(1):9–17.
2. Darley FL, Aronson AE, Brown JR. *Motor speech disorders*. Philadelphia: WB Saunders; 1975.
3. Pinto S, Ozsancak C, Tripoliti E, Thobois S, Limousin-Dowsey P, Auzou P. Treatments for dysarthria in Parkinson's disease. *Lancet Neurol*. 2004;3(9):547–556.
4. Yorkston KM. The degenerative dysarthrias: a window into critical clinical and research issues. *Folia Phoniatr Logop*. 2007;59(3):107–117.
5. Duffy JR. *Motor Speech Disorders: substrates, differential diagnosis, and management*. St. Louis, Mo: Elsevier Mosby; 2005.
6. Ziegler W, von Cramon D. Spastic dysarthria after acquired brain injury: an acoustic study. *Br J Disord Commun*. 1986;21(2):173–187.
7. Wildgruber D, Ackermann H, Grodd W. Differential contributions of motor cortex, basal ganglia, and cerebellum to speech motor control: effects of syllable repetition rate evaluated by fMRI. *Neuroimage*. 2001;13(1):101–109.
8. Murdoch BE. Subcortical brain mechanisms in speech and language. *Folia Phoniatr Logop*. 2001;53(2):233–251.
9. Bohland JW, Guenther FH. An fMRI investigation of syllable sequence production. *Neuroimage*. 2006;32(2):821–841.
10. Riecker A, Mathiak K, Wildgruber D, et al. fMRI reveals two distinct cerebral networks subserving speech motor control. *Neurology*. 2005;64(4):700–706.
11. Wise RJ, Greene J, Büchel C, Scott SK. Brain regions involved in articulation. *Lancet*. 1999;353(9158):1057–1061.

12. Ackermann H, Ziegler W. Articulatory deficits in parkinsonian dysarthria: an acoustic analysis. *J Neurol Neurosurg Psychiatry*. 1991;54(12):1093–1098.

13. Logemann JA, Fisher HB, Boshes B, Blonsky ER. Frequency and co-occurrence of vocal tract dysfunctions in the speech of a large sample of Parkinson patients. *J Speech Hear Res*. 1978;43(1):47–57.

14. Ackermann H, Hertrich I, Daum I, Scharf G, Spieker S. Kinematic analysis of articulatory movements in central motor disorders. *Mov Disord*. 1997;12(6):1019–1027.

15. Wildgruber D, Kischka U, Ackermann H, Klose U, Grodd W. Dynamic pattern of brain activation during sequencing of word strings evaluated by fMRI. *Brain Res Cogn Brain Res*. 1999;7(3):285–294.

16. Fiez JA, Raichle ME. Linguistic processing. *Int Rev Neurobiol*. 1997;41:233–254.

17. Square PA, Martin RE. The nature and treatment of neuromotor speech disorders in aphasia. In: Chapey R, ed. *Language intervention strategies in adult aphasia*. Baltimore: Williams &Wilkins; 1994.

18. Levelt WJM. Spoken word production: A theory of lexical access. *Proc Natl Acad Sci U S A*. 2001;98(23):13464–13471.

19. Levelt WJM, Roelofs A, Meyer AS. A theory of lexical access in speech production. *Behav Brain Sci*. 1999;22:1–75.

20. Jonas S. The supplementary motor region and speech emission. *J Commun Disord*. 1981;14(5):349–373.

21. Gerloff C, Corwell B, Chen R, Hallett M, Cohen LG. Stimulation over the human supplementary motor area interferes with the organization of future elements in complex motor sequences. *Brain*. 1997;120(9):1587–1602.

22. Krainik A, Lehéricy S, Duffau H, et al. Role of the supplementary motor area in motor deficit following medial frontal lobe surgery. *Neurology*. 2001;57(5):871–878.

23. Bennett S, Netsell RW. Possible roles of the insula in speech and language processing: directions for research. *J Med Speech Lang Pathol*. 1999;7(4):255–272.

24. Ackermann H, Riecker A. The contribution of the insula to motor aspects of speech production: a review and a hypothesis. *Brain Lang*. 2004;89(2):320–328.

25. McNeil MR, Robin DA, Schmidt RA. Apraxia of speech: Definition, differentiation, and treatment. In: McNeil MR, ed. *Clinical management of sensorimotor speech disorders*. New York: Thieme; 1997.

26. Dronkers NF. A new brain region for coordinating speech articulation. *Nature*. 1996;384(6605):159–161.

27. Cereda C, Ghika J, Maeder P, Bogousslavsky J. Strokes restricted to the insular cortex. *Neurology*. 2002;59(12):1950–1955.

28. Jiang J, O'Mara T, Chen HJ, Stern JI, Vlagos D, D H. Aerodynamic measurements of patients with Parkinson's disease. *J Voice*. 1999;13(4):583–591.

29. Gallena S, Smith PJ, Zeffiro T, Ludlow CL. Effects of levodopa on laryngeal muscle activity for voice onset and offset in Parkinson disease. *J Speech Hear Res*. 2001;44(6):1284–1299.

30. Sanabria J, Ruiz PG, Gutierrez R, et al. The effect of levodopa on vocal function in Parkinson's disease. *Clin Neuropharmacol*. 2001;24(2):99–102.

31. Braak H, Del Tredici K, Bratzke H, Hamm-Clement J, Sandmann-Keil D, Rüb U. Staging of the intracerebral inclusion body pathology associated with

idiopathic Parkinson's disease (preclinical and clinical stages). *J Neurol.* 2002;249 (Suppl 3):III/1–5.

32. Braak H, Bohl JR, Müller CM, Rüb U, de Vos RA, Del Tredici K. Stanley Fahn Lecture 2005: The staging procedure for the inclusion body pathology associated with sporadic Parkinson's disease reconsidered. *Mov Disord.* 2006;21(12):2042–2051.

33. Bonnet AM, Loria Y, Saint-Hilaire MH, Lhermitte F, Agid Y. Does long-term aggravation of Parkinson's disease result from nondopaminergic lesions? *Neurology.* 1987;37:1539–1542.

34. Pinto S, Thobois S, Costes N, et al. Subthalamic nucleus stimulation and dysarthria in Parkinson's disease: a PET study. *Brain.* 2004;127(Pt 3):602–615.

35. Liotti M, Ramig LO, Vogel D, et al. Hypophonia in Parkinson's disease: neural correlates of voice treatment revealed by PET. *Neurology.* 2003;60(3):432–440.

36. Rektorova I, Barrett J, Mikl M, Rektor I, Paus T. Functional abnormalities in the primary orofacial sensorimotor cortex during speech in Parkinson's disease. *Mov Disord.* 2007;22(14):2043–2051.

37. Dias AE, Barbosa ER, Coracini K, Maia F, Marcolin MA, Fregni F. Effects of repetitive transcranial magnetic stimulation on voice and speech in Parkinson's disease. *Acta Neurol Scand.* 2006;113(2):92–99.

38. Logemann JA, Fisher HB. Vocal tract control in Parkinson's disease: phonetic feature analysis of misarticulations. *J Speech Hear Res.* 1981;46(4):348–352.

39. Lim EC, Wilder-Smith E, Ong BK, Seet RC. Adult-onset re-emergent stuttering as a presentation of Parkinson's disease. *Ann Acad Med Singapore.* 2005;34(9):579–581.

40. Kent RD, Read C. *The Acoustic Analysis of Speech.* San Diego: Singular; 1992.

41. Fant G. *Acoustic theory of speech production (2nd edition).* Mouton De Gruyter: The Hague; 1970.

42. Solomon NP, Hixon TJ. Speech breathing in Parkinson's disease. *J Speech Hear Res.* 1993;36(2):294–310.

43. Murdoch BE, Chenery HJ, Bowler S, Ingram JC. Respiratory function in Parkinson's subjects exhibiting a perceptible speech deficit: a kinematic and spirometric analysis. *J Speech Hear Res.* 1989;54(4):610–626.

44. Goberman AM, Coelho C, Robb M. Phonatory characteristics of Parkinsonian speech before and after morning medication: the ON and OFF states. *J Commun Disord.* 2002;35(3):217–239.

45. Kent RD, Vorperian HK, Kent JF, Duffy JR. Voice dysfunction in dysarthria: application of the Multi-Dimensional Voice Program. *J Commun Disord.* 2003;36(4):281–306.

46. Hertrich I, Ackermann H. Gender-specific vocal dysfunctions in Parkinson's disease: electroglottographic and acoustic analyses. *Ann Otol Rhinol Laryngol.* 1995;104(3):197–202.

47. Midi I, Dogan M, Koseoglu M, Can G, Sehitoglu MA, Gunal DI. Voice abnormalities and their relation with motor dysfunction in Parkinson's disease. *Acta Neurol Scand.* 2008;117(1):26–34.

48. Perez KS, Ramig LO, Smith ME, Dromey C. The Parkinson larynx: tremor and videostroboscopic findings. *J Voice.* 1996;10(4):354–361.

49. Shulz GM, Peterson T, Sapienza CM, Greer M, Friedman W. Voice and speech characteristics of persons with Parkinson's disease pre and post-pallidotomy surgery: Preliminary findings. *J Speech Lang Hear Res.* 1999;42(5):1176–1194.

50. Holmes RJ, Oates JM, Phyland DJ, Hughes AJ. Voice characteristics in the progression of Parkinson's disease. *Int J Lang Commun Disord.* 2000;35(3):407–418.

51. Ludlow C, Bassich C. Relationships between perceptual ratings and acoustic measures of hypokinetic speech. In: McNeil MR, Rosenbeck JC, Aronson AE, eds. *The Dysarthrias.* San Diego: College-Hill Press; 1984.

52. Hoodin RB, Gilbert HR. Parkinsonian dysarthria: an aerodynamic and perceptual description of velopharyngeal closure for speech. *Folia Phoniatr (Basel).* 1989;41(6):249–258.

53. Kent RD, Rosenbek JC. Prosodic disturbance and neurologic lesion. *Brain Lang.* 1982;15(2):259–291.

54. Hirose H. Pathophysiology of motor speech disorders (dysarthria). *Folia Phoniatr (Basel).* 1986;38(2–4):61–88.

55. Moreau C, Ozsancak C, Blatt JL, Derambure P, Destee A, Defebvre L. Oral festination in Parkinson's disease: biomechanical analysis and correlation with festination and freezing of gait. *Mov Disord.* 2007;22(10):1503–1506.

56. Illes J, Metter EJ, Hanson WR, Iritani S. Language production in Parkinson's disease: acoustic and linguistic considerations. *Brain Lang.* 1988;33(1):146–160.

57. Bayles KA, Tomoeda CK, Wood JA, Cruz RF, Azuma T, Montgomery EB. The effect of Parkinson's disease on language. *J Med Speech Lang Pathol.* 1997;5:157–166.

58. Enderby P, Philipp R. Speech and language handicap: towards knowing the size of the problem. *Br J Disord Commun.* 1986;21(2):151–165.

59. Blumin JH, Pcolinsky DE, Atkins JP. Laryngeal findings in advanced Parkinson's disease. *Ann Otol Rhinol Laryngol.* 2004;113(4):253–258.

60. De Letter M, Santens P, Van Borsel J. The effects of levodopa on word intelligibility in Parkinson's disease. *J Commun Disord.* 2005;38(3):187–196.

61. Miller N, Allcock L, Jones D, Noble E, Hildreth AJ, Burn DJ. Prevalence and pattern of perceived intelligibility changes in Parkinson's disease. *J Neurol Neurosurg Psychiatry.* 2007;78(11):1188–1190.

62. Skodda S, Schlegel U. Speech rate and rhythm in Parkinson's disease. *Mov Disord.* 2008;23(7):985–992.

63. Goberman AM. Correlation between acoustic speech characteristics and non-speech motor performance in Parkinson Disease. *Med Sci Monit.* 2005;11(3):CR109–116.

64. Mutch WJ, Strudwick A, Roy SK, Downie AW. Parkinson's disease: disability, review, and management. *Br Med J (Clin Res Ed).* 1986;293(6548):675–677.

65. Ho AK, Iansek R, Marigliani C, Bradshaw JL, Gates S. Speech impairment in a large sample of patients with Parkinson's disease. *Behav Neurol.* 1998;11(3):131–137.

66. Coates C, Bakheit AM. The prevalence of verbal communication disability in patients with Parkinson's disease. *Disabil Rehabil.* 1997;19(3):104–107.

67. Hartelius L, Elmberg M, Holm R, Lovberg AS, Nikolaidis S. Living with dysarthria: evaluation of a self-report questionnaire. *Folia Phoniatr Logop.* 2008;60(1):11–19.

68. Ludlow CL, Bassich CJ. The Results of Acoustic and Perceptual Assessment of Two Types of Dysarthria. In: Berry WR, ed. *Clinical Dysarthria.* San Diego: College-Hill Press; 1983.

69. Ozsancak C, Auzou P, Jan M, Defebvre L, Derambure P, A D. The place of perceptual analysis of dysarthria in the differential diagnosis of corticobasal degeneration and Parkinson's disease. *J Neurol*. 2006;253(1):92–97.

70. Darley FL, Aronson AE, Brown JR. Clusters of deviant speech dimensions in the dysarthrias. *J Speech Hear Res*. 1969;12(3):462–496.

71. Darley FL, Aronson AE, Brown JR. Differential diagnostic patterns of dysarthria. *J Speech Hear Res*. 1969;12(2):246–269.

72. Hirano M. *Clinical Examination of Voice*. New York: Springer-Verlag; 1981.

73. Enderby P. *Frenchay Dysarthria Assessment*. San Diego: College-Hill Press; 1983.

74. Forrest K, Weismer G, Turner GS. Kinematic, acoustic, and perceptual analyses of connected speech produced by parkinsonian and normal geriatric adults. *J Acoust Soc Am*. 1989;85(6):2608–2622.

75. Robertson SJ. *Dysarthria Profile*. Chesterfield: Winslow Press; 1982.

76. Robertson SJ, Thomson F. Speech therapy in Parkinson's disease: a study of the efficacy and long term effects of intensive treatment. *Br J Disord Commun*. 1984;19(3): 213–224.

77. Yorkston KM, Beukelman DR. *Assessment of Intelligibility of Dysarthric Speech (AIDS)*. Austin, TX: Pro-Ed; 1984.

78. Kompoliti K, Wang QE, Goetz CG, Leurgans S, Raman R. Effects of central dopaminergic stimulation by apomorphine on speech in Parkinson's disease. *Neurology*. 2000;54(2):458–462.

79. Yorkston KM, Hammen VL, Beukelman DR, Traynor CD. The effect of rate control on the intelligibility and naturalness of dysarthric speech. *J Speech Hear Res*. 1990;55(3):550–560.

80. Hammen VL, Yorkston KM, Minifie FD. Effects of temporal alterations on speech intelligibility in parkinsonian dysarthria. *J Speech Hear Res*. 1994;37(2):244–253.

81. Hustad KC, Cahill MA. Effects of presentation mode and repeated familiarization on intelligibility of dysarthric speech. *Am J Speech Lang Pathol*. 2003;12(2):198–208.

82. Ho AK, Iansek R, Bradshaw JL. The effect of a concurrent task on Parkinsonian speech. *J Clin Exp Neuropsychol*. 2002;24(1):36–47.

83. Rosen KM, Kent RD, Duffy JR. Task-based profile of vocal intensity decline in Parkinson's disease. *Folia Phoniatr Logop*. 2005;57(1):28–37.

84. Kempler D, Van Lancker D. Effect of speech task on intelligibility in dysarthria: a case study of Parkinson's disease. *Brain Lang*. 2002;80(3):449–464.

85. Eadie TL, Yorkston KM, Klasner ER, et al. Measuring communicative participation: a review of self-report instruments in speech-language pathology. *Am J Speech Lang Pathol*. 2006;15(4):307–320.

86. Jacobson BH, Johnson A, Grywalski C, et al. The Voice Handicap Index (VHI): Development and validation. *Am J Speech Lang Pathol*. 1997;6:66–70.

87. Sewall GK, Jiang J, Ford CN. Clinical evaluation of Parkinson's-related dysphonia. *Laryngoscope*. 2006;116(10):1740–1744.

88. Hogikyan ND, Sethuraman G. Validation of an instrument to measure voice-related quality of life (V-RQOL). *J Voice*. 1999;13(4):557–569.

89. Gómez-Esteban JC, Zarranz JJ, Lezcano E, et al. Influence of motor symptoms upon the quality of life of patients with Parkinson's disease. *Eur Neurol*. 2007;57(3): 161–165.

90. Rahman S, Griffin HJ, Quinn NP, Jahanshahi M. Quality of life in Parkinson's disease: the relative importance of the symptoms. *Mov Disord.* 2008;23(10):1428–1434.

91. Peto V, Jenkinson C, Fitzpatrick R. PDQ-39: a review of the development, validation and application of a Parkinson's disease quality of life questionnaire and its associated measures. *J Neurol.* 1998;245(Suppl 1):S10–14.

92. de Boer AG, Wijker W, Speelman JD, de Haes JC. Quality of life in patients with Parkinson's disease: development of a questionnaire. *J Neurol Neurosurg Psychiatry.* 1996;61(1):70–74.

93. Haapaniemi TH, Sotaniemi KA, Sintonen H, Taimela E. The generic 15D instrument is valid and feasible for measuring health related quality of life in Parkinson's disease. *J Neurol Neurosurg Psychiatry.* 2004;75(7):976–983.

94. Rigrodsky S, Morrison EB. Speech changes in parkinsonism during L-dopa therapy: preliminary findings. *J Am Geriatr Soc.* 1970;18(2):142–151.

95. Mawdsley C, Gamsu CV. Periodicity of speech in Parkinsonism. *Nature.* 1971;231(5301):315–316.

96. Wolfe VI, Garvin JS, Bacon M, Waldrop W. Speech changes in Parkinson's disease during treatment with L-dopa. *J Commun Disord.* 1975;8(3):271–279.

97. Goberman AM, Blomgren M. Parkinsonian speech dysfluencies: effects of L-dopa-related fluctuations. *J Fluency Disord.* 2003;28(1):55–70.

98. Leanderson R, Persson A, Ohman S. Electromyographic studies of facial muscle activity in speech. *Acta Otolaryngol.* 1971;72(5):361–369.

99. Leanderson R, Meyerson BA, Persson A. Effect of L-dopa on speech in parkinsonism: an EMG study of labial articulatory function. *J Neurol Neurosurg Psychiatry.* 1971;34(6):679–681.

100. Leanderson R, Meyerson BA, Persson A. Lip muscle function in Parkinsonian dysarthria. *Acta Otolaryngol.* 1972;74(4):350–357.

101. Nakano KK, Zubick H, Tyler HR. Speech defects of parkinsonian patients: effects of levodopa therapy on speech intelligibility. *Neurology.* 1973;23(8):865–870.

102. Cahill LM, Murdoch BE, Theodoros DG, Triggs EJ, Charles BG, Yao AA. Effect of oral levodopa treatment on articulatory function in Parkinson's disease: preliminary results. *Motor Control.* 1998;2:161–172.

103. Jeanty P, Van den Kerchove M, Lowenthal A, De Bruyne H. Pergolide therapy in Parkinson's disease. *J Neurol.* 1984;231(3):148–152.

104. Gauthier G, Martins da Silva A. Bromocriptine combined with levodopa in Parkinson's disease. *Eur Neurol.* 1982;21(4):217–226.

105. Selby G. The addition of bromocriptine to long-term dopa therapy in Parkinson's disease. *Clin Exp Neurol.* 1989;26:129–139.

106. Quaglieri CE, Celesia GG. Effect of thalamotomy and levodopa therapy on the speech of Parkinson patients. *Eur Neurol.* 1977;15(1):34–39.

107. Poluha PC, Teulings HL, Brookshire RH. Handwriting and speech changes across the levodopa cycle in Parkinson's disease. *Acta Psychol (Amst).* 1998;100(1–2):71–84.

108. Ho AK, Bradshaw JL, Iansek R. For better or worse: The effect of levodopa on speech in Parkinson's disease. *Mov Disord.* 2008;23(4):574–580.

109. Brumlik J, Canter G, Delatorre R, Mier M, Petrovick M, Boshes B. A critical analysis of the effects of trihexyphenidyl (Artane) on the components of the parkinsonian syndrome. *J Nerv Ment Dis*. 1964;138:424–431.

110. Critchley EM. Speech disorders of Parkinsonism: a review. *J Neurol Neurosurg Psychiatry*. 1981;44(9):751–758.

111. Mardsen CD, Parkes JD. "On-off" effects in patients with Parkinson's disease on chronic levodopa therapy. *Lancet*. 1976;1(7954):292–296.

112. Critchley EM. Peak-dose dysphonia in parkinsonism. *Lancet*. 1976;1(7958):544.

113. Higuchi Y, Iacono RP. Surgical complications in patients with Parkinson's disease after posteroventral pallidotomy. *Neurosurgery*. 2003;52(3):558–571.

114. Tröster AI, Woods SP, Fields JA, Hanisch C, Beatty WW. Declines in switching underlie verbal fluency changes after unilateral pallidal surgery in Parkinson's disease. *Brain Cogn*. 2002;50(2):207–217.

115. Barlow SH, Iacono RP, Paseman LA, Biswas A, D'Antonio L. The effects of posteroventral pallidotomy on force and speech aerodynamics in Parkinson's disease. In: Cannito MP, Yorkston CM, Beukelman DR, eds. *Neuromotor Speech Disorders: Nature, Assessment and management*. Baltimore: Brookes Publishing Co; 1998.

116. Ghika J, Villemure JG, Fankhauser H, Favre J, Assal G, Ghika-Schmid F. Efficiency and safety of bilateral contemporaneous pallidal stimulation (deep brain stimulation) in levodopa-responsive patients with Parkinson's disease with severe motor fluctuations: a 2-year follow-up review. *J Neurosurg*. 1998;89(5):713–718.

117. Krause M, Fogel W, Heck A, et al. Deep brain stimulation for the treatment of Parkinson's disease: subthalamic nucleus versus globus pallidus internus. *J Neurol Neurosurg Psychiatry*. 2001;70(4):464–470.

118. Hariz MI, Rehncrona S, Quinn NP, Speelman JD, Wensing C. Multicentre Advanced Parkinson's Disease Deep Brain Stimulation Group. Multicenter study on deep brain stimulation in Parkinson's disease: an independent assessment of reported adverse events at 4 years. *Mov Disord*. 2008;23(3):416–421.

119. Lyons KE, Wilkinson SB, Troster AI, Pahwa R. Long-term efficacy of globus pallidus stimulation for the treatment of Parkinson's disease. *Stereotact Funct Neurosurg*. 2002;79(3–4):214–220.

120. Parkin S, Nandi D, Giladi N, et al. Lesioning the subthalamic nucleus in the treatment of Parkinson's disease. *Stereotact Funct Neurosurg*. 2001;77(1–4):68–72.

121. Rousseaux M, Krystkowiak P, Kozlowski O, Ozsancak C, Blond S, Destee A. Effects of subthalamic nucleus stimulation on parkinsonian dysarthria and speech intelligibility. *J Neurol*. 2004;251(3):327–334.

122. Limousin P, Krack P, Pollak P, et al. Electrical stimulation of the subthalamic nucleus in advanced Parkinson's disease. *N Engl J Med*. 1998;339(16):1105–1111.

123. Wang E, Verhagen Metman L, Bakay R, Arzbaecher J, Bernard B. The effect of unilateral electrostimulation of the subthalamic nucleus on respiratory/phonatory subsystems of speech production in Parkinson's disease–a preliminary report. *Clin Linguist Phon*. 2003;17(4–5):283–289.

124. Wang EQ, Metman LV, Bakay RA, Arzbaecher J, Bernard B, Corcos DM. Hemisphere-specific effects of subthalamic nucleus deep brain stimulation on speaking

rate and articulatory accuracy of syllable repetitions in Parkinson's disease. *J Med Speech Lang Pathol.* 2006;14(4):323–334.

125. Santens P, De Letter M, Van Borsel J, De Reuck J, Caemaert J. Lateralized effects of subthalamic nucleus stimulation on different aspects of speech in Parkinson's disease. *Brain Lang.* 2003;87(2):253–258.

126. Pinto S, Gentil M, Fraix V, Benabid AL, Pollak P. Bilateral subthalamic stimulation effects on oral force control in Parkinson's disease. *J Neurol.* 2003;250(2): 179–187.

127. Gentil M, Tournier CL, Pollak P, Benabid AL. Effect of bilateral subthalamic nucleus stimulation and dopatherapy on oral control in Parkinson's disease. *Eur Neurol.* 1999;42(3):136–140.

128. Dromey C, Kumar R, Lang AE, Lozano AM. An investigation of the effects of subthalamic nucleus stimulation on acoustic measures of voice. *Mov Disord.* 2000;15(6):1132–1138.

129. D'Alatri L, Paludetti G, Contarino MF, Galla S, Marchese MR, Bentivoglio AR. Effects of bilateral subthalamic nucleus stimulation and medication on parkinsonian speech impairment. *J Voice.* 2008;22(3):365–372.

130. Taha JM, Janszen MA, Favre J. Thalamic deep brain stimulation for the treatment of head, voice, and bilateral limb tremor. *J Neurosurg.* 1999;91(1):68–72.

131. Koller W, Pahwa R, Busenbark K, et al. High frequency unilateral thalamic stimulation in the treatment of essential and parkinsonian tremor. *Ann Neurol.* 1997;42(3): 292–299.

132. Obwegeser AA, Uitti RJ, Witte RJ, Lucas JA, Turk MF, Wharen RE Jr. Quantitative and qualitative outcome measures after thalamic deep brain stimulation to treat disabling tremors. *Neurosurgery.* 2001;48(2):274–281.

133. Putzke JD, Wharen RE Jr, Wszolek ZK, Turk MF, Strongosky AJ, Uitti RJ. Thalamic deep brain stimulation for tremor-predominant Parkinson's disease. *Parkinsonism Relat Disord.* 2003;10(2):81–88.

134. Petrovici JN. Speech disturbances following stereotaxic surgery in ventrolateral thalamus. *Neurosurg Rev.* 1980;3(3):189–195.

135. Canter GJ, van Lancker DR. Disturbances of the temporal organization of speech following bilateral thalamic surgery in a patient with Parkinson's disease. *J Commun Disord.* 1985;18(5):329–349.

136. Tasker RR, Siqueira J, Hawrylyshyn P, Organ LW. What happened to VIM thalamotomy for Parkinson's disease? *Appl Neurophysiol.* 1983;46(1–4):68–83.

137. Oxtoby M. *Parkinson's disease patients and their social needs.* London: Parkinson's Disease Society; 1982.

138. Clarke CE, Zobkiw RM, Gullaksen E. Quality of life and care in Parkinson's disease. *Br J Clin Pract.* 1995;49(6):288–293.

139. Yarrow S, ed. *1998 survey of members of a Parkinson's Disease Society of the United Kingdom. Parkinson's Disease: Studies in psychological and social care.* Leicester, UK: BPS Books; 1998.

140. Noble E, Jones D, Miller N, Burn D. Speech and Language therapy provision for people with Parkinson's disease. *International Journal of Therapy and Rehabilitation.* 2006;13:323–327.

141. Sarno MT. Speech impairment in Parkinson's disease. *Arch Phys Med Rehabil.* 1968;49(5):269–275.
142. Erb E. Improving speech in Parkinson's disease. *Am J Nurs.* 1973;73(11):1910–1911.
143. Allan CM. Treatment of non fluent speech resulting from neurological disease-treatment of dysarthria. *Br J Disord Commun.* 1970;5(1):3–5.
144. Deane KHO, Whurr R, Clarke CE, Playford ED, Ben-Shlomo Y. Non-pharmacological therapies for dysphagia in Parkinson's disease. *Cochrane Database Syst Rev.* 2001;1(1):CD002816.
145. Lang AE, Fishbein V. The "pacing board" in selected speech disorders of Parkinson's disease. *J Neurol Neurosurg Psychiatry.* 1983;46(8):789.
146. Scott S, Caird FI. Speech therapy for Parkinson's disease. *J Neurol Neurosurg Psychiatry.* 1983;46(2):140–144.
147. Yorkston KM, Beukelman DR, Bell KR. *Clinical management of dysarthric speakers.* Boston, MA: College-Hill Press; 1988.
148. Johnson JA, Pring TR. Speech therapy and Parkinson's disease: a review and further data. *Br J Disord Commun.* 1990;25(2):183–194.
149. Scott S, Caird FI. Speech therapy for patients with Parkinson's disease. *Br Med J (Clin Res Ed).* 1981;283(6299):1088.
150. Robertson SJ, Thomson F. Speech therapy and Parkinson's disease. *The College of Speech Therapists Bulletin.* 1983;370:10–12.
151. Ramig LO, Countryman S, Thompson LL, Horii Y. Comparison of two forms of intensive speech treatment for Parkinson disease. *J Speech Hear Res.* 1995;38(6):1232–1251.
152. Ramig LO, Countryman S, O'Brien C, Hoehn M, Thompson L. Intensive speech treatment for patients with Parkinson's disease: short-and long-term comparison of two techniques. *Neurology.* 1996;47(6):1496–1504.
153. Ramig LO, Fox C, Sapir S. Speech treatment for Parkinson's disease. *Expert Rev Neurother.* 2008;8(2):297–309.

Chapter 3

Lesions Associated with Eye Movements

Andrew W. Michell, Roger A. Barker,
and Glenda M. Halliday

Eye movements are necessary to acquire, fixate and track visual stimuli in order to stabilize images on the retina, especially against movements of the head and body (image-stabilization system), to image important details of the visual world on the fovea (foveation system), and to align the retinal images in the two eyes in order to promote single vision and stereopsis (vergence-accommodation system). There are 6 basic types of eye movements to achieve these 3 principal functions,[1] as well as eyelid movement to open the eyes for sight and protect the eyes from dryness, foreign bodies, and bright light (Table 3-1). Image stabilization occurs through the vestibulocular reflex (stabilizes images on the retina during head movement by producing eye movements in the opposite direction to the head movement) and the optokinetic reflex (allows the eyes to follow objects in motion when the head remains stationary).[1] Foveation occurs through fixation that maintains the visual gaze on a single location, smooth pursuit that smoothly follows a moving object, and saccades that rapidly move both eyes simultaneously in the same direction.[1] Binocular alignment occurs through vergence that simultaneously moves both eyes in opposite directions to maintain binocular vision.[1] The eyes are protected by a thin sheet of skin (eyelid), which is voluntarily elevated to open the eyes by a single muscle, the levator palpebrae superioris, and lower the eyelid by passive downward forces and a decrease in muscle activity.[2] This muscle

50

Table 3-1. Basic Types of Eye and Eyelid Movements.

System	Eye/Eyelid Movement	Function
Image-stabilization	1.Vestibulocular reflex	Stabilizes images on the retina during head movement by producing eye movements in the opposite direction to the head movement
	2. Optokinetic reflex	Allows the eyes to follow objects in motion when the head remains stationary
Foveation	3. Fixation	Maintains the visual gaze on a single location
	4. Smooth pursuit	Smoothly follows a moving object
	5. Saccade	Rapidly moves both eyes simultaneously in the same direction
Binocular alignment	6. Vergence	Simultaneously moves both eyes in opposite directions
Protection	7. Blink reflex	Protects the eyes from dryness, foreign bodies and bright light

is also active in the involuntary blink reflex necessary to protect the eyes from dryness, foreign bodies, and bright light.[2]

Eye and eyelid movements are both voluntary and reflex, and can be abnormal in Parkinson's disease (PD), although rarely cause symptoms and substantive disability.[3] Significant eye movement abnormalities are most commonly used to differentiate the atypical parkinsonian conditions, especially progressive supranuclear palsy (PSP) and to a lesser extent multiple system atrophy (MSA), from PD.[4]

Neural Control of Eyelid Movement

The motoneurons innervating the levator palpebrae superioris muscle are located in the trochlear and oculomotor nuclei of the midbrain and receive tonic input during waking (from hypothalamic and limbic regions) to keep the eyes open (Figure 3-1), with a decrease in this input resulting in lid lowering during drowsiness.[5] A decrease in tonic input to these motoneurons is also achieved through inhibitory neurons in the nuclei of the posterior commissure and the deep layers of the superior colliculi[5,6] (Figure 3-1). Superimposed on the tonic input are excitatory signals from premotor

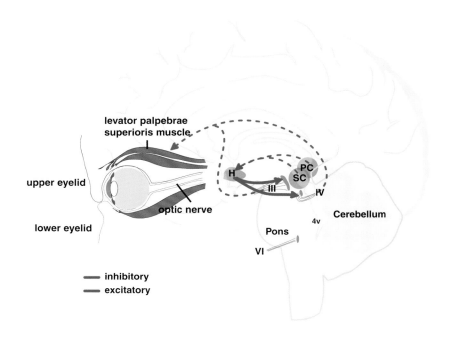

Figure 3-1. Primary neural circuit for eyelid movements. The motoneurons innervating the levator palpebrae superioris muscle are located in the trochlear (IV) and oculomotor (III) nuclei of the midbrain. These neurons receive tonic input during waking from hypothalamic (H) and limbic regions to keep the eyes open. Inhibitory neurons in the nuclei of the posterior commissure (PC) and the deep layers of the superior colliculi (SC) can reduce the tonic firing of the hypothalamic neurons, resulting in lid lowering during drowsiness.

neurons in the M group medial to the rostral interstitial nucleus of the medial longitudinal fasciculus (contains the premotor burst neurons for vertical saccades).[5] Neurons of the M group couple the lid to the eye during vertical eye movements by integrating information from the premotor burst neurons, the medial superior colliculi and inhibitory neurons in the interstitial nuclei of Cajal.[5]

Neural Control of Eye Movements

All eye movements share a common final pathway through 3 cranial nerve nuclei (oculomotor, trochlear and abducens) and the 6 pairs of eye muscles they control (superior, inferior, medial and lateral rectus muscles, and the superior and inferior oblique muscles) (Figure 3-2). These cranial nuclei are linked via the medial longitudinal fasciculus and associated with a range of other brainstem nuclei involved in gaze and saccadic movements. The trochlear nucleus is unique amongst cranial nerve nuclei since its axons cross the midline before leaving the brainstem (Figure 3-2), thus its neurons innervate the contralateral superior oblique. Abducens neurons innervate the ipsilateral lateral rectus, and oculomotor neurons innervate the remaining 4 muscles as well as the eyelid.

The neural circuits generating the different types of eye movements are widely separated structurally and converge on oculomotor neurons through various brainstem premotor oculomotor nuclei (see Figure 3-2 and[7,8]). The premotor oculomotor nuclei are highly interconnected and guarantee the generation and modulation of distinct aspects of all types of eye movements.

The premotor neurons responsible for binocular alignment, or the synchronous movement required to maintain congruent retinal images, are located dorsal and dorsolateral to the oculomotor nucleus.[1,7] The two principal cues for vergence movements are retinal disparity and retinal blur, signals processed through the cortex and cerebellum. While the exact brain regions involved in the control of binocular alignment are still poorly defined, they include the primary visual cortex, lateral suprasylvian area, lateral interparietal area, and frontal eye fields (Figure 3-2), which relay information through the nucleus reticularis pontine tegmenti to brainstem and cerebellar regions.[1,7] The cerebellar flocculus, dorsal vermis, and deep nuclei discharge prior to the onset of vergence movements.[7,9]

The premotor neurons responsible for foveation are located in a variety of brainstem regions.[7] All premotor neurons send collaterals to paramedian tract neurons (Figure 3-2). Premotor neurons responsible for fixation of eye position in the horizontal plane are located in the nucleus prepositus hypoglossi (Figure 3-2), while those for fixation in the vertical plane or with torsional movement are located in the interstitial nucleus of Cajal (Figure 3-2).[7] Paramedian tract neurons project exclusively to the flocculus of the cerebellum, providing eye position feedback signals essential for gaze holding.[7] The flocculus directly innervates the premotor neurons responsible for fixation. Premotor neurons for smooth pursuit are located in the vestibular nuclei (Figure 3-2), while those for horizontal saccades are found in the paramedian pontine reticular formation (Figure 3-2) and

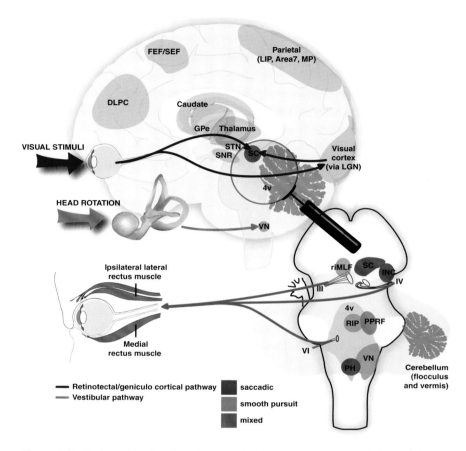

Figure 3-2. Brain regions involved in the control of eye movements. The 3 cranial nerve nuclei innervating eye muscles are the oculomotor, trochlear and abducens nuclei. These cranial nuclei are linked via the medial longitudinal fasciculus and receive input through highly connected brainstem premotor neurons which guarantee the generation and modulation of distinct aspects of all types of eye movements. The exact brain regions involved in the control of binocular alignment are still poorly defined, but include the primary visual cortex, lateral suprasylvian area (LIP), lateral interparietal area (Area7), and frontal eye fields (FEF/SEF), which relay information through the pons to brainstem and cerebellar regions for relay to premotor neurons. The central brainstem regulator for foveation is the paramedian pontine reticular formation (PPRF) which receives input from all premotor neurons and relays this through to the cerebellum for direct feedback to the premotor neurons. Premotor neurons responsible for fixation of eye position in the horizontal plane are located in the nucleus prepositus hypoglossi (PH), while those for fixation in the vertical plane or with torsional movement are located in the interstitial nucleus of Cajal (INC). Premotor neurons for smooth pursuit are located in the vestibular nuclei (VN), while those for horizontal saccades are found in the paramedian pontine reticular formation (PPRF) and those for vertical and torsional saccades are in the rostral interstitial nucleus of the medial longitudinal fasciculus (riMLF). Saccadic omnipause neurons are located in the nucleus raphe interpositus (RIP). Cortical (DPLC, FEF/SEF, parietal, visual cortices),

those for vertical and torsional saccades are in the rostral interstitial nucleus of the medial longitudinal fasciculus (Figure 3-2).[7] Saccadic omnipause neurons are located in the nucleus raphe interpositus (Figure 3-2). The vestibular nuclei receive visual information from neurons with smooth pursuit activity in the middle temporal and medial superior temporal cortices, as well as from lateral interparietal area, precuneus, frontal, and supplementary eye fields through cerebellar relays. These latter cortical regions also process information necessary for saccades. Temporal lobe neurons project through the pons to the ventral paraflocculus of the cerebellum, whereas frontal neurons project through the nucleus reticularis tegmenti pontis to the oculomotor vermis and fastigial regions of the cerebellum.[7] These cerebellar regions project directly to the premotor neurons for smooth pursuit and saccades to adapt eye movements to changing circumstances. The cortical regions also project to the thalamus (ventral anterior and lateral regions) and importantly for our discussion here, to the caudate nucleus, which relays goal selection information to the superior colliculus through the substantia nigra pars reticularis.[7] The superior colliculus projects to the premotor neurons to influence saccades and smooth pursuit.

The premotor neurons responsible for image stabilization are located in the vestibular nuclei and nucleus prepositus hypoglossi (Figure 3-2).[7] The vestibulocular reflex depends on afferents from the vestibular nerve to the vestibular nuclei (Figure 3-2) and output to the oculomotor nuclei with an important arm of this reflex passing through the cerebellum which conveys plasticity to the vestibulocular reflex in the event of altered parameter relationships. The vestibular nuclei have extensive reciprocal connections with the premotor nuclei responsible for fixation, as well as receiving diverse cerebellar input.[7] The optokinetic reflex has 2 components, a direct component that involves smooth pursuit mechanisms and an indirect component which receives retinal input through the nuclei of the accessory optic tract and the pretectal nucleus of the optic tract that is relayed to the vestibular nuclei and the nucleus prepositus hypoglossi.[7]

Figure 3-2. (continued)
basal ganglia (caudate, GPe, STN, SNR) and thalamic brain regions influence these nuclei largely through the superior colliculi (SC) or cerebellum, although some also innervate the premotor nuclei directly. The premotor neurons responsible for image stabilization are located in the vestibular nuclei (VN) and nucleus prepositus hypoglossi (PH). The vestibulocular reflex depends on afferents from the vestibular nerve to the vestibular nuclei and output to the oculomotor nuclei with an important arm of this reflex passing through the cerebellum. The optokinetic reflex has two components, a direct component that involves smooth pursuit mechanisms (see above) and an indirect component which receives retinal input through the nuclei of the accessory optic tract and the pretectal nucleus of the optic tract that is relayed to the premotor neurons.

Eye and Eyelid Movement Abnormalities in PD

Gross eye movement abnormalities obvious at the bedside are rarely seen in patients with PD, and their presence should always raise the possibility of another parkinsonian disorder, especially PSP or parkinsonism secondary to metabolic disorders such as Gaucher's disease.[4] However, several subtle abnormalities are common, particularly affecting saccades and smooth pursuit due to the influence of the basal ganglia on foveation (see above).

Abnormal saccadic and smooth pursuit eye movements are reported in about 75% of patients,[10] although it is important to clarify whether one is measuring reaction time, velocity, accuracy or some other parameter of the movement. Slow reaction times and horizontal saccadic velocity are common, and are thought to be a consequence of akinesia plus, in the case of reaction times, slowed central decision time. A relatively consistent abnormality is saccade hypometria, in which the primary saccade undershoots,[3] while smooth pursuit movements may be interrupted by small saccades.[11] Hypometric predictive, anticipatory, and memory-guided saccades also occur,[3] showing a basic deficit across all types of saccade generation when reflective choice is involved. These saccadic and smooth pursuit abnormalities occur early in the disease and are under some level of dopaminergic control,[12–14] although the relationship between saccades and dopamine is not straightforward.[15] In addition, recent studies have shown that subthalamic stimulation reduces saccade latencies in association with improvement in akinesia, and that dopamine replacement therapies share a common mechanism in reducing saccadic latencies in PD by changing basal ganglia excitability.[16] Of course, subtle differences are seen with respect to eye movement changes and these different therapies for PD.[15] While it has been thought that there is relatively little abnormality in reflexive saccades[3,14] and that it is the volitional component of saccade and smooth pursuit generation that is affected in PD, this has recently been questioned using meta-analyses to show hypometric reflexive saccades in PD.[17] In this context it is of interest to note that levodopa significantly increases response time for reflexive saccades while allowing patients with PD to better plan and execute voluntary eye movements.[14,18]

Convergence insufficiency occurs with increasing disease severity in patients with PD [19] and can result in diplopia over time.[13,20,21]

Even more common than eye movement abnormalities are complaints about ocular surface irritation in PD,[13] suggestive of difficulties with eyelid movement. As described above, the main role of blinking is to protect the eyes from dryness, foreign bodies, and bright light.[2] Patients with PD have a reduced blink rate, an increased blink duration, and a reduced habituation of the blink reflex.[10] The decrease in blink rate occurs in early untreated patients, is masked with effective treatment, and re-emerges in advanced disease where medications are no longer as effective.[13,22] In advanced stages, apraxia of eyelid opening may occur,[23] which can be prominent and disabling in some cases.

Pathology and Pathophysiology of Eye and Eyelid Movement Abnormalities in PD

Despite the brainstem predominance of early Lewy pathology in PD,[24] the brainstem motor and premotor oculomotor nuclei are not directly affected by the disease process. Neither is the cerebellum or the cerebellar relays involved in oculomotor control affected by PD pathology. At early disease stages there is also no PD pathology in any cortical regions involved in the control of eye or eyelid movements. The only region affected early in PD that is involved in the regulation of oculomotor function and eyelid movement is the dopaminergic substantia nigra which contains Lewy pathology and demonstrates significant neuronal loss. Although there is a substantive loss of dopaminergic nigrostriatal neurons early in PD, this loss is primarily restricted to the ventrolateral nigra which innervates the putamen, with the dopaminergic innervation of the caudate nucleus relatively intact until later in the disease course.[25] However, the basal ganglia regulation of foveation occurs through the caudate nucleus (see above), suggesting that early dopamine dysregulation in the caudate nucleus is not the cause of early eye movement abnormalities in PD, with this pathway affected only with disease progression.[25] The early deficits in foveation are therefore likely to be due to abnormalities in other regions.

The principal parkinsonian symptoms of bradykinesia and rigidity are caused by activity changes in the putamen due to its early dopamine depletion,[26] and are most likely responsible for the eyelid movement abnormalities observed in PD. In laboratory primates, this deficit increases synchronous oscillations in the subthalamic nucleus within a 2 to 3 week period,[26] and decreasing subthalamic activity has proven to be an effective treatment for parkinsonian bradykinesia and rigidity. Recent evidence has shown that the subthalamic nucleus also mediates the cortical signal from the presupplementary motor region to switch from reflexive to volitional eye movements by either directly stimulating inhibitory reticulata projection neurons to the superior colliculus, or by stimulating inhibitory pallidal neurons projecting to these reticulata neurons.[27] Abnormal activity in this pathway is likely to be responsible for the early eye and eyelid movement abnormalities in PD (Figure 3-3) with the ongoing loss of dopamine in the caudate nucleus contributing further to these deficits over time. The effective

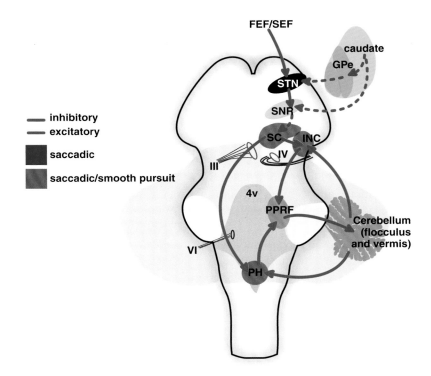

Figure 3-3. Abnormal eye movement circuits in Parkinson's disease. Early increased activity in the cortical signal from the presupplementary motor eye regions (FEF/SEF) to subthalamic neurons (STN) increases the stimulation of inhibitory reticulata projection neurons (SNR) to the superior colliculus (SC), affecting downstream premotor neurons (INC, PH, PPRF) for eye and eyelid movements. The loss of dopamine in the caudate nucleus contributes further to this deficit over time. GPe=external globus pallidus.

treatment of these eye movement abnormalities by subthalamic stimulation shows that there is a common mechanism of motor preparation for both eyes and limb movements through this circuit in PD.[16,28]

As vergence control is not under the regulation of the basal ganglia, abnormalities in vergence in patients with PD are more likely to be due to retinal or cortical changes. Loss of retinal dopamine neurons occurs in PD and may cause deficits in visual acuity and the ability to detect blur.[29] Patients with PD have also been reported to have a reduction in glucose metabolism in primary and association visual cortices that relates to the severity of their dopaminergic deficit.[30] However, neither the retina nor visual cortices have Lewy pathology, although over time Lewy pathology occurs in frontal and eventually parietal cortices[24] and may contribute to more substantive difficulties with eye movements late in the disease course in patients with PD.

How Oculomotor Examination can Assist in the Differential Diagnosis of Parkinsonian Syndromes

As may be expected, the most significant abnormalities on an oculomotor examination are observed in patients with PSP where the oculomotor anomalies are one of the cardinal signs of the condition: particularly paralysis of vertical ocular saccades (downbeat and upbeat) or downbeat saccades, ocular pursuit also being perturbed but not reflex movements (preservation of oculocephalic reflexes).[31] This dissociation between palsy of saccade and pursuit movements and preservation of oculocephalic reflexes is the sign of the supranuclear origin of the oculomotor disorder in PSP. In the early stage of PSP before the full expression of eye signs, oculomotor recordings are required to see more subtle supranuclear abnormalities.[31] Over time PSP also involves other less specific anomalies such as a perturbation of the antisaccade movements (related to a frontal syndrome), anomalous ocular pursuit (becoming saccadic), and presence of square wave eye movements.[31] A rigorous clinical examination of oculomotor function at a more advanced stage of PSP, or oculomotor recordings at an early stage of PSP, can contribute significantly to the diagnosis of the condition. However, as part of the aging process a loss of vertical upgaze is seen and thus patients with PD may appear superficially to have a vertical gaze palsy. Furthermore, some patients with PSP do not exhibit much in the way of eye movement abnormalities, at least in the early stages of disease, which again can create diagnostic problems.

Although eye movement abnormalities occur in PD and MSA, the minimal anomalies found at the onset of these conditions, both clinically and on oculomotor recordings, may not contribute significantly to diagnosis. Recent findings suggest that spontaneous nystagmus or positioning downbeat nystagmus, the presence of excessive square wave jerks and/or impaired suppression of the vestibulocular reflex may indicate the presence of MSA[32] and that measurement of pursuit tracking can go some way to differentiating this disorder from PD.[33] Difficulties with foveation are, of course, likely in all parkinsonian conditions due to the common loss of dopamine innervation to the putamen, with differences in the severity of symptoms related to the more substantial basal ganglia involvement in PSP and MSA.

It is important, though, to be cautious of studies claiming to have demonstrated diagnostic disease markers, be they measures of eye movement or other parameters. One of the more common pitfalls is to compare values of the chosen marker in a cohort with PD versus controls. The groups are defined clinically, albeit by experts, since that is currently the gold standard method to diagnose PD, yet this, by definition, means the groups may be readily distinguished at the bedside—there is no need for a 'diagnostic' biomarker even if the parameter measured is indeed different in the two groups. The diagnostic difficulty comes in those cases where it is not clear whether the patient has true PD or one of its mimics, and it is therefore in this far more challenging environment that a true diagnostic disease marker must prove its worth.

Finally, other rarer causes of parkinsonism can cause eye movement abnormalities, including Gaucher's disease, Huntington's disease, spinocerebellar ataxias, Niemann-Pick disease type C, and so on.

Why Measure Eye Movements in PD?

The abnormalities of eye movement in PD are subtle, and in general the bedside assessment of eye movement has little, if any, role in the diagnosis of PD, which tends to be made on the basis of a more global motor deficit. So what is the point in studying eye movements in this disease if they are not going to help in diagnosis?

The answer, at least from a clinician's perspective, is there is great hope they may be able to accurately quantify disease progression, and thus help demonstrate a change in the trajectory of disease over time in response to new therapies. From a more basic science perspective they offer a powerful way to learn about neural control of motor function and the effects of disease on this process.

Eye movements are an appealing way to study motor phenotype because they are unaffected by load bearing or arthritis, which alter how a patient moves their limbs in response to neural commands, generating undesired noise for the neuroscientist. The eyes thus provide a unique window into the brain's true output that goes to determine motor behavior, both in health and in disease. Furthermore, there is now new equipment allowing the accurate recording of hundreds of eye movements in just a few minutes using infra-red reflectance[34] or video technology. This permits easy and rapid data collection, and does not require head stabilization, which is impossible in the latter stages of PD.

From the perspective of disease progression there is reasonable hope that some eye movement parameters will indeed change over time, perhaps thereby helping us to track and understand the evolution of disease. Using sensitive measurements and analysis, rather than bedside assessment, it is possible to detect abnormalities of eye movement early in

PD, and there appears to be a worsening of the eye movement dysfunction in patients more severely affected by disease,[14,35] although at present the evidence from time-consuming longitudinal trials is more limited.[36]

But which of the many types of eye movement should we study, and how should they be measured? If we are interested in disease progression it might be expected that those parameters of eye movement determined largely by brainstem nuclei, which are relatively unaffected by the pathology in PD,[24] will be relatively unrewarding. This would include, for example, saccadic velocity and duration. On the other hand it might be anticipated that eye movement parameters influenced by higher basal ganglia and cortical circuits would be more rewarding since over time these regions take the brunt of the pathology in PD.[24] Examples would include saccadic latency, especially volitional tasks where the brain must make a decision about when and where to move, and perhaps accuracy of response.

However, as an illustration of the complexity and challenge of studying eye movements in PD, plus the difficulty in comparing the numerous studies, it is worth considering the measurement of saccadic latencies, or reaction times, in more detail. Firstly, it is important to know about the population studied since the stage of PD and type of medication will affect eye movement response. Secondly, the testing paradigm will determine how abnormal the eye movement parameter measured really is—in general 'reflexive' saccades seem to be rather less affected in PD than those requiring a more 'voluntary' decision process about when to move or in which direction. The type of target stimulus, timing of its appearance, and so on will also affect saccadic latency. Thirdly, but by no means finally, the type of data analysis chosen varies, with many researchers presenting mean values of a relatively small number of responses, whilst others analyze hundreds of latency measures and find they are non-Gaussian in distribution, and that this distribution itself can inform us about the neural decision process.[37] Thus it is difficult, although not impossible, to directly compare results from different groups, and it is crucial in longitudinal studies that recording protocols remain unchanged.

Conclusion

Eye movement abnormalities are not a major symptom or sign of patients with PD, although a variety of subtle deficits that particularly affect foveation and eyelid movements are seen. In more advanced disease, apraxia of eyelid opening can be disabling and difficult to treat. However, whilst complaints of eye movement problems are rare in PD, they can be commonly detected and as such provide useful insights into the role of the basal ganglia in motor control and decision making. There is hope that accurate quantification of eye movement abnormality over time may inform us about disease progression in PD, but it is not yet clear to what extent, and what type of testing paradigm to use.

References

1. Bruce CJ, Friedman HR. Eye movements. In: Ramachandran VS, ed. *Encyclopedia of the Human Brain.* Vol 2. San Diego: Academic Press; 2002:269–297.
2. Zucker JL. The eyelids: some common disorders seen in everyday practice. *Geriatrics.* Apr 2009;64(4):14–19, 28.
3. Kennard C, Lueck CJ. Oculomotor abnormalities in diseases of the basal ganglia. *Rev Neurol (Paris).* 1989;145(8–9):587–595.
4. Litvan I, Bhatia KP, Burn DJ, et al. Movement Disorders Society Scientific Issues Committee report: SIC Task Force appraisal of clinical diagnostic criteria for Parkinsonian disorders. *Mov Disord.* May 2003;18(5):467–486.
5. Horn AK, Buttner-Ennever JA. Brainstem circuits controlling lid-eye coordination in monkey. *Prog Brain Res.* 2008;171:87–95.
6. Esteban A, Traba A, Prieto J. Eyelid movements in health and disease. The supranuclear impairment of the palpebral motility. *Neurophysiol Clin.* Feb 2004;34(1):3–15.
7. Buttner U, Buttner-Ennever JA. Present concepts of oculomotor organization. *Prog Brain Res.* 2006;151:1–42.
8. Buttner-Ennever JA. Mapping the oculomotor system. *Prog Brain Res.* 2008;171:3–11.
9. Nitta T, Akao T, Kurkin S, Fukushima K. Vergence eye movement signals in the cerebellar dorsal vermis. *Prog Brain Res.* 2008;171:173–176.
10. Armstrong RA. Visual signs and symptoms of Parkinson's disease. *Clin Exp Optom.* Mar 2008;91(2):129–138.
11. Waterston JA, Barnes GR, Grealy MA, Collins S. Abnormalities of smooth eye and head movement control in Parkinson's disease. *Ann Neurol.* Jun 1996;39(6):749–760.
12. Bares M, Brazdil M, Kanovsky P, et al. The effect of apomorphine administration on smooth pursuit ocular movements in early Parkinsonian patients. *Parkinsonism Relat Disord.* Jan 2003;9(3):139–144.
13. Biousse V, Skibell BC, Watts RL, Loupe DN, Drews-Botsch C, Newman NJ. Ophthalmologic features of Parkinson's disease. *Neurology.* Jan 27 2004;62(2):177–180.
14. Michell AW, Xu Z, Fritz D, et al. Saccadic latency distributions in Parkinson's disease and the effects of L-dopa. *Exp Brain Res.* Sep 2006;174(1):7–18.
15. Barker RA, Michell AW. "The eyes have it." Saccadometry and Parkinson's disease. *Exp Neurol.* Oct 2009;219(2):382–384.
16. Temel Y, Visser-Vandewalle V, Carpenter RH. Saccadometry: a novel clinical tool for quantification of the motor effects of subthalamic nucleus stimulation in Parkinson's disease. *Exp Neurol.* Apr 2009;216(2):481–489.

17. Chambers JM, Prescott TJ. Response times for visually guided saccades in persons with Parkinson's disease: A meta-analytic review. *Neuropsychologia*. Nov 11 2009.

18. Hood AJ, Amador SC, Cain AE, et al. Levodopa slows prosaccades and improves antisaccades: an eye movement study in Parkinson's disease. *J Neurol Neurosurg Psychiatry*. Jun 2007;78(6):565–570.

19. Repka MX, Claro MC, Loupe DN, Reich SG. Ocular motility in Parkinson's disease. *J Pediatr Ophthalmol Strabismus*. May-Jun 1996;33(3):144–147.

20. Davidsdottir S, Cronin-Golomb A, Lee A. Visual and spatial symptoms in Parkinson's disease. *Vision Res*. May 2005;45(10):1285–1296.

21. Lepore FE. Parkinson's disease and diplopia. *Neuro-ophthalmol*. 2006;30:37–40.

22. Karson CN, LeWitt PA, Calne DB, Wyatt RJ. Blink rates in parkinsonism. *Ann Neurol*. Dec 1982;12(6):580–583.

23. Lepore FE, Duvoisin RC. "Apraxia" of eyelid opening: An involuntary levator inhibition. *Neurology*. 1985;35:423–427.

24. Braak H, Del Tredici K, Rüb U, de Vos RAI, Jansen Steur ENH, Braak E. Staging of brain pathology related to sporadic Parkinson's disease. *Neurobiol Aging*. 2003;24:197–211.

25. Nurmi E, Ruottinen HM, Bergman J, et al. Rate of progression in Parkinson's disease: A 6-[^{18}F]fluoro-L-dopa PET study. *Mov. Disord*. 2001;16:608–615.

26. Mallet N, Pogosyan A, Sharott A, et al. Disrupted dopamine transmission and the emergence of exaggerated beta oscillations in subthalamic nucleus and cerebral cortex. *J Neurosci*. Apr 30 2008;28(18):4795–4806.

27. Isoda M, Hikosaka O. Role for subthalamic nucleus neurons in switching from automatic to controlled eye movement. *J Neurosci*. Jul 9 2008;28(28):7209–7218.

28. Sauleau P, Pollak P, Krack P, et al. Subthalamic stimulation improves orienting gaze movements in Parkinson's disease. *Clin Neurophysiol*. Aug 2008;119(8):1857–1863.

29. Archibald NK, Clarke MP, Mosimann UP, Burn DJ. The retina in Parkinson's disease. *Brain*. May 2009;132(Pt 5):1128–1145.

30. Bohnen NI, Minoshima S, Giordani B, Frey KA, Kuhl DE. Motor correlates of occipital glucose hypometabolism in Parkinson's disease without dementia. *Neurology*. Feb 1999;52(3):541–546.

31. Pierrot-Deseilligny C, Rivaud-Pechoux S. [Contribution of oculomotor examination for the etiological diagnosis of parkinsonian syndromes]. *Rev Neurol (Paris)*. May 2003;159(5 Pt 2):3S75–81.

32. Anderson T, Luxon L, Quinn N, Daniel S, Marsden CD, Bronstein A. Oculomotor function in multiple system atrophy: clinical and laboratory features in 30 patients. *Mov Disord*. May 15 2008;23(7):977–984.

33. Pinkhardt EH, Kassubek J, Sussmuth S, Ludolph AC, Becker W, Jurgens R. Comparison of smooth pursuit eye movement deficits in multiple system atrophy and Parkinson's disease. *J Neurol*. Sep 2009;256(9):1438–1446.

34. Ober JK, Przedpelska-Ober E, Gryncewicz W, Dylak J, Carpenter RS, Ober JJ. Hand-held system for ambulatory measurement of saccadic durations of neurological patients. In: Gadja J, ed. *Modelling and Measurement in Medicine*. Warsaw: PAN; 2003:187–198.

35. Mosimann UP, Muri RM, Burn DJ, Felblinger J, O'Brien JT, McKeith IG. Saccadic eye movement changes in Parkinson's disease dementia and dementia with Lewy bodies. *Brain*. Jun 2005;128(Pt 6):1267–1276.

36. Gordon PH, Yu Q, Qualls C, et al. Reaction time and movement time after embryonic cell implantation in Parkinson disease. *Arch Neurol*. Jun 2004;61(6):858–861.

37. Carpenter RH, Williams ML. Neural computation of log likelihood in control of saccadic eye movements. *Nature*. Sep 7 1995;377(6544):59–62.

Chapter 4

Olfactory Dysfunction in Parkinson's Disease and Related Disorders

Richard L. Doty, Christopher H. Hawkes,
and Henk W. Berendse

Approximately half of the population between the ages of 65 and 80 years, and nearly three-quarters of those over the age of 80 years, experience measurable smell loss.[1] Such dysfunction adversely impacts quality of life, the flavor and palatability of foods and beverages, nutrition, and safety. In one study of 445 patients tested for olfactory function, at least one hazardous event, such as food poisoning or failure to detect fire or leaking natural gas, was reported by 45.2% of those with anosmia, 34.1% of those with severe hyposmia, 32.8% of those with moderate hyposmia, 24.2% of those with mild hyposmia, and 19.0% of those with normal olfactory function.[2] In a study of 750 consecutive patients presenting to the University of Pennsylvania Smell and Taste Center with primarily olfactory problems, 68 % experienced altered quality of life, 46 % changes in appetite or body weight, and 56 % adverse influences on daily living or psychological well-being.[3] Given that olfaction plays a significant role in monitoring the quality of air that enters the body, it is noteworthy that even small amounts of pollutants can pose a significant burden on the olfactory and respiratory systems, given that the average adult breathes in about 12,000 L of air each day, in contrast to taking in only ~1.5 kg of food and 2 kg of water.[4]

Among the causes of olfactory dysfunction in the elderly are the cumulative damage incurred by the olfactory epithelium from environmental insults, age-related ossification of the foramina of the cribriform plate, and the onset of neurodegenerative disease, as reflected by age-related increases in neurofibrillary tangles and neuritic plaques in olfaction-related brain structures.[5] It is now well established that olfactory dysfunction is among the first clinical signs of such neurodegenerative diseases as Alzheimer's disease and Parkinson's disease (PD).[6–8]

In this chapter we review the functional and pathological olfactory changes that occur in patients with PD and related syndromes, including familial-, idiopathic-, and toxin-related forms of parkinsonism. We consider evidence suggesting that olfactory dysfunction precedes the onset of the motor symptoms and describe disease-specific pathological lesions within olfactory structures that may cause the olfactory impairment. While some of these changes may involve dopamine, the majority do not, in accord with the concept that PD is not solely a dopamine-related disorder.

Classical Parkinson's Disease

In keeping with its first description by James Parkinson in 1817, Parkinson's disease has been considered mainly a somatic motor disorder. However, as illustrated by a number of the chapters of this volume, it has become apparent over the course of the last four decades that a number of sensory changes are present in PD, most notably changes in vision and olfaction.

Odor Perception in Parkinson's Disease

Since first described in 1975, over 60 empirical studies have appeared in the peer-reviewed literature demonstrating an altered ability to smell in patients with PD.[6] The vast majority of these studies have used forced-choice odor identification tests, although odor threshold, recognition, and memory tests have also been used. At least 15 generalizations can be made from this literature. *First*, the olfactory deficits are robust, with nearly all p values in published studies being less than 0.001. In one meta-analysis, effect sizes >3.00 were observed for both odor identification and odor detection threshold scores (effect sizes >0.80 are considered "enormous").[9] *Second*, while the olfactory dysfunction is generally bilateral, there can be slight individual differences in the degree to which the left and right sides of the nose are involved. However, no association is present between the side of the relatively greater impairment and the side of hemiparkinsonism, as might be expected if asymmetrical damage to striatal dopamine systems is the basis of the olfactory problem.[10] *Third*, female PD patients generally have less dysfunction than male PD patients.[11] *Fourth*, total anosmia is not present in most cases and many patients are unaware of their deficit until formal testing. Thus, in one study only 13% of 38 patients who received an odor detection threshold test were unable to detect the highest odorant concentration presented, and only 38.3% of 81 patients had scores on the standardized University of Pennsylvania Smell Identification Test (UPSIT) suggestive of anosmia.[12] Moreover, all but one of 41 PD patients indicated that some odor was present on 35 or more of the 40 items, even though the majority were unable to identify most of the odors or felt that the perceived sensation did not correspond to the response alternatives. *Fifth*, although there are reports that some odorants may be more sensitive to the PD-related deficits than others, little consistency has been found among laboratories and the relative influences of culture, odorant intensity, odorant type, and response alternatives provided in testing are unknown and likely complicate the issue.[13–17] *Sixth*, the smell dysfunction of PD appears indistinguishable from that of AD and the Parkinson-dementia complex of Guam, with UPSIT scores averaging around 20.[9,18,19] *Seventh*, the smell loss in well-established PD appears to be relatively stable over time and is unrelated to the magnitude of the motor symptoms or disease stage,[10,12,20,21] although subtle variations among so-called benign vs. malignant forms may be present[11] and this generalization may not apply to patients in the earliest stages of the disease.[8,22] *Eighth*, the dysfunction is unrelated to numerous neuropsychological measures, such as the Randt memory test and selected verbal and performance subsets of the Wechsler Adult Intelligence Scale–Revised.[20] *Ninth*, smell loss is present in some familial and sporadic forms of parkinsonism and may be a sign of the preclinical state of the disease.[23–25] *Tenth*, anti-PD medications (e.g., L-dopa, dopamine agonists, anticholinergic compounds) have no influence on the smell deficit, which occurs as severely in non- or never-medicated patients as in medicated ones.[10,26,27] Although odor event-related potential latencies have been reported to be longer in medicated than non-medicated PD patients, this is likely due to other factors, including non-specific drug influences on evoked potentials and the fact that the more severely disabled patients are more likely to be receiving medication. *Eleventh*, suboptimal sniffing behavior may contribute to the olfactory problem seen in PD, although the degree of contribution is relatively small, particularly in early stage cases.[28] *Twelfth*, olfactory testing is useful in the differential diagnosis of idiopathic PD from other neurodegenerative diseases with motor symptoms, including disorders often misdiagnosed as PD (e.g., PSP, MPTP-induced PD, and essential tremor).[29–33] *Thirteenth*, some asymptomatic first-degree relatives of patients with either familial or sporadic forms of PD appear to exhibit olfactory dysfunction.[23,34,35] *Fourteenth*, a strong correlation exists between olfactory test scores and cardiac[123] I-metaiodobenzylguanidine (MIBG) uptake in patients with PD which is independent of disease duration and clinical ratings of motor function, implying that functional losses of the olfactory and cardiac sympathetic systems are closely coupled.[36] *Fifteenth*, longitudinal studies also suggest that the olfactory deficit precedes the classical clinical signs by several years, serving as a 'pre-clinical' marker.[37–39] For example, in one study of 361 asymptomatic relatives of PD patients who were administered olfactory tests, those with test scores in the top and bottom 10% of the group underwent [123I]ß-CIT labeled dopamine transporter functional imaging within the striatum, a measure of the health of this motor control brain region.[23] At the 5-year follow-up, 5 of the 40 relatives with olfactory test scores in the bottom 10%, all of whom exhibited substantial reduction in transporter uptake at baseline, had developed clinically defined PD, while none of the 38 relatives with test scores in the top 10% did so.[38]

A number of studies have examined the sensitivity and specificity of olfactory testing in discriminating between PD and controls or other forms of parkinsonism. For example, in a study of 180 PD patients and 612 non-PD controls, the sensitivity and specificity of the UPSIT in distinguishing between PD patients and controls was found to be 91% and 88%, respectively, for males 60 years of age or less.[31] The corresponding values for females 60 years of age or less were 79% and 85%. The sensitivity and specificity of this test for individuals 61 to 70 years of age were 81% and 82% for men and 80% and 88% for women. Katzenschlager et al reported the overall sensitivity and specificity of the UPSIT in distinguishing between older persons with PD (mean = 72.6 yrs) and vascular parkinsonism (mean = 74.1 yrs) to be 85.7% and 88.9%, respectively.[40] When the data were divided into two age categories (65–75 and 76–88 yrs), the sensitivity and specificity values were 100% and 85.7% and 85.7% and 80%, respectively. Comparable sensitivity and specificity estimates have been noted by others.[15,41]

Pathology within the Olfactory System of Patients with Classical PD

The cause of the olfactory dysfunction of PD is not known, although presumably it relates to the degree of neuropathology within olfaction-related brain structures, as described below. As noted above, repletion of dopamine does not influence the functional deficit.[10,26,27] Thus, the PD-related olfactory problem is not due to decreased dopamine as such.

Olfactory Epithelium

PD-related pathology within the olfactory epithelium seems no more apparent in patients with PD than in healthy elderly controls and patients with AD, Lewy body disease, or multiple system atrophy (MSA).[42] Nonetheless, dystrophic neurites without Lewy bodies, amyloid precursor protein fragments, and all varieties of synuclein (α, β, γ) are present within the olfactory receptor neurons of PD patients[43] but so far no one has found abnormal α-synuclein deposits or Lewy bodies in the nasal olfactory epithelium.

Olfactory Bulb and Anterior Olfactory Nucleus

Unlike the olfactory epithelium, considerable disease-specific alterations are present in the olfactory bulbs and tracts of patients with PD. In a pioneering study of 8 PD patients and 8 controls, all of the PD cases contained Lewy bodies which were most numerous in the anterior olfactory nucleus (AON) but also present in mitral cells, cells which receive direct input from the bipolar olfactory cells.[44] The Lewy body morphology at this site resembled that observed in the cortex, although inclusions showing a classical tri-laminar structure were rarely present. Within the AON, the loss of neurons correlates with the number of Lewy bodies, as well as with disease duration.[45]

It should be noted that the human olfactory bulb contains at least 20 different neurotransmitters in addition to dopamine. Dopamine deficiency within the bulb has not been observed in PD at autopsy. Indeed, there is one report suggesting a significant increase of dopaminergic neurons in the olfactory bulbs of patients with PD,[46] although more recent work employing a larger sample found the increase to be gender-related.[47] A doubling of tyrosine hydroxylase expression was reported in the olfactory bulbs of 3 Macaca monkeys who had been injected with the proneurotoxin 1-methyl-4-phenyl-1,2,3,6-tetrahydropyride (MPTP) relative to 3 controls.[48] In a MPTP mouse model of PD, a 4-fold *increase* of dopamine expression in the olfactory bulb has also been reported.[49] Such increases in dopamine may reflect attempts to compensate for loss of a dopamine-responsive substrate, conceivably via increased migration of dopamine-secreting cells from the subventricular zone/rostral migratory stream into the olfactory bulb (see[50]).

Olfactory Cortex and Medulla

The primary olfactory cortex, i.e., cortical brain regions that receive direct projections from the olfactory bulb, includes the piriform cortex, the entorhinal cortex, the corticomedial nucleus of the amygdala, and the posterior sector of the anterior olfactory nucleus. It is well established that high

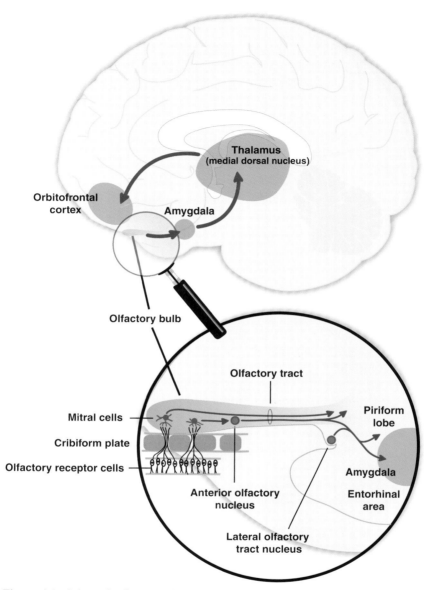

Figure 4-1. Schematic diagram of the main olfactory pathways affected in Parkinson's disease. Olfactory receptor neurons are located in the olfactory epithelium in the roof of the nasal cavity and send their axons through the cribriform plate to the olfactory bulb. Mitral cells in the olfactory bulb send their axons through the olfactory nerve to innervate 5 main areas: the anterior olfactory nucleus, the lateral olfactory nucleus (olfactory tubercle), the amygdala, the piriform cortex, and the entorhinal cortex. The piriform cortex and amygdala project to the medial dorsal nucleus of the thalamus, which then projects to the orbitofrontal cortex. The orbitofrontal cortex mediates conscious perception of the odor. The anterior olfactory nucleus is not a true nucleus but a transition zone of grey substance, sectors of which are located within the posterior olfactory bulb and in brain regions anterior to the piriform cortex within the olfactory peduncle.

concentrations of dopamine receptors and dopaminergic fibers are present in the piriform cortex. The main innervation of the piriform cortex is the olfactory tubercle, which has markedly decreased dopamine levels in PD.[51] However, as discussed above, dopamine repletion has no influence on the olfactory deficit of PD, implying that if the dopamine system is involved the receptive substrate must be entirely dysfunctional.

Histopathologic studies of postmortem PD tissue have found neurofibrillary tangles and Lewy bodies within lamina II of the entorhinal cortex.[52] In one study, Lewy bodies were detected in this region in 48% of the cases examined (20/42), whereas neurofibrillary tangles were positively identified in 98% of the cases (41/42).[53] In a study of brains from 45 PD patients, Mattila et al identified α-synuclein-immunoreactive cortical Lewy bodies in the amygdala (primary olfactory cortex), hippocampus (secondary olfactory processing center), or cortical gyrus of 43 of 45 PD patients.[54] This study further demonstrated that α-synuclein-positive cortical Lewy bodies were associated with cognitive impairment in PD that was independent of any AD-type pathology.

In a landmark series of neuropathological studies, Braak et al. found PD-related pathology to extend from the AON into more central olfactory sites (olfactory tubercle, piriform and periamygdalar cortex, entorhinal cortex of the ambient gyrus) without advancing into non-olfactory cortical areas.[55–57] In this research, a careful examination of PD-related brain neuropathology, including α-synuclein immunostaining, was made in 41 cases of PD, 69 'incidental' cases that displayed no extra-pyramidal signs in life but were found to have Lewy neurites and/or Lewy bodies at autopsy, and 58 age- and gender-matched cases that had no Lewy bodies or Lewy neurites and no history of neurological or psychiatric illness. Based on these specimens, Braak et al. theorized that the pathological process of PD advances in a predictable sequence, with the earliest changes occurring within the olfactory bulb, the associated AON, and the dorsal motor nuclear complex of the glossopharyngeal and vagus nerves (DMC) before the onset of motor manifestations.[58] When Lewy bodies were found in the substantia nigra, similar and more severe changes were invariably observed in the olfactory bulb, the anterior olfactory nucleus, and the dorsal medulla. The involvement of DMC led to the proposal that PD-related pathology starts in the enteric plexus (Auerbach's submucosal plexus) and that a pathogen, possibly viral or chemical, ascends the motor vagal fibers in retrograde fashion to the dorsal medulla.[59] However, this theory does not explain the olfactory bulb changes or the early pathology in the sympathetic ganglia.[60] An alternative theory is that a pathogen enters both the olfactory bulb and the enteric nervous system, the latter from swallowed secretions.[61]

The sequential changes in PD-related pathology proposed by Braak et al have received support from the majority of other neuropathologists. Muller et al asked 6 observers from 5 different institutions to classify 21 cases of the original pathological material upon which the Braak staging was based.[62] A near perfect correlation was obtained for inter- and intra-rater reliability. Duda et al examined 126 brains taken from the Honolulu Asia Aging Study.[63] Twenty-three had clinically diagnosed PD and 35 had incidental Lewy bodies. The vast majority of cases were consistent with the Braak classification. However, Parkkinen et al conducted post mortem assessment of 904 brains that had α-synuclein pathology in the dorsal motor nucleus of the vagus, substantia nigra, and/or basal forebrain nuclei.[64] Only 32 (30%) of 106 α-synuclein-positive cases had been diagnosed with a neurodegenerative disorder in life and the distribution of α-synuclein pathology did not allow a reliable diagnosis of an extrapyramidal syndrome. Some neurologically unimpaired cases had a moderate burden of alpha-synuclein pathology in both brainstem and cortical areas, suggesting that α-synuclein-positive structures outside olfactory system-related structures are not unequivocal markers of neuronal dysfunction. Recently, Kalaitzakis et al examined the topography of α-synuclein pathology in 57 PD brains, excluding the olfactory bulb.[65] There were 4/57 (7%) cases of PD without medullary involvement, which led them to conclude that the medulla is not always the induction site of pathology in sporadic PD. Halliday et al used Braak staging to group an autopsy cohort into *pre-clinical* (stages 1–2), *early* (stages 3–4, 35% with clinical PD), and *late* (stages 5–6, 86% with clinical PD) cases.[66] These authors theorized that preclinical compared to early or late-stage cases should progressively be more elderly at the time of sampling, but this feature was not observed.

In light of evidence that at least 50% of substantia nigra cells must die before clinical symptoms arise,[67,68] the clinical motor manifestations of PD would seem to represent later stages of an ongoing pathological process. This is in accord with reports from PD patients that their smell dysfunction occurred years before their first motor symptoms. In summary, all of the above studies support the idea that PD-related olfactory dysfunction reflects peripheral pathology that occurs before the onset of the motor phenotype.

Familial Parkinson's Disease

There is convincing evidence that smell dysfunction occurs in some first degree relatives of patients with monogenetic forms of parkinsonism, but relatively small numbers of individuals have been tested. Markopoulou et al found, in the initial Michigan study of familial parkinsonism, 6 kindreds,

3 of whom had typical PD and 3 a 'parkinsonism-plus' syndrome.[25] In the typical families there were 4 apparently healthy individuals at 50% risk, of whom 3 were microsmic on the UPSIT. Of the 8 at-risk subjects in the PD-plus families, 2 had abnormal UPSIT scores. The typical PD families are now known to have had the PARK 1, 3 and 8 mutations.[69] The single case of PARK1 was anosmic and the two PARK3 families had variable findings but were mostly normal. There were 7 cases of genetically confirmed pallidopontonigral degeneration (probably a form of frontotemporal dementia) in the atypical group and their mean UPSIT score was indicative of anosmia (mean = 10.5). Four cases with the PARK8 mutation scored an average of 29.7 on the UPSIT, which was lower than the mean of those at risk (34). There was no clear relationship between olfaction and parkinsonian phenotype.

It is now clear that the PARK8 mutation (LRRK2/Dardarin) is the most prevalent cause of familial PD, accounting for 2–5% of all PD in Europe with a much higher level in Spain, Portugal and North Africa.[70] Khan et al reported a Lincolnshire kindred with the PARK8 mutation and found slight olfactory impairment in 2 of 4 individuals.[71] More recently, olfaction in PARK8 families was assessed in 5 patients from London and 16 from Lisbon.[70,72] There was severe impairment in both London and Lisbon populations and the UPSIT scores and clinical phenotype were indistinguishable from their idiopathic PD subjects. In PARK2 (Parkin disease), a dominant form of parkinsonism, the sense of smell appeared relatively preserved on a culturally-modified UPSIT in 27 subjects, an observation that would be in keeping with the absence of Lewy bodies in this condition.[71] In a study of PARK1, 2 of 7 patients from separate families were found to be anosmic (Bostantjopoulou et al 2001).

Parkinsonism

Olfactory dysfunction is present in some conditions that resemble PD but differ from it on clinical, genetic, or pathological grounds. Diseases included under the general category of "parkinsonism" or "Parkinson-plus syndromes" are Lewy body disease, multiple system atrophy (MSA), progressive supranuclear palsy (PSP), corticobasal degeneration (CBD), drug-induced PD (DPD), the PD-dementia complex of Guam (PDC), X-linked dystonia-parkinsonism ('Lubag'), and vascular parkinsonism (VP). What little is known about the olfactory function of these disorders is indicated in the following sections. With rare exception, little pathological study of the olfactory bulbs and other olfaction-related structures has been performed in these syndromes.

Lewy Body Disease

Lewy body disease (LBD) is a term applied to diseases in which Lewy bodies are widely deposited in the brain. Classic PD is, in a strict sense, a form of Lewy body disease given its defining pathology of widespread Lewy body deposition. Several forms of Lewy body disease are associated with dementia. If dementia comes on before, during, or within one year of the motor symptom onset, then dementia with Lewy bodies is a preferred designation (DLB[73]). If dementia develops more than a year after well-established PD, the disorder is classified as Parkinson disease dementia (PDD). Many patients with classical PD develop dementia after 10 or more years, leading to the diagnosis of PDD. Pathologically DLB, PDD, and PD are largely indistinguishable[74,75] and clinically it is difficult to distinguish PDD from DLB; hence, the common use of the generic term Lewy body disease. Numerous alternative names have been employed, leading to further confusion. For example, DLB has been termed diffuse Lewy body disease, Lewy body dementia, Lewy body variant of AD, senile dementia of Lewy body type, and dementia associated with cortical Lewy bodies.[76] The sole published histological study of olfactory bulbs from patients with DLB found 9 of 10 cases with tau pathology, Lewy bodies, and α-synuclein deposits.[77]

Severe impairment of olfactory identification and detection was observed in a study of clinically defined DLB, but without pathological verification. As with PD, the olfactory test scores were unrelated to disease stage and duration.[78] In another investigation, McShane et al assessed simple smell perception to one odor (lavender water) in 92 patients with autopsy-confirmed dementia, of whom 22 had DLB and 43 had only AD pathology.[79] They were compared to 94 age-matched controls. Impaired smell perception was observed in the DLB group, but not in the patients with AD. This study affords pathological confirmation for the clinically-based conclusion of Liberini et al that impairment of smell is significant in DLB,[80] given that we are dealing with a disorder separate from PD. In an autopsy confirmed study by Olichney et al of DLB (which they termed Lewy body variant of PD), anosmia was found to be common and its presence was thought useful to improve the sensitivity for detecting DLB, but it did not improve discrimination between AD and DLB because of false positives.[81]

Multiple System Atrophy

Akinesia and rigidity predominate in the most common, predominantly parkinsonian, variety of multiple system atrophy (MSA), which comprises 80% of the total cases (MSA-P; Shy-Drager syndrome). In the remaining 20%, cerebellar ataxia is dominant (MSA-C). These two varieties of MSA are associated with comparatively rapidly evolving parkinsonism with dysautonomia that affects orthostatic blood pressure and the bladder. In both forms of MSA, pathological changes are found in the olfactory bulbs, characterized by cytoplasmic inclusions in oligodendrocytes which are sometimes called Papp-Lantos filaments.[82]

In an initial study of olfactory function in 29 patients with a clinical diagnosis of MSA-P, mild impairment was noted, with a mean UPSIT score of 26.7 compared to the control mean of 33.5.[83] There were no differences between the parkinsonian and cerebellar types. Similarly, Nee et al and Muller et al found reduced smell function in 7 of 8 MSA patients (in both publications) which did not differ for MSA-P and MSA-C.[84,85] More recently, Abele et al focused particularly on MSA-C in comparison to other ataxias of unknown etiology, and found no meaningful difference in olfactory test scores between the two categories.[86] Unlike PD, no correlation appears to exist between odor identification test scores and cardiac (123)I-metaiodobenzylguanidine (MIBG) uptake in MSA.[38] Taken together, these studies suggest that mild to moderate olfactory impairment is present in MSA, but that the overall dysfunction is less than, and perhaps qualitatively distinct from, that observed in PD.

Corticobasal Degeneration

In corticobasal degeneration (CBD), parkinsonian features are observed along with limb dystonia, ideomotor apraxia, myoclonus and ultimately, cognitive decline. This disorder reflects the accumulation of tau protein mainly in the fronto-parietal cortex and basal ganglia. In one study of 7 patients with clinically suspected CBD, UPSIT scores were in the low normal range with a mean of 27, a value not significantly different from their age-matched controls.[83] A more recent study of another 7 patients with clinically defined CBD showed mild impairment of odor naming and odor picture matching in the presence of normal discrimination.[87] Provisionally, the finding of normal or near-normal smell function in suspected CBD may permit differentiation from typical PD and AD. Unlike most other disorders accompanied by olfactory loss, tau pathology appears to be absent in the olfactory bulbs of CBD,[77] conceivably explaining why olfaction is preserved.

Progressive Supranuclear Palsy

Progressive supranuclear palsy, also known as Steele-Richardson-Olszewski syndrome, is a disorder characterized by failure of voluntary vertical gaze, rapid progression of motor dysfunction, imbalance, and advancing cognitive decline. Although the characteristic pathology in PSP is the widespread accumulation of tau protein in degenerating neurons, tau and α-synuclein pathology to be absent in the olfactory bulbs, as in the case of CBD.[77]

In the first major study of olfactory function in PSP, no significant difference was observed either in UPSIT scores or phenyl ethyl alcohol threshold values between 21 patients and 21 matched controls, although there was a trend towards higher threshold values (p=0.085).[30] Similar UPSIT findings were found in a subsequent study of 15 cases of PSP by Wenning et al.[83] The relative absence of tau or α-synuclein pathology in the olfactory bulbs of such patients may explain why no meaningful olfactory dysfunction is present in this disorder. It should be noted that all of these studies were undertaken prior to the division of PSP into two varieties—a typical 'Richardson' variant with parkinsonian features and a more subtle variant with imbalance.[88] Presumably most relate to the parkinsonian (Richardson) variant.

Vascular Parkinsonism

Vascular parkinsonism (VP) is a syndrome that mimics PD, but the response to levodopa is variable. This disorder occurs in patients with cerebrovascular disease involving the basal ganglia, particularly the putamen and striatum. Its diagnosis is relatively straight-forward when unilateral parkinsonism develops acutely in someone with significant cerebrovascular disease. However, when the onset is insidious or stepwise, diagnosis is difficult. Although vascular lesions may be noted on a brain MRI, in some cases this can be coincidental, especially in the presence of known cerebrovascular disease. In one study, cases of acute onset displayed lesions in the subcortical grey nuclei (striatum, globus pallidus and thalamus), whereas cases of insidious onset had lesions distributed diffusely in watershed areas.[89] Usually striatal dopamine transporter imaging is normal in VP,[90] although a 'punched out' appearance may be present, reflecting local ischemia.

One study of 14 patients fulfilling strictly defined clinical criteria for VP exhibited UPSIT scores equivalent to those of age-matched controls (respective means = 25.5 & 27.5).[40] This finding suggests that olfactory testing may be of value in differentiating VP from idiopathic PD.

Drug-induced Parkinson's Disease

Drug-induced Parkinson's disease (DPD), which is often clinically indistinguishable from classic PD, was common when broad-spectrum dopamine antagonists were popular in the treatment of psychotic disorders. Its prevalence subsided dramatically following the introduction of selective D2 dopamine receptor blockers in the 1980s (e.g., clozapine, olanzepine, quetiapine).

Hensiak et al administered the UPSIT to 10 non-demented patients with DPD induced by a range of phenothiazine preparations that had been administered for at least 2 weeks.[91] Five had an abnormal UPSIT score for their age and none made a complete recovery from DPD even when the offending medication was changed or stopped. Of the remaining 5 who did regain normal motor function after withdrawing treatment, all but one had normal smell function. Lee et al compared Brief Smell Identification Test (B-SIT) scores of 15 patients whose DPD was induced by levosulpiride, haloperidone, flunarizine, perphenazine, metoclopramide, or risperidone to B-SIT scores of controls and patients with PD.[92] The DPD scores did not differ from those of the controls and were significantly higher than those of the PD patients. A problem with both of these studies is confounding by the presence of a psychotic disorder which in itself can be associated with olfactory dysfunction. It should also be noted that, at least theoretically, some individuals with drug-induced PD may be predisposed to develop PD and that exposure to a dopamine depleting drug may unmask underlying disease and the associated olfactory dysfunction.

The pesticide rotenone, which is a complex I inhibitor, reproduces features of PD in animals, including selective nigrostriatal dopaminergic degeneration and α-synuclein-positive cytoplasmic inclusions.[93,94] Oxidative damage has been noted in brains from rotenone-treated animals in the same midbrain and olfactory bulb dopaminergic regions that are affected by PD.[95] Rotenone is freely available and has the potential to cause a form of parkinsonism, although there are no documented cases of rotenone-induced PD in humans.

The most notorious compound known to induce parkinsonism is 1-methyl-4-phenyl-1, 2, 3, 6-tetrahydropyridine (MPTP). This agent is metabolically converted to the neurotoxin MPP+, which selectively damages dopamine neurons within the striatum. Six young drug abusers who came down with MPTP-induced parkinsonism (MPTP-P) were administered the UPSIT and a detection threshold test for phenyl ethyl alcohol (PEA).[96] Comparison groups consisted of 13 young PD patients and 10 normal subjects. The MPTP-P patients evidenced no major decrements in olfactory function and did not differ from normal controls. They could sniff adequately and could respond verbally to the examiner's questions without difficulty. The young PD patients, on the other hand, had olfactory dysfunction, differing significantly from controls. This study suggests that the functional integrity of the olfactory system of patients with MPTP-induced parkinsonism is greater than that of similarly-aged PD patients and supports the notion that olfactory dysfunction is not a concomitant element of all parkinsonian syndromes.

That being said, animal studies are conflicting regarding the influences of MPTP on the olfactory system, suggesting more work is needed on this topic. Non-human primate studies have reported an MPTP-related increase in dopamine and tyrosine hydroxylase expression in the olfactory bulbs[48] and, in one study, 3 marmosets systemically treated with MPTP had difficulty locating bananas by smell. These animals would eat bananas tainted with skatole (putrid, fecal) or isovaleric acid (dirty socks, rancid cheese), which was not the case prior to the MPTP-treatment or in 3 untreated marmosets.[97] In rats, MPTP introduced intranasally, but not systemically, produces a syndrome which mimics key elements of human PD, including smell loss, although the smell loss is transient.[98] In mice, systemically-administered MPTP induces olfactory bulb microgliosis and increased expression of pro-inflammatory cytokines interleukin (IL)-1α, IL-1β, and IL-1ra mRNA within a day of administration.[99] A reduction in MPTP-induced microgliosis was found in both the olfactory bulbs and the striatum of IL-1α/β knockout mice, implicating IL-1 in mediating the microglia activation.

Parkinsonism Dementia Complex of Guam

The Parkinsonism dementia complex of Guam (PDC) is typified by coexistence of Alzheimer's disease (AD), parkinsonism, and amyotrophic lateral sclerosis (ALS; motor neuron disease), either singly or in combination. Individuals with this disorder, which is largely confined to the Chamorro population on the Pacific Island of Guam, exhibit smell loss analogous to that observed in AD and PD. In the first of 2 studies of PDC, 24 patients were administered the UPSIT.[19] Half were from Umatac and Merizo, two southern villages associated with a high prevalence of PDC. The others were from Guamanian villages with lower PDC prevalence rates. For comparison, UPSIT data from 24 AD and 24 PD North American patients matched to the PDC data on the basis of smoking behavior, gender, and age. The UPSIT scores of the 3 groups, which were lower than normal controls, did not differ significantly from one another. Each participant was asked whether he or she suffered from smell or taste problems prior to olfactory testing. Three of the PDC patients reported such problems (13%), as compared to 2 of the AD (8%) and 3 of the PD (13%) patients, suggesting that the level of awareness of the problem is similar and low in these 3 groups.

Subsequent to this work, Ahlskog et al administered an abbreviated version of the UPSIT to 9 Guamanians with symptoms of ALS, 9 with symptoms of pure parkinsonism, 11 patients with pure dementia, and 31 patients with PDC, as well as to neurologically normal Guamanians and 25 North American controls. The UPSIT scores were markedly depressed in the

4 disease groups relative to the controls, and did not differentiate among the 4 phenotypes. Some control subjects had lower scores than their North American counterparts, suggesting the possibility that subclinical neuro-degeneration may be occurring.

X-linked Recessive Dystonia-parkinsonism

X-linked recessive dystonia-parkinsonism, also termed 'Lubag', affects Filipino male adults with maternal roots from the Philippine Island of Panay. A single study of 20 affected males and 20 controls using a cultur-ally modified UPSIT suggested that olfaction was moderately impaired (respective mean scores = 18 & 20.5, p = 0.003), even early in the disorder.[101] The smell loss was unrelated to disease duration, severity, and the degree of dystonia.

Essential Tremor

Classical essential tremor (ET) is typically diagnosed without difficulty, particularly when a strong family history is present. There can be confu-sion between ET and benign tremulous PD when cogwheeling is absent or equivocal, and in a minority of cases when the tremor appears to be dys-tonic or there is co-existing rigidity. No pathological studies have been made of the olfactory pathways of ET, and only a few on the rest of the brain.[102]

The first study to assess olfaction in this condition evaluated UPSIT scores in 15 ET patients and found all to be within the normal range.[29] A decade later, Louis et al reported that a significant proportion of ET patients had mild impairment on the UPSIT,[103] leading to the suggestion that the defect may relate to a role of the cerebellum in olfactory function. However, a subsequent study of ET patients with isolated rest tremor found UPSIT scores to be no different from typical ET patients.[104] In accord with the findings of Busenbark et al, recent studies have found normal UPSIT scores in ET[33,105] and the suggestion was made that errors may occur if apparent ET is confused with benign tremulous PD, a condition associated with smell dysfunction. Shah et al recently compared UPSIT scores of 59 healthy persons with ET to those from 64 persons with tremor-dominant PD.[106] Nearly complete separation of the two groups was made on the basis of UPSIT scores and to lesser degree on measures from odor event-related potentials (OERPs). When ET subjects were separated by family history of tremor in a first degree relative (FET), this group scored significantly better than age- and gender-matched controls. There was a suggestion of resis-tance to the effects of aging in FET as well. These unexpected findings need to be verified, but it is likely that patients with ET have no important disorder of olfaction.

Cerebellar Ataxia

Functional imaging studies suggest that the cerebellum plays some role in olfaction,[107] an observation that has prompted investigations into cerebellar disorders. Given the possibility of confusion between cerebellar tremor and parkinsonism, olfactory testing could conceivably aid in their differential diagnosis.

In an early study on this topic, mild abnormalities in UPSIT scores were found in Friedreich's ataxia and some other ataxic disorders.[108] No correlation was seen between UPSIT scores and trinucleotide repeat length, disease duration, or walking disability. In another study, mild UPSIT impairment was found in autosomal dominant spinocerebellar ataxia type 2 (SCA2), but not in Machado-Joseph syndrome (SCA3).[109] In contrast, Hentschel et al found normal UPSIT scores in 7 individuals with the SCA2 mutation.[110] Patients with SCA2 or SCA3 mutations may have parkinsonian tremor or dystonia (SCA3), which can cause diagnostic difficulty; hence the finding of normal olfaction in suspected PD could indicate an inherited cerebellar syndrome. It is important to note that the aforementioned observations are based on relatively small numbers of subjects and that little is specifically known about cerebellar involvement, if any, in olfactory function.

Huntington's Disease

Huntington's disease (HD) is a late presenting autosomal dominant disorder of basal ganglia function typified by choreic movement, dementia, and, in rare cases, muscular rigidity similar to that of PD (Westphal variant). An initial study of 38 patients and 38 controls found deficits in their ability to remember odor qualities.[111] Subsequent studies using tests of odor identification and detection have found moderate olfactory impairment in HD patients with established disease, but of less severity than PD.[112–115] In one study, UPSIT scores and phenyl ethyl alcohol thresholds were normal in 12 at-risk relatives, but abnormal in 25 probands.[114] In another, 20 healthy subjects with the HD mutation exhibited normal UPSIT scores, whereas 20 of those expressing the HD phenotype were mildly abnormal.[112] A significant delay in the 'P3' components of the OERP was noted by Wetter and Murphy in 8 subjects with established HD.[116]

The aforementioned studies, while demonstrating that smell loss is present at the time of HD phenotypic expression, shed little light on when the olfactory loss first appears. A provocative recent report suggests that subtle smell dysfunction may occur, along with mild cognitive and motor changes, in HD gene carriers 10 to 15 years before phenotypic HD expression.[117]

A number of other conditions are now recognized that can simulate the HD phenotype, including neuroacanthocytosis, spinocerebellar atrophy type 17 (SCA- 17), benign hereditary chorea, and Huntington disease-like disorder (HDL1 and HDL2). In all of these disorders, a molecular diagnosis can be made, but presently it is unknown if they are accompanied by olfactory dysfunction.

Conclusion and Future Needs

It is apparent from the studies reviewed in this chapter that smell dysfunction is an integral component of PD and some other movement disorders. Olfactory dysfunction is also found in a number of other neurological diseases (Table 4-1) and the same olfactory phenotype appears to be present

Table 4-1. Relative Degree of Olfactory Dysfunction in Various 'Neurodegenerative' Conditions on an Arbitrary Scale.

Disease	Relative Severity of Smell Loss
Idiopathic Parkinson's disease, Alzheimer's disease, dementia with Lewy bodies, Guam PD-dementia complex.	++++
Huntington's disease, Down's syndrome, PARK6, PARK8	+++
Multiple system atrophy (type-P), PARK1, pallidopontonigral degeneration (probably a form of frontotemporal dementia), drug induced PD?, schizophrenia, semantic dementia, X-linked dystonia-parkinsonism (Lubag).	++
Motor neuron disease, SCA2, Friedreich's ataxia	+
PARK3, essential tremor?, corticobasal degeneration?, frontotemporal dementia	+
Vascular parkinsonism, MPTP parkinsonism, idiopathic dystonia, SCA3, progressive supranuclear palsy, PARK2?	0

Key: ++++ marked damage; + mild; 0 normal. SCA = spinocerebellar atrophy. NB. Most of these scores, except for idiopathic Parkinson's disease, are based on relatively small patient numbers and should be interpreted conservatively.

Table 4-2. Relative Degree of Olfactory Lewy Body, Alzheimer Pathology, and Smell Loss in 3 Major Neurodegenerative Diseases.

Diagnosis	Lewy Bodies	Alzheimer Pathology	Severity of Smell Loss
Parkinson's disease (PD)	++++	+	++++
Dementia with Lewy bodies (DLB)	++++	++	++++
Alzheimer's disease (AD)	+	++++	++++

Key: ++++ marked severity or damage; + mild severity or damage.

even in the presence of different underlying major neuropathology (Table 4-2). In the case of PD, the olfactory dysfunction is little influenced by anti-PD drug therapy. Moreover, individuals with MPTP-induced PD seem to have relatively normal smell function.[96]

The association between the changes in olfactory function and other non-motor changes that may occur in the PD prodome, such as sleep disturbance, constipation, and dysautonomia, also requires more study. Like olfactory dysfunction, cardiac sympathetic dysfunction is present prior to the onset of the motor symptoms of PD.[118] One group reported a 0.56 positive correlation between 123-I-metaiodobenzylguanidine (MIGB) cardiac uptake and B-SIT scores in patients with PD (mean H&Y score 2.1), but not in patients with multiple system atrophy.[38] In another study, increased olfactory thresholds were observed in nearly all 30 patients with a REM sleep behavioral disorder (RBD), 8 of whom had evidence of parkinsonism[119]; see also Iranzo et al.[120] However, RBD-related pathological changes are more in keeping with those of parkinsonism than with those of classical PD,[121] and acute sleep deprivation *per se* has a specific but mild adverse influence on smell identification ability.[122]

Presently the time between the onset of smell dysfunction and the motor symptom phenotype of PD is unknown and marked individual variation may be the norm (for recent review, see Hawkes).[123] Many studies likely underestimate this interval because the olfactory and dopamine transporter deficits are already present at the time of the first assessment of the olfactory loss. Anecdotally, some patients recall having smell loss 3 decades or more before the onset of their motor symptoms.[123]

The basis for the olfactory loss associated with PD is unclear, although 3 non-mutually exclusive hypotheses are worthy of consideration. *First*, if one accepts the pathological staging of Braak et al. and the possibility that xenobiotics may be causally related to PD, the smell loss may well reflect damage from a pathogenic agent that directly enters the brain via the olfactory system (the 'olfactory vector' hypothesis).[124] Recent studies suggest that environmental agents, most notably nanoparticles, may enter the brain of even young children exposed to extreme air pollution, inducing smell dysfunction, olfactory bulb inflammation, and neuropathological changes within the bulb similar to those observed in AD and PD.[125] Given the early pathology within the dorsomotor nucleus of the vagus, such agents could also enter the brain via swallowed secretions that invade the vagal enteric motor fibers within the stomach (the 'dual hit' hypothesis).[61] Since olfactory receptor cell entry ultimately occurs for some systemically-introduced viruses and neurotoxins in rodents,[126, 127] such entry still could cause olfactory loss in marmosets given systemic MPTP.[97] *Second*, damage to the olfactory system, per se, may be the precipitating event (the 'olfactory damage' hypothesis). Thus, any factor that damages the olfactory nerve fibers, including xenobiotics, head trauma, or occlusion of the foramina of the cribriform plate, may set the disease process into motion in genetically or otherwise susceptible individuals. Evidence for such a possibility is reviewed elsewhere.[124] *Third*, a more orthodox and conceivably parsimonious explanation is that cells within the olfactory pathways are genetically selectively vulnerable to the earliest stages of the PD-related disease.

Whatever the cause of the olfactory loss of PD, the studies reviewed in this chapter clearly demonstrate that such loss is an integral component of this disorder, occurring more frequently than tremor and at frequencies equivalent to the classic diagnostic signs. These studies also indicate that such loss is of potential value in differential diagnosis, since such disorders as PSP and essential tremor exhibit little or no olfactory dysfunction.

References

1. Doty RL, Shaman P, Applebaum SL, Giberson R, Siksorski L, Rosenberg L. Smell identification ability: changes with age. *Science*. 1984;226:1441–3.
2. Santos DV, Reiter ER, DiNardo LJ, Costanzo RM. Hazardous events associated with impaired olfactory function. *Arch Otolaryngol Head Neck Surg*. 2004;130:317–9.
3. Deems DA, Doty RL, Settle RG et al. Smell and taste disorders, a study of 750 patients from the University of Pennsylvania Smell and Taste Center. *Arch Otolaryngol Head Neck Surg*. 1991;117(5):519–28.
4. Andersen IB. The ambient air. In: Brain JD, Procter DF, Reid LM, editors. *Respiratory defense mechanisms*. New York: Marcel Dekker; 1977. p. 25–62.
5. Doty RL. Olfaction and gustation in normal aging and Alzheimer's disease. In: Hof PR, Mobbs CV, editors. *Functional Neurobiology of Aging*. San Diego: Academic Press; 2001. p. 647–58.

6. Doty RL. Odor perception in neurodegenerative diseases. In: Doty RL, editor. *Handbook of Olfaction and Gustation*. 2nd ed. New York: Marcel Dekker; 2003. p. 479–502.

7. Hawkes CH, Shephard BC, Daniel SE. Is Parkinson's disease a primary olfactory disorder? *QJM*. 1999;92(8):473–80.

8. Tissingh G, Berendse HW, Bergmans P et al. Loss of olfaction in de novo and treated Parkinson's disease: possible implications for early diagnosis. *Movement Dis*. 2001;16:41–6.

9. Mesholam RI, Moberg PJ, Mahr RN, Doty RL. Olfaction in neurodegenerative disease: a meta-analysis of olfactory functioning in Alzheimer's and Parkinson's diseases. *Arch Neurol*. 1998;55(1):84–90.

10. Doty RL, Stern MB, Pfeiffer C, Gollomp SM, Hurtig HI. Bilateral olfactory dysfunction in early stage treated and untreated idiopathic Parkinson's disease. *J Neurol Neurosurg Psychiat*. 1992;55(2):138–42.

11. Stern MB, Doty RL, Dotti M et al. Olfactory function in Parkinson's disease subtypes. *Neurology*. 1994;44(2):266–8.

12. Doty RL, Deems DA, Stellar S. Olfactory dysfunction in parkinsonism: a general deficit unrelated to neurologic signs, disease stage, or disease duration. *Neurology*. 1988;38(8):1237–44.

13. Hawkes C. Olfaction in neurodegenerative disorder. *Movement Dis*. 2003;18(4):364–72.

14. Silveira-Moriyama L, Williams D, Katzenschlager R, Lees AJ. Pizza, mint, and licorice: Smell testing in Parkinson's disease in a UK population. *Movement Dis*. 2005;20:S139.

15. Double KL, Rowe DB, Hayes M et al. Identifying the pattern of olfactory deficits in Parkinson disease using the brief smell identification test. *Arch Neurol*. 2003; 60(4):545–9.

16. Bohnen NI, Gedela S, Kuwabara H et al. Selective hyposmia and nigrostriatal dopaminergic denervation in Parkinson's disease. *J Neurol*. 2007;254(1):84–90.

17. Boesveldt S, Verbaan D, Knol DL, Visser M, Van Rooden SM, Van Hilten JJ, Berendse HW. A comparative study of odor identification and odor discrimination deficits in Parkinson's disease. *Mov. Disord*. 2008;23:1984–90.

18. Doty RL, Perl DP, Steele JC et al. Olfactory dysfunction in three neurodegenerative diseases. *Geriatrics*. 1991;46 Suppl 1:47–51.

19. Doty RL, Perl DP, Steele JC et al. Odor identification deficit of the parkinsonism-dementia complex of Guam: Equivalence to that of Alzheimer's and idiopathic Parkinson's disease. *Neurology*. 1991;41(5 Suppl 2):77–80.

20. Doty RL, Riklan M, Deems DA, Reynolds C, Stellar S. The olfactory and cognitive deficits of Parkinson's disease: evidence for independence. *Ann Neurol*. 1989;25(2): 166–71.

21. Barz S, Hummel T, Pauli E, Majer M, Lang CJ, Kobal G. Chemosensory event-related potentials in response to trigeminal and olfactory stimulation in idiopathic Parkinson's disease. *Neurology*. 1997;49(5):1424–31.

22. Siderowf A, Newberg A, Chou KL et al. [99mTc]TRODAT-1 SPECT imaging correlates with odor identification in early Parkinson disease. *Neurology*. 2005;64(10): 1716–20.

23. Ponsen MM, Stoffers D, Booij J, van Eck-Smit BL, Wolters EC, Berendse HW. Idiopathic hyposmia as a preclinical sign of Parkinson's disease. *Ann Neurol.* 2004;56(2):173–81.

24. Berendse HWB. Subclinical dopaminergic dysfunction in asymptomatic Parkinson's disease patients' relatives with a decreased sense of smell. *Ann Neurol.* 2001;50(1): 34–41.

25. Markopoulou K, Larsen KW, Wszolek EK et al. Olfactory dysfunction in familial parkinsonism. *Neurology.* 1997;49(5):1262–7.

26. Quinn NP, Rossor MN, Marsden CD. Olfactory threshold in Parkinson's disease. *J Neurol Neurosurg Psychiat.* 1987;50:88–9.

27. Roth J, Radil T, Ruzicka E, Jech R, Tichy J. Apomorphine does not influence olfactory thresholds in Parkinson's disease. *Funct Neurol.* 1998;13(2):99–103.

28. Sobel N, Thomason ME, Stappen I et al. An impairment in sniffing contributes to the olfactory impairment in Parkinson's disease. *Proc Nat Acad Sci USA.* 2001 27;98(7):4154–9.

29. Busenbark KL, Huber SI, Greer G, Pahwa R, Koller WC. Olfactory function in essential tremor. *Neurology.* 1992;42:1631–2.

30. Doty RL, Golbe LI, McKeown DA, Stern MB, Lehrach CM, Crawford D. Olfactory testing differentiates between progressive supranuclear palsy and idiopathic Parkinson's disease. *Neurology.* 1993;43(5):962–5.

31. Doty RL, Bromley SM, Stern MB. Olfactory testing as an aid in the diagnosis of Parkinson's disease: development of optimal discrimination criteria. *Neurodegeneration.* 1995;4(1):93–7.

32. Ondo WG, Lai D. Olfaction testing in patients with tremor-dominant Parkinson's disease: is this a distinct condition? *Movement Dis.* 2005;20(4):471–5.

33. Shah M, Muhammed N, Findley LJ, Hawkes CH. Olfactory tests in the diagnosis of essential tremor. *Parkinsonism Relat Disord.* 2008;14(7):563–8.

34. Montgomery EB, Jr., Baker KB, Lyons K, Koller WC. Abnormal performance on the PD test battery by asymptomatic first-degree relatives. *Neurology.* 1999 10; 52(4):757–62.

35. Montgomery EB, Jr., Lyons K, Koller WC. Early detection of probable idiopathic Parkinson's disease: II. A prospective application of a diagnostic test battery. *Movement Dis.* 2000;15(3):474–8.

36. Lee PH, Yeo SH, Kim HJ, Youm HY. Correlation between cardiac 123I-MIBG and odor identification in patients with Parkinson's disease and multiple system atrophy. *Movement Dis.* 2006;21(11):1975–7.

37. Ross GW, Petrovitch H, Abbott RD, Tanner CM, Popper J, Masaki K. et al. Association of olfactory dysfunction with risk for future Parkinson's disease. *Ann. Neurology.* 2008;63:167–73.

38. Ponsen MM, Stoffers D, Wolters ECh, Booij J, Berendse HW . Olfactory testing combined with dopamine transporter imaging as a method to detect prodromal Parkinson's disease. *J Neurol Neurosurg Psychiat.* 2010;81:396–399.

39. Haehner A, Hummel T, Hummel C, Sommer U, Junghanns S, Reichmann H. Olfactory loss may be a first sign of idiopathic Parkinson's disease. *Movement Dis.* 2007;22(6):839–42.

40. Katzenschlager R, Zijlmans J, Evans A, Watt H, Lees AJ. Olfactory function distinguishes vascular parkinsonism from Parkinson's disease. *J Neurol Neurosurg Psychiat*. 2004;75(12):1749–52.

41. Muller A, Reichmann H, Livermore A, Hummel T. Olfactory function in idiopathic Parkinson's disease (IPD): results from cross-sectional studies in IPD patients and long-term follow-up of de-novo IPD patients. *J Neural Transm*. 2002;109(5–6): 805–11.

42. Duda JE, Shah U, Arnold SE, Lee VM, Trojanowski JQ. The expression of alpha-, beta-, and gamma-synucleins in olfactory mucosa from patients with and without neurodegenerative diseases. *Exp Neurol*. 1999;160(2):515–22.

43. Crino PB, Martin JA, Hill WD, Greenberg B, Lee VM, Trojanowski JQ. Beta-amyloid peptide and amyloid precursor proteins in olfactory mucosa of patients with Alzheimer's disease, Parkinson's disease, and Down syndrome. *Ann Otol Rhinol Laryngol*. 1995;104(8):655–61.

44. Daniel SE, Hawkes CH. Preliminary diagnosis of Parkinson's disease by olfactory bulb pathology [letter]. *Lancet*. 1992 18;340(8812):186.

45. Pearce RK, Hawkes CH, Daniel SE. The anterior olfactory nucleus in Parkinson's disease. *Movement Dis*. 1995;10(3):283–7.

46. Huisman E, Uylings HBM, Hoogland PV. A 100% increase of 687 dopaminergic cells in the olfactory bulb may explain hyposmia in Parkinson's disease. *Movement Dis*. 2004;19(6):687–92.

47. Huisman E, Uylings HBM, Hoogland PV. Gender-related changes in increase of dopaminergic neurons in the olfactory bulb of Parkinson's disease patients. *Movement Dis*. 2008;23(10):1407–13.

48. Belzunegui S, Sebastian WS, Garrido-Gil P. The number of dopaminergic cells is increased in the olfactory bulb of monkeys chronically exposed to MPTP. *Synapse*. 2007;61:1006–12.

49. Yamada M, Onodera M, Mizuno Y, Mochizuki H. Neurogenesis in olfactory bulb identified by retroviral labeling in normal and 1-methyl-4-phenyl-1,2,3,6-tetrahydropyridine-treated adult mice. *Neuroscience. 124(1):173–81, 2004*.

50. Bedard A, Parent A. Evidence of newly generated neurons in the human olfactory bulb. *Dev Brain Res*. 2004;151(1–2):159–68.

51. Bogerts B, Hantsch J, Herzer M. A morphometric study of the dopamine-containing cell groups in the mesencephalon of normals, Parkinson patients, and schizophrenics. *Biol Psychiat*. 1983;18(9):951–69.

52. Braak H, Braak E. Cognitive impairment in Parkinson's disease: amyloid plaques, neurofibrillary tangles, and neuropil threads in the cerebral cortex. *J Neural Transm Park Dis Dement Sect*. 1990;2(1):45–57.

53. Mattila PM, Roytta M, Torikka H, Dickson DW, Rinne JO. Cortical Lewy bodies and Alzheimer-type changes in patients with Parkinson's disease. *Acta Neuropathol*. 1998;95(6):576–82.

54. Mattila PM, Rinne JO, Helenius H, Dickson DW, Roytta M. Alpha-synuclein-immunoreactive cortical Lewy bodies are associated with cognitive impairment in Parkinson's disease. *Acta Neuropath*. 2000;100(3):285–90.

55. Braak H, Del TK, Rub U, De Vos RA, Jansen Steur EN, Braak E. Staging of brain pathology related to sporadic Parkinson's disease. *Neurobiol Aging.* 2003;24(2):197–211.

56. Braak H, Ghebremedhin E, Rub U, Bratzke H, Del TK. Stages in the development of Parkinson's disease-related pathology. *Cell Tissue Res.* 2004;318(1):121–34.

57. Del Tredici K, Rub U, De Vos RA, Bohl JR, Braak H. Where does Parkinson disease pathology begin in the brain? *J Neuropathol Exp Neurol.* 2002;61(5):413–26.

58. Braak H, Rub U, Gai WP, Del TK. Idiopathic Parkinson's disease: possible routes by which vulnerable neuronal types may be subject to neuroinvasion by an unknown pathogen. *J Neural Trans.* 2003;110(5):517–36.

59. Braak H, de Vos RAI, Bohl J, Del Tredici K. Gastric alpha-synuclein immunoreactive inclusions in Meissner's and Auerbach's plexuses in cases staged for Parkinson's disease-related brain pathology. *Neurosci Letters.* 2006;396(1):67–72.

60. Kaufmann H, Nahm K, Purohit D, Wolfe D. Autonomic failure as the initial presentation of Parkinson disease and dementia with Lewy bodies. *Neurology.* 2004;63(6): 1093–5.

61. Hawkes CH, Del Tredici K, Braak H. Parkinson's disease: a dual-hit hypothesis. *Neuropathol Appl Neurobiol.* 2007;33(6):599–614.

62. Muller CM, de Vos RAI, Maurage CA, Thal DR, Tolnay M, Braak H. Staging of sporadic Parkinson disease-related alpha-synuclein pathology: Inter- and intra-rater reliability. *J Neuropathol Exp Neurol.* 2005;64(7):623–8.

63. Duda JE, Noorigian JV, Petrovitch H, White LR, Ross WR. One-third of elderly men without a history of Parkinson's disease or dementia with Lewy bodies have Lewy pathology in the olfactory bulb. *Mov Disord.* 2008;23(Suppl. 1):S60.

64. Parkkinen L, Kauppinen T, Pirttila T, Autere JM, Alafuzoff I. alpha-Synuclein pathology does not predict extrapyramidal symptoms or dementia. *Ann Neurol.* 2005;57(1):82–91.

65. Kalaitzakis ME, Graeber MB, Gentleman SM, Pearce RKB. The dorsal motor nucleus of the vagus is not an obligatory trigger site of Parkinson's disease: a critical analysis of alpha-synuclein staging. *Neuropathol Appl Neurobiol.* 2008;34(3):284–95.

66. Halliday GM, Del Tredici K, Braak H. Critical appraisal of brain pathology staging related to presymptomatic and symptomatic cases of sporadic Parkinson's disease. *Journal of Neural Transmission-Supplement.* 2006;(70):99–103.

67. Fearnley JM, Lees AJ. Ageing and Parkinson's disease: substantia nigra regional selectivity. *Brain.* 1991;114(Pt 5):2283–301.

68. Ross GW, Petrovitch H, Abbott RD et al. Parkinsonian signs and substantia nigra neuron density in descendents' elders without PD. *Ann Neurol.* 2004;56(4):532–9.

69. Hentschel K, Furtado S, Markopoulou K, Doty RL, Uitti RJ, Wszolek ZK. Differences in olfactory dysfunction between sporadic PD and familial Parkinson's disease kindreds by UPSIT subgroup analysis. *Movement Dis.* 2005;20:S55.

70. Ferreira JJ, Guedes LC, Rosa MM et al. High prevalence of LRRK2 mutations in familial and sporadic Parkinson's disease in Portugal. *Movement Dis.* 2007;22(8): 1194–201.

71. Khan NL, Katzenschlager R, Watt H et al. Olfaction differentiates parkin disease from early-onset parkinsonism and Parkinson disease. *Neurology.* 2004;62(7):1224–6.

72. Silveira-Moriyama L, Guedes L, Kingsbury A, et al. Olfaction in dardarin/LRRK2 associated Parkinsonism. *Movement Dis.* 22 (Suppl 16), S258. 2007.

73. McKeith IG, Dickson DW, Lowe J et al. Diagnosis and management of dementia with Lewy bodies - Third report of the DLB consortium. *Neurology.* 2005;65(12): 1863–72.

74. Ballard C, Ziabreva I, Perry R et al. Differences in neuropathologic characteristics across the Lewy body dementia spectrum. *Neurology.* 2006;67(11):1931–4.

75. Galvin JE, Pollack J, Morris JC. Clinical phenotype of Parkinson disease dementia. *Neurology.* 2006;67(9):1605–11.

76. Geser F, Wenning GK, Poewe W, McKeith I. How to diagnose dementia with Lewy bodies: State of the art. *Movement Dis.* 2005;20:S11–S20.

77. Tsuboi Y, Wszolek ZK, Graff-Radford NR, Cookson N, Dickson DW. Tau pathology in the olfactory bulb correlates with Braak stage, Lewy body pathology and apolipo-protein epsilon4. *Neuropathol Appl Neurobiol.* 2003;29(5):503–10.

78. Liberini P, Parola S, Spano PF, Antonini L. Olfaction in Parkinson's disease: methods of assessment and clinical relevance. *J Neurol.* 2000;247(2):88–96.

79. McShane RH, Nagy Z, Esiri MM et al. Anosmia in dementia is associated with Lewy bodies rather than Alzheimer's pathology. *J Neurol, Neurosurg Psychiat.* 2001;70(6):739–43.

80. Liberini P, Parola S, Spano PF, Antonini L. Olfaction in Parkinson's disease: methods of assessment and clinical relevance. *J Neurol.* 2000;247(2):88–96.

81. Olichney JM, Murphy C, Hofstetter CR, et al. Anosmia is very common in the Lewy body variant of Alzheimer's disease. *J Neurol Neurosurg Psychiat.* 2005;76(10):1342–7.

82. Kovacs T, Papp MI, Cairns NJ, Khan MN, Lantos PL. Olfactory bulb in multiple system atrophy. *Movement Dis.* 2003;18(8):938–42.

83. Wenning GK, Shephard B, Hawkes C, Petruckevitch A, Lees A, Quinn N. Olfactory function in atypical parkinsonian syndromes. *Acta Neurol Scand.* 1995;91(4):247–50.

84. Nee LE, Scott J, Polinsky RJ. Olfactory dysfunction in the Shy-Drager syndrome. *Clin Auton Res.* 3, 281–282. 1993.

85. Muller A, Mungersdorf M, Reichmann H, Strehle G, Hummel T. Olfactory function in Parkinsonian syndromes. *J Clin Neurosci.* 2002;9(5):521–4.

86. Abele M, Riet A, Hummel T, Klockgether T, Wullner U. Olfactory dysfunction in cerebellar ataxia and multiple system atrophy. *J Neurol.* 2003;250(12):1453–5.

87. Luzzi S, Snowden JS, Neary D, Coccia M, Provinciali L, Ralph MAL. Distinct patterns of olfactory impairment in Alzheimer's disease, semantic dementia, frontotemporal dementia, and corticobasal degeneration. *Neuropsychologia.* 2007;45(8):1823–31.

88. Williams DR, de Silva R, Paviour DC et al. Characteristics of two distinct clinical phenotypes in pathologically proven progressive supranuclear palsy: Richardson's syndrome and PSP-parkinsonism. *Brain.* 2005;128:1247–58.

89. Zijlmans JCM, Thijssen HOM, Vogels OJM et al. MRI in patients with suspected vascular parkinsonism. *Neurology.* 1995;45(12):2183–8.

90. Tzen KY, Lu CS, Yen TC, Wey SP, Ting C. Differential diagnosis of Parkinson's disease and vascular parkinsonism by Tc-99m-TRODAT-1. *J Nuclear Med.* 2001;42(3):408–13.

91. Hensiek AE, Bhatia K, Hawkes CH. Olfactory function in drug induced parkinsonism. *J Neurol.* 247 (Suppl. 3), 82. 2000.

92. Lee PH, Yeo SH, Yong SW, Kim YJ. Odour identification test and its relation to cardiac I-123-metaiodobenzylguanidine in patients with drug induced parkinsonism. *J Neurol Neurosurg Psychiat.* 2007;78(11):1250–2.

93. Betarbet R, Sherer TB, MacKenzie G, Garcia-Osuna M, Panov AV, Greenamyre JT. Chronic systemic pesticide exposure reproduces features of Parkinson's disease. *Nat Neurosci.* 2000;3(12):1301–6.

94. Betarbet R, Canet-Aviles RA, Sherer TB et al. Intersecting pathways to neurodegeneration in Parkinson's disease: Effects of the pesticide rotenone on DJ-1, alpha-synuclein, and the ubiquitin-proteasome system. *Neurobiol Dis.* 2006;22(2):404–20.

95. Sherer TB, Betarbet R, Testa CM et al. Mechanism of toxicity in rotenone models of Parkinson's disease. *J Neurosci.* 2003;23(34):10756–64.

96. Doty RL, Singh A, Tetrud J, Langston JW. Lack of Major Olfactory Dysfunction in MPTP-Induced Parkinsonism. *Ann Neurol.* 1992;32(1):97–100.

97. Miwa T, Watanabe A, Mitsumoto Y, Furukawa M, Fukushima N, Moriizumi T. Olfactory impairment and Parkinson's disease-like symptoms observed in the common marmoset following administration of 1-methyl-4-phenyl-1,2,3,6-tetrahydropyridine. *Acta Otolaryngol (Stockh).* 2004;124:80–4.

98. Prediger RDS, Batista LC, Medeiros R, Pandolfo P, Florio JC, Takahashi RN. The risk is in the air: Intranasal administration of MPTP to rats reproducing clinical features of Parkinson's disease. *Exp Neurol.* 2006;202(2):391–403.

99. Vroon A, Drukarch B, Bol JGJM et al. Neuroinflammation in Parkinson's patients and MPTP-treated mice is not restricted to the nigrostriatal system: Microgliosis and differential expression of interleukin-1 receptors in the olfactory bulb. *Exp Gerontol.* 2007;42(8):762–71.

100. Ahlskog JE, Waring SC, Petersen RC et al. Olfactory dysfunction in Guamanian ALS, parkinsonism, and dementia. *Neurology.* 1998;51(6):1672–7.

101. Evidente VG, Esteban RP, Hernandez JL et al. Smell testing is abnormal in 'Lubag' or X-linked dystonia-parkinsonism: a pilot study. *Parkinsonism Rel Dis.* 2004;10(7):407–10.

102. Louis ED, Vonsattel JPG, Honig LS, Ross GW, Lyons KE, Pahwa R. Neuropathologic findings in essential tremor. *Neurology.* 2006;66(11):1756–9.

103. Louis ED, Bromley SM, Jurewicz EC, Watner D. Olfactory dysfunction in essential tremor: a deficit unrelated to disease duration or severity. *Neurology.* 2002 26;59(10):1631–3.

104. Louis ED, Jurewicz EC. Olfaction in essential tremor patients with and without isolated rest tremor. *Movement Dis.* 2003;18(11):1387–9.

105. Shah M, Findley L, Muhammed N, Hawkes C. Olfaction is normal in essential tremor and can be used to distinguish it from Parkinson's disease. *Neurology.* 2005;64(6):A261.

106. Shah M, Muhammed N, Findley LJ, Hawkes CH. Olfactory tests in the diagnosis of essential tremor. 13, 143. 2007. *Parkinsonism Rel Dis* 14(7):563–568.

107. Sobel N, Prabhakaran V, Hartley CA, Desmond JE, Zhao Z, Glover GH, Gabrieli JD, Sullivan EV. Odor-induced and sniff-induced activation in the cerebellum of the human. *J Neurosci.* 1998;18(21):8990–9001.

108. Connelly T, Farmer JM, Lynch DR, Doty RL. Olfactory dysfunction in degenerative ataxias. J Neurol Neurosurg Psychiat. 2003;74(10):1435–7.

109. Fernandez-Ruiz J, Diaz R, Hall-Haro C et al. Olfactory dysfunction in hereditary ataxia and basal ganglia disorders. *Neuroreport.* 2003 18;14(10):1339–41.

110. Hentschel K, Baba Y, Williams LN, Doty RL, Uitti RJ, Wszolek ZK. Olfaction in familial Parkinsonism (FP). *Movement Dis.* 2005;20:S52.

111. Moberg PJ, Pearlson GD, Speedie LJ, Lipsey JR, Strauss ME, Folstein SE. Olfactory recognition: differential impairments in early and late Huntington's and Alzheimer's diseases. *J Clin Exp Neuropsychol.* 1987;9(6):650–64.

112. Bylsma FW, Moberg PJ, Doty RL, Brandt J. Odor identification in Huntington's disease patients and asymptomatic gene carriers. *J Neuropsychiatry Clin Neurosci.* 1997;9(4):598–600.

113. Hamilton JM, Murphy C, Paulsen JS. Odor detection, learning, and memory in Huntington's disease. *J Internat Neuropsychol Soc.* 1999;5(7):609–15.

114. Moberg PJ, Doty RL. Olfactory function in Huntington's disease patients and at-risk offspring. *Int J Neurosci.* 1997;89(1–2):133–9.

115. Nordin S, Paulsen JS, Murphy C. Sensory- and memory-mediated olfactory dysfunction in Huntington's disease. *J Internat Neuropsychol Soc.* 1995;1(3):281–90.

116. Wetter S, Murphy C. Apolipoprotein E epsilon4 positive individuals demonstrate delayed olfactory event-related potentials. *Neurobiol Aging.* 2001;22(3):439–47.

117. Paulsen JS, Langbehn DR, Stout JC, et al. Detection of Huntington's disease decades before diagnosis: the predict-HD study. *J Neurol Neurosurg Psychiat.* 2008;79: 874–80.

118. Fujishiro H, Frigerio R, Burnett M et al. Cardiac sympathetic denervation correlates with clinical and pathologic stages of Parkinson's disease. *Mov Disord.* 2008;23(8):1085–92.

119. Stiasny-Kolster K, Doerr Y, Moller JC et al. Combination of 'idiopathic' REM sleep behaviour disorder and olfactory dysfunction as possible indicator for alpha-synucleinopathy demonstrated by dopamine transporter FP-CIT-SPECT. *Brain.* 2005;128:126–37.

120. Iranzo A, Molinuevo J, Santamaria J et al. REM sleep behaviour disorder as an early marker for a neurodegenerative disease. *J Sleep Res.* 2006;15:213.

121. Boeve B, Silber MH, Parisi JE et al. Synucleinopathy pathology and REM sleep behavior disorder plus dementia or parkinsonism. *Neurology.* 2003;61(1): 40–5.

122. Killgore WD, McBride SA. Odor identification accuracy declines following 24 h of sleep deprivation. *J Sleep Res.* 2006;15(2):111–6.

123. Hawkes CH. The prodromal phase of sporadic Parkinson's disease: Does it exist and if so how long is it? *Movement Dis.* 2008;23(1):994.

124. Doty RL. The olfactory vector hypothesis of neurodegenerative disease: Is it viable? *Ann Neurol.* 2008;63:7–15.

125. Calderón-Garcidueñas L, Franco-Lira M, Henríquez-Roldán C, Osnaya N et al. Urban air pollution: influences on olfactory function and pathology in exposed children and young adults. *Exp Toxicol Pathol.* 2010;62(1):91–102.

126. Monath TP, Croop CB, Harrison AK. Mode of entry of a neurotropic virus into the central nervous system: Reinvestigation of an old controversy. *Lab Invest.* 1983;48:399–410.

127. Gillner M, Brittebo EB, Brandt I, Soderkvist P, Appelgren LE, Gustafsson JA. Uptake and specific binding of 2,3,7,8-tetrachlorodibenzo-p-dioxin in the olfactory mucosa of mice and rats. *Cancer Res.* 1987;47(15):4150–9.

Chapter 5A

Lesions Associated with Autonomic Dysfunction: Swallowing Disorders and Drooling

Maria G. Cersosimo and Eduardo E. Benarroch

Overview

Swallowing is a stereotyped and complex sequential motor act that includes an oropharyngeal stage and a subsequent esophageal stage. Swallowing is controlled by a medullary central pattern generator that includes the nucleus of the solitary tract and ventromedullary reticular formation, and several effector nuclei, including the nucleus ambiguus (NAmb) and dorsal motor nucleus of the vagus (DMV), which control the muscles involved in the pharyngeal and esophageal phases. Swallowing is frequently affected in Parkinson disease (PD). Whereas the DMV is affected in early stages of PD, the other components of the medullary central pattern generator for swallowing are relatively spared. On the other hand, the pedunculopontine tegmental nucleus (PPT), which may modulate the medullary swallowing central pattern generator, is affected in PD. Although drooling is a common complaint in PD, salivary production is reduced in these patients and improves with dopamine therapy. This chapter summarizes current concepts on the neural control of swallowing and salivary production and potential clinicopathological correlations of dysphagia and salivation difficulties in PD.

Introduction

Excessive drooling and dysphagia are important manifestations of PD.[1-6] Drooling is a consequence of dysphagia and reflects impaired control of the central pattern generator network for swallowing, located in the medulla.[7] The output of this central pattern generator originates primarily from the nucleus ambiguus (NAmb), which controls the striate muscles of the pharynx and upper esophagus; and the dorsal motor nucleus of the vagus (DMV), which controls the intrinsic neurons of the myenteric plexus controlling the motility of the esophageal smooth muscle. Whereas the myenteric neurons and the DMV are affected in the early stages of PD, there is relative sparing of the NAmb, which suggests that abnormalities in the oral and pharyngeal phases of swallowing reflect supramedullary control of the swallowing pattern generator network.

Neural Control of Swallowing

Medullary Pattern Generator and its Effectors
Swallowing is a complex and sequential motor act that is initiated and coordinated by a motor pattern generator located in the medulla.[7] The interneurons of this central pattern generator are located in the nucleus of the solitary tract (NTS), adjacent reticular formation, and the reticular formation of the ventrolateral medulla located just above the NAmb. Neurons in the NTS (dorsal swallowing group) receive inputs from the pharynx and esophagus and organize the sequential motor pattern for swallowing. The neurons in the ventrolateral medulla (ventral swallowing group) may coordinate and distribute the drive generated in the NTS to the various pools of effector nuclei.[7] Swallowing includes an oropharyngeal stage and a subsequent esophageal stage. All the muscles involved in the oropharyngeal phase are striate and driven by several pools of motoneurons (Figure 5A-1). The main motor nuclei involved are the hypoglossal nucleus, which innervates the tongue muscles; and the NAmb, which innervates the pharynx, larynx, and upper esophagus. The motor neurons of the NAmb are organized topographically. Those innervating the esophagus are located in the most rostral portion of the NAmb, followed by those innervating the pharynx, and finally those innervating the larynx, which occupy the most caudal portion of the nucleus.[8]

The esophageal phase is controlled by the vagus nerve. The striate muscle of the upper esophagus receives vagal inputs from neurons of the NAmb, whereas the smooth muscle of the rest of the esophagus is controlled by the DMV. The DMV provides preganglionic parasympathetic

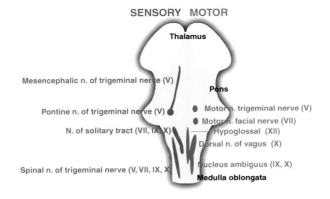

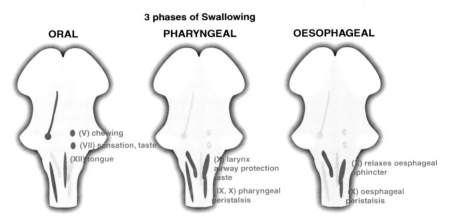

Figure 5A-1. Sensory and motor cranial nerve nuclei involved in swallowing mechanisms.

input to the myenteric neurons controlling the motility of the smooth muscle of the esophagus. All vagal efferents utilize acetylcholine (ACh) as their primary neurotransmitter. The DMV gives rise to excitatory and inhibitory pathways that control visceral smooth muscles via different subtypes of myenteric neurons. The vagal excitatory pathway is mediated by myenteric neurons that primarily utilize ACh as well as substance P and elicit smooth muscle contraction; the inhibitory pathway involves myenteric neurons that primarily utilize nitric oxide (NO) and vasoactive intestinal polypeptide (VIP).[9]

Sequential Motor Activation During Swallowing

Normal swallowing depends on a complex, sequential and coordinated activation of oropharyngeal and esophageal muscles.[7] Some muscles, called obligate muscles, always participate in the fundamental stereotyped sequence of excitatory and inhibitory events that characterize the oropharyngeal stage of swallowing. The coordinated activation of several muscles, including primarily those innervated by the hypoglossal nerve, invariably initiates the act of swallowing. The sequence continues with a pattern of excitation and inhibition involving the pharyngeal and laryngeal muscles innervated by the NAmb. The oropharyngeal phase ends when the wave of contraction reaches the upper esophageal sphincter. There is a tonic excitatory input from neurons of the NAmb to the cricopharyngeal and inferior pharyngeal constrictor muscles that is responsible for the basal closure of the upper esophageal sphincter. Inhibition of the tonic contraction of the cricopharyngeal muscle starts at the onset of swallowing and lasts until this muscle becomes active again and propels the bolus into the esophagus. Opening of this sphincter during swallowing requires central inhibition of these NAmb neurons and stimulation of NAmb neurons innervating the suprahyoid muscles. Sequential activation of NAmb motor neurons under the control of the central subnucleus of the NTS initiates peristalsis of the striated muscle portion of the esophagus. The duration of the whole oropharyngeal sequence is in the range of 0.6 to 1 s.[7]

The esophageal phase of swallowing is relatively simple and consists of a wave of contraction that propagates down the esophagus at a speed of 2 to 4 cm/s. The esophageal phase ends when the wave of contraction reaches the lower esophageal sphincter and propels the bolus to the stomach. Peristalsis of the esophageal smooth muscle is controlled by extrinsic and intrinsic reflexes. Primary peristalsis is the consequence of a vago-vagal reflex that involves inputs to the NTS and outputs from the preganglionic neurons of the DMV. The intrinsic esophageal peristalsis, called secondary peristalsis, involves local reflexes mediated by myenteric neurons.[9]

Peripheral and Central Inputs to the Medullary Swallowing Pattern Generator

Peripheral sensory inputs have an essential role in inducing the swallowing motor sequence. Although the afferents involved in the initiation of swallowing are in the trigeminal, glossopharyngeal, and vagal nerves, the only afferent input that specifically triggers the whole motor sequence arises from the superior laryngeal branch of the vagus nerve that provides input to the NTS. The swallowing interneurons of the NTS and ventrolateral medulla and the motoneurons in the NAmb, DMV, and other nuclei involved in swallowing also participate in many other types of motor behavior, including elementary reflexes and more complex patterns such as mastication, respiration, vocalization, or vomiting.[7]

The supramedullary control of swallowing depends on descending cortical and subcortical inputs to the medullary pattern generator. There is activation of several premotor, motor, and associative areas of the cerebral cortex,[10–12] basal ganglia, and cerebellum[13] during swallowing. The pedunculopontine tegmental nucleus (PPT) consists of cholinergic and glutamatergic neurons that receive inputs from the cerebral cortex, have reciprocal connections with the basal ganglia, and project to the lower brainstem and spinal cord. The PPT is thought to be involved in initiation, timing, and modulation of stereotyped sequential motor automatisms such as locomotion.[14]

Motility of the Lower Esophagus

The lower esophageal sphincter (LES) consists of tonically active smooth muscles with intrinsic myogenic properties that keep the sphincter closed in basal conditions. Both the vagal excitatory and the vagal inhibitory pathway from the DMV exert a tonic influence on the LES and are selectively activated in several motor reflexes involving the LES. For example, selective activation of the inhibitory pathway is critical for reflex relaxation of the LES associated with swallowing.[9]

Dysphagia and Drooling in PD

Dysphagia

Dysphagia is common in PD and typically occurs at late stages of disease and correlates with motor disability.[15,1,2,16] This is unlike the cases of multiple system atrophy (MSA) and progressive supranuclear palsy (PSP), where dysphagia may be prominent and early manifestation.[16] Swallowing dysfunction may be symptomatic in up to 50% of PD patients but videofluoroscopy may detect abnormalities in more than 90% of cases.[15,1] In PD, impairment of oral, pharyngeal, and esophageal phases of deglutition may occur in isolation or in various combinations.[17–21] Abnormalities found during the oral phase include poor bolus formation and lingual festination or repetitive tongue elevation. During the pharyngeal phase there may be delay of the swallow reflex, slowing of pharyngeal transit and pooling in the valleculae and pyriform sinuses. Abnormalities in the esophageal phase include incomplete relaxation of the upper esophageal sphincter, abnormal esophageal peristalsis, and gastroesophageal reflux.[17–22] All these factors increase the risk of laryngeal penetration and aspiration in PD patients. A recent electrophysiological study[23]showed that the most typical abnormalities found in PD were prolongation of the interval between electromyographic (EMG) activity of suprahyoid/submental muscles and onset of laryngeal-pharyngeal mechanogram and prolongation of the swallowing reaction time.[23]

Dopaminergic stimulation produces a variable degree of improvement of swallowing dysfunction in PD.[22] Subthalamic nucleus stimulation improves the timing and muscle excursion for some aspects of the pharyngeal phase without affecting the oral phase of swallowing in PD.[24] Thus, like gait disturbances and other late manifestations of PD, dysphagia cannot be solely explained by the loss of the dopaminergic input to the basal ganglia but likely reflects involvement of other central neurochemical systems and long-term changes in the function of the medullary central pattern generators.

Esophageal dysmotility also occurs frequently in PD.[1,25–27] Manifestations include slowed esophageal transit, aperistalsis, and reduced pressure of the LES, segmental esophageal spasm, and achalasia.

Drooling

Sialorrhea is prevalent in patients with PD.[28,1] Eadie and Tirer[28] reported that 78% of parkinsonian patients experienced increased saliva in the mouth and drooling. Sialorrhea in PD does not result from excess saliva production but from a combination of infrequent or impaired swallowing. Drooling is present in 86% of PD subjects with dysphagia, but only 44% of subjects without dysphagia.

Salivary production is reduced in PD in the "off" and "on" conditions.[29] Levodopa increases both basal and reflex activated salivary flow rate, even in PD patients pretreated with the peripheral D2 antagonist domperidone.[31] The assessment and therapeutic approaches to sialorrhea in PD have been recently reviewed.[32] Two anticholinergic agents, sublingual atropine and ipratropium bromide, have been investigated as a treatment for drooling in parkinsonian patients. Clonidine, an alpha-2 receptor agonist, improved sialorrhea in a small double-blind placebo-controlled trial, and there have also been several trials of botulinum toxin for the treatment of sialorrhea in PD.[32] Overall, botulinum toxin appears to be a well-tolerated treatment for sialorrhea in PD. However, more studies are needed to establish the optimal injection technique, doses, and botulinum toxin serotype that is most effective.

Pathological Basis

Oropharyngeal Dysphagia

Impairment of the oral and pharyngeal phases of swallowing in PD reflects impaired function of the medullary pattern generator network. In PD there

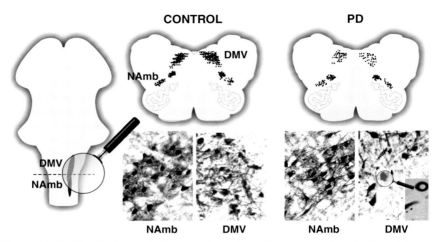

Figure 5A-2. Distribution of choline-acetyltransferase immunoreactive (cholinergic) neurons in the nucleus ambiguus (NAmb) and dorsal motor nucleus of the vagus (DMV) in a control and in a patient with Parkinson's disease (PD). Note the loss of neurons and accumulation of Lewy bodies (insert) in the DMV and preservation of neurons in the compact portion of the NAmb in PD.

is sparing of the motor neurons of the NAmb innervating the pharynx and upper esophagus[33–35] (Figure 5A-2). It has been hypothesized that dysphagia in parkinsonian syndromes may reflect involvement of the PPT as it may have an important role in modulating the activity of the medullary swallowing pattern generator. The PPT provides cholinergic inputs to the NTS, a critical component of the medullary pattern generator. The PPT is affected in PD[14,33,34] as well as in other parkinsonian syndromes where dysphagia is a prominent manifestation, such as PSP[36] and MSA.[37]

Esophageal Dysmotility

Esophageal dysmotility in PD reflects involvement of both the DMV and the myenteric plexus of the esophagus. These areas are affected at early stages of the disease.[38,39] In PD, there is accumulation of alpha-synuclein immunoreactive Lewy bodies and Lewy neurites as well as neuronal loss in the DMV[34,40,35] (Figure 5A-1). There is also prominent Lewy body pathology in both the Auerbach and Meissner plexuses along the entire gastrointestinal tract, particularly in neurons of the Auerbach plexus in the lower esophagus.[39,41] In a series of 98 post mortem cases with no history of PD-associated symptoms, alpha-synuclein pathology was found in the peripheral autonomic nervous system, including the myenteric plexus of esophagus, in 17.3% of cases.[42] This study indicates that the peripheral autonomic nuclei are among the earliest regions affected by Lewy body pathology. Braak et al proposed that enteric nervous system neurons may provide the first pathogenic link in Lewy body pathology,[43] leading to involvement of the DMV at the earliest stage of disease. According to this intriguing, but yet unproven hypothesis, a putative environmental neurotoxin capable of passing the gut epithelium might induce alpha-synuclein misfolding and aggregation in enteric neurons and, via retrograde axonal transport, involve the DMV.[43]

The abundant Lewy body pathology and loss of DMV neurons in PD (Figure 5A-1) may have a prominent consequence in the control of motility of the esophagus and stomach in PD. Slowed esophageal transit, aperistalsis, and reduced pressure of the LES may reflect impairment of the vagal motor excitatory pathway, whereas segmental esophageal spasm and achalasia may reflect impairment of the vagal inhibitory pathway. For example, achalasia may be associated with Lewy bodies in the esophageal myenteric plexus [44] and may result from loss of NO neurons.[45]

Decreased Salivary Production

Reduction of salivary production in PD may reflect involvement of brainstem salivatory nuclei, cranial autonomic ganglia, or both, but the exact mechanism remains to be elucidated. The output for salivation involves preganglionic neurons in the salivatory nucleus at the level of the pons, which are cholinergic and express markers for NO synthesis.[46] These neurons, like those of the DMV, form part of the general visceral efferent column of the brainstem and send unmyelinated axons that innervate the submaxillary, submandibular, and otic ganglia. Whereas there is evidence of Lewy body pathology in peripheral autonomic ganglia in PD, involvement of these cranial parasympathetic ganglia, to our knowledge, has not been established. The fact that dopamine stimulates salivation in PD patients even in the presence of peripheral D^2 receptor blockade with domperidone[31] suggests that involvement of this system at the level of the basal ganglia or brainstem circuit may contribute to the reduced salivation in these patients.

Conclusions

Dysphagia is a prominent manifestation of PD and its pathophysiology is multifactorial. Impaired modulation of the medullary swallowing pattern generator, by both dopaminergic and non-dopaminergic mechanisms, affects the oropharyngeal phase of swallowing despite preservation of the motor neurons of the NAmb innervating the pharynx and upper esophagus. An important consequence of oropharyngeal dysphagia is drooling, which may be a disabling symptom in PD. Impaired esophageal peristalsis reflects loss of vagal preganglionic neurons in the DMV and myenteric neurons in the esophagus, which are prominently affected by Lewy body pathology at early stages of disease. Careful clinico-pathological correlations and physiological studies will likely provide further insights into the basic mechanism of dysphagia and impaired salivation in PD; well-designed, large, controlled clinical trials are necessary to better define the appropriate treatment of these disorders.

References

1. Edwards LL, Quigley EM, Pfeiffer RF. Gastrointestinal dysfunction in Parkinson's disease: frequency and pathophysiology. *Neurology*. Apr 1992;42(4):726–732.
2. Pfeiffer RF. Gastrointestinal dysfunction in Parkinson's disease. *Lancet Neurol*. Feb 2003;2(2):107–116.
3. Dubow JS. Autonomic dysfunction in Parkinson's disease. *Dis Mon*. May 2007;53(5):265–274.
4. Chaudhuri KR, Healy DG, Schapira AH. Non-motor symptoms of Parkinson's disease: diagnosis and management. *Lancet Neurol*. Mar 2006;5(3):235–245.
5. Jost WH. Gastrointestinal motility problems in patients with Parkinson's disease. Effects of antiparkinsonian treatment and guidelines for management. *Drugs Aging*. Apr 1997;10(4):249–258.
6. Verbaan D, Marinus J, Visser M, van Rooden SM, Stiggelbout AM, van Hilten JJ. Patient-reported autonomic symptoms in Parkinson disease. *Neurology*. Jul 24 2007;69(4):333–341.
7. Jean A. Brainstem control of swallowing: neuronal network and cellular mechanisms. *Physiol Rev*. Apr 2001;81(2):929–969.
8. Hopkins DA, Bieger D, deVente J, Steinbusch WM. Vagal efferent projections: viscerotopy, neurochemistry and effects of vagotomy. *Prog Brain Res*. 1996;107:79–96.
9. Chang HY, Mashimo H, Goyal RK. Musings on the wanderer: what's new in our understanding of vago-vagal reflex? IV. Current concepts of vagal efferent projections to the gut. *Am J Physiol Gastrointest Liver Physiol*. Mar 2003;284(3):G357–366.
10. Harris ML, Julyan P, Kulkarni B, et al. Mapping metabolic brain activation during human volitional swallowing: a positron emission tomography study using [18F]fluorodeoxyglucose. *J Cereb Blood Flow Metab*. Apr 2005;25(4):520–526.
11. Martin RE, MacIntosh BJ, Smith RC, et al. Cerebral areas processing swallowing and tongue movement are overlapping but distinct: a functional magnetic resonance imaging study. *J Neurophysiol*. Oct 2004;92(4):2428–2443.
12. Watanabe Y, Abe S, Ishikawa T, Yamada Y, Yamane GY. Cortical regulation during the early stage of initiation of voluntary swallowing in humans. *Dysphagia*. Spring 2004;19(2):100–108.
13. Suzuki M, Asada Y, Ito J, Hayashi K, Inoue H, Kitano H. Activation of cerebellum and basal ganglia on volitional swallowing detected by functional magnetic resonance imaging. *Dysphagia*. Spring 2003;18(2):71–77.

14. Pahapill PA, Lozano AM. The pedunculopontine nucleus and Parkinson's disease. *Brain*. Sep 2000;123 (Pt 9):1767–1783.

15. Bushmann M, Dobmeyer SM, Leeker L, Perlmutter JS. Swallowing abnormalities and their response to treatment in Parkinson's disease. *Neurology*. Oct 1989;39(10): 1309–1314.

16. Muller J, Wenning GK, Verny M, et al. Progression of dysarthria and dysphagia in postmortem-confirmed parkinsonian disorders. *Arch Neurol*. Feb 2001;58(2): 259–264.

17. Ali GN, Wallace KL, Schwartz R, DeCarle DJ, Zagami AS, Cook IJ. Mechanisms of oral-pharyngeal dysphagia in patients with Parkinson's disease. *Gastroenterology*. Feb 1996;110(2):383–392.

18. Born LJ, Harned RH, Rikkers LF, Pfeiffer RF, Quigley EM. Cricopharyngeal dysfunction in Parkinson's disease: role in dysphagia and response to myotomy. *Mov Disord*. Jan 1996;11(1):53–58.

19. Ertekin C, Tarlaci S, Aydogdu I, et al. Electrophysiological evaluation of pharyngeal phase of swallowing in patients with Parkinson's disease. *Mov Disord*. Sep 2002;17(5):942–949.

20. Nilsson H, Ekberg O, Olsson R, Hindfelt B. Quantitative assessment of oral and pharyngeal function in Parkinson's disease. *Dysphagia*. Spring 1996;11(2):144–150.

21. Potulska A, Friedman A, Krolicki L, Spychala A. Swallowing disorders in Parkinson's disease. *Parkinsonism Relat Disord*. Aug 2003;9(6):349–353.

22. Hunter PC, Crameri J, Austin S, Woodward MC, Hughes AJ. Response of parkinsonian swallowing dysfunction to dopaminergic stimulation. *J Neurol Neurosurg Psychiatry*. Nov 1997;63(5):579–583.

23. Alfonsi E, Versino M, Merlo IM, et al. Electrophysiologic patterns of oral-pharyngeal swallowing in parkinsonian syndromes. *Neurology*. Feb 20 2007;68(8):583–589.

24. Ciucci MR, Barkmeier-Kraemer JM, Sherman SJ. Subthalamic nucleus deep brain stimulation improves deglutition in Parkinson's disease. *Mov Disord*. Dec 28 2007.

25. Lin WY, Kao CH, Wang SJ, et al. Radionuclide esophageal transit test in the detection of esophageal dysmotility in Parkinson's disease. *Gaoxiong Yi Xue Ke Xue Za Zhi*. Aug 1994;10(8):438–443.

26. Leopold NA, Kagel MC. Pharyngo-esophageal dysphagia in Parkinson's disease. *Dysphagia*. Winter 1997;12(1):11–18; discussion 19–20.

27. Castell JA, Johnston BT, Colcher A, Li Q, Gideon RM, Castell DO. Manometric abnormalities of the oesophagus in patients with Parkinson's disease. *Neurogastroenterol Motil*. Aug 2001;13(4):361–364.

28. Eadie MJ, Tyrer JH. Alimentary disorder in parkinsonism. *Australas Ann Med*. Feb 1965;14:13–22.

29. Cersosimo MG, Tumilasci OR, Raina GB, et al. Hyposialorrhea as an early manifestation of Parkinson disease. *Auton Neurosci*. May 4 2009.

30. Proulx M, de Courval FP, Wiseman MA, Panisset M. Salivary production in Parkinson's disease. *Mov Disord*. Feb 2005;20(2):204–207.

31. Tumilasci OR, Cersosimo MG, Belforte JE, Micheli FE, Benarroch EE, Pazo JH. Quantitative study of salivary secretion in Parkinson's disease. *Mov Disord*. May 2006;21(5):660–667.

32. Chou KL, Evatt M, Hinson V, Kompoliti K. Sialorrhea in Parkinson's disease: a review. *Mov Disord.* Dec 2007;22(16):2306–2313.

33. Jellinger KA. Pathology of Parkinson's disease. Changes other than the nigrostriatal pathway. *Mol Chem Neuropathol.* Jun 1991;14(3):153–197.

34. Braak E, Sandmann-Keil D, Rub U, et al. alpha-synuclein immunopositive Parkinson's disease-related inclusion bodies in lower brain stem nuclei. *Acta Neuropathologica.* 2001;101(3):195–201.

35. Benarroch EE, Schmeichel AM, Sandroni P, Low PA, Parisi JE. Involvement of vagal autonomic nuclei in multiple system atrophy and Lewy body disease. *Neurology.* Feb 14 2006;66(3):378–383.

36. Warren NM, Piggott MA, Perry EK, Burn DJ. Cholinergic systems in progressive supranuclear palsy. *Brain.* Feb 2005;128(Pt 2):239–249.

37. Schmeichel AM, Buchhalter LC, Low PA, et al. Mesopontine cholinergic neuron involvement in Lewy body dementia and multiple system atrophy. *Neurology.* Jan 29 2008;70(5):368–373.

38. Wakabayashi K, Takahashi H. Neuropathology of autonomic nervous system in Parkinson's disease. *Eur Neurol.* 1997;38 Suppl 2:2–7.

39. Braak H, Del Tredici K. Invited Article: Nervous system pathology in sporadic Parkinson disease. *Neurology.* May 13 2008;70(20):1916–1925.

40. Gai WP, Blumbergs PC, Geffen LB, Blessing WW. Age-related loss of dorsal vagal neurons in Parkinson's disease. *Neurology.* Nov 1992;42(11):2106–2111.

41. Wakabayashi K, Takahashi H, Ohama E, Takeda S, Ikuta F. Lewy bodies in the visceral autonomic nervous system in Parkinson's disease. *Adv Neurol.* 1993;60: 609–612.

42. Bloch A, Probst A, Bissig H, Adams H, Tolnay M. Alpha-synuclein pathology of the spinal and peripheral autonomic nervous system in neurologically unimpaired elderly subjects. *Neuropathol Appl Neurobiol.* Jun 2006;32(3):284–295.

43. Braak H, Bohl JR, Muller CM, Rub U, de Vos RA, Del Tredici K. Stanley Fahn Lecture 2005: The staging procedure for the inclusion body pathology associated with sporadic Parkinson's disease reconsidered. *Mov Disord.* Dec 2006;21(12):2042–2051.

44. Qualman SJ, Haupt HM, Yang P, Hamilton SR. Esophageal Lewy bodies associated with ganglion cell loss in achalasia. Similarity to Parkinson's disease. *Gastroenterology.* Oct 1984;87(4):848–856.

45. Takahashi T. Pathophysiological significance of neuronal nitric oxide synthase in the gastrointestinal tract. *J Gastroenterol.* 2003;38(5):421–430.

46. Gai WP, Blessing WW. Human brainstem preganglionic parasympathetic neurons localized by markers for nitric oxide synthesis. *Brain.* Aug 1996;119 (Pt 4):1145–1152.

Chapter 5B

Lesions Associated with Autonomic Dysfunction: Gastrointestinal Disorders

Adolfo Mínguez-Castellanos and Dominic B. Rowe

The bowels, which had been all along torpid, now in most cases, demand stimulating medicines of very considerable power: the expulsion of the faeces from the rectum sometimes requiring mechanical aid...

—(Parkinson 1817)

Introduction

Gastrointestinal dysfunction, mainly constipation, is an almost universal manifestation of Parkinson's disease (PD), referred to by some pundits as the original 'movement disorder'. Although recognized by James Parkinson in his monograph,[1] it has become a subject of growing interest in recent years. Gastrointestinal symptoms have a major impact on daily activities and require proper evaluation and treatment. Furthermore, gastrointestinal dysfunction appears to develop at an early stage of the disease process, sometimes many years before onset of the classical motor features, which may have potential implications for the pathogenesis and early diagnosis of PD. We will review the major gastrointestinal clinical manifestations of constipation, gastroparesis and weight loss. The related pathological findings of these conditions and their therapeutic options will be discussed in detail. Other gastrointestinal problems that occur in PD will be considered in passing.

Definitions

While constipation, gastroparesis, and weight loss are common in PD, definitions of each of these are sometimes problematic for both the patient with PD and the clinician. Constipation can be defined as unsatisfactory defecation with infrequent stool, difficult defecation, or both.[2] Diagnostic criteria for constipation according to the Rome III consensus includes 2 or more of the following symptoms: straining, lumpy or hard stools, sensation of anorectal obstruction, manual maneuvers to assist defecation more than 25% of the time, and fewer than 3 unassisted defecations per week. The symptoms need to be present for more than 3 days a month, with onset at least 6 months previously.[3] Gastroparesis, or delayed emptying of the stomach, is even more difficult to define symptomatically, as it can give rise to a plethora of symptoms including postprandial fullness, bloating, abdominal distension, nausea, and vomiting, all of which can also be attributed to many other problems. Unintended weight loss is a common manifestation of all neurodegenerative diseases and is very common in PD, recently the subject of a comprehensive review.[4] Measurement of weight and calculation of the body mass index (BMI) is part of the assessment of the patient with PD to detect unintended weight loss. A BMI of $<20kg/m^2$, or unintentional weight loss of greater than 5% in 3 months is significant in the clinical management of PD. Weight loss results from an imbalance between caloric intake and expenditure, and there are many factors that influence both sides of this equation in PD.

Clinical Features

Constipation and other disturbances of defecation are very common problems in PD, perhaps occurring in more than 50% of all PD patients,[5-8] and the subject of a recent review.[9] The exact extent of constipation in PD is difficult to determine for several reasons, including the definition of constipation and the high prevalence of constipation in the elderly due to diet, exercise, and age-related degeneration of the enteric nervous system,[10] among many other factors. Compared to age- and sex-matched controls, constipation is more common in patients with PD.[5,8,11] Constipation is associated with future risk of PD[12] and with incidental Lewy bodies in the locus coeruleus or substantia nigra,[13] and is considered one of the major manifestations of the pre-motor phase of PD.[8] Abbott et al reported a prospective study which followed the bowel habits of nearly 7000 men for 24 years and reported that those with initial constipation (<1 bowel movement/day) had a threefold risk of developing PD after a mean interval of

10 years from initial constipation.[12] Constipation can be present early in the course of PD, and patients with PD can present to a general physician or gastroenterologist with constipation before the diagnosis of PD is made, especially in the absence of tremor. Constipation is more common in advanced PD, although no studies exist to predict the severity of constipation in PD. Disturbances of defecation, incontinence, and diarrhea are also described in PD, more common in patients in later stages of PD.[5,14,15] An uncommon enteric manifestation of PD is intestinal pseudo-obstruction, presenting with abdominal bloating, pain, nausea, and/or vomiting,[14] which can uncommonly lead to volvulus and death.[16] The objective measurement of constipation is usually by survey, but also by the measurement of the colonic transit time (CTT) via several methods.[17] Slow colonic transport is the most common cause for decreased stool frequency in PD. CTT is prolonged beyond the normal threshold in >80% of patients with PD, and is also significantly prolonged in de novo PD patients,[18] however PD patients with prolonged CTT need not necessarily have subjective symptoms of constipation.[19]

Anorectal dysfunction also occurs in PD, leading to urgency, tenesmus, diarrhea, and fecal incontinence. These disturbances severely disrupt the life of patients with PD, and in later stages lead to a significant impairment in the quality of life.[20] Mathers et al described two small series of patients with severe anorectal dysfunction in PD.[21,22] The dysfunction was so severe that it produced obstruction at the pelvic outlet (anismus) due to paradoxical contraction of the striated muscles of the anal sphincter during defecation. This paradoxical contraction was postulated to be a form of focal dystonia that responded to dopamine agonist therapy. Anorectal manometry, video-manometry and electromyography are among some of the methods used in the assessment of anorectal dysfunction in PD,[14,18,22,23] although these methods are uncommonly used in routine clinical practice.

The clinical features of gastroparesis in PD are variable and include bloating or abdominal discomfort or distention, early satiety, nausea, and weight loss. Edwards and co-workers reported nausea in 24% of PD patients, with 45% reporting a sense of bloating or abdominal distension.[5] A significant number of PD patients in this survey were not taking dopamine replacement therapy, concordant with involvement of the upper gastrointestinal tract early in the course of PD, perhaps in the premotor phase of PD. Although there are only a few studies on the objective measurement of gastroparesis in PD, it appears that symptoms of upper gastrointestinal dysfunction do not correlate with objective measures of gastroparesis.[24] This cross-sectional study in a group of PD patients with mild to moderate disease severity evaluated predictors of delayed gastric emptying of both solids and liquids in patients with PD. In comparison with a control group, the study demonstrated delayed gastric emptying in 88% of PD patients for solids, consistent with prior studies[25,26] and only 38% of PD patients for liquids. The only predictor of delayed gastric emptying was motor impairment as assessed by UPDRS, with no correlation with symptoms, demographic feature, or PD medication. However, gastroparesis can have repercussions for the absorption of oral medication, nutritional status, as well as producing pseudo-obstruction that in PD can uncommonly lead to death.[27]

Body weight in PD is the subject of a recent comprehensive review.[4] Essentially, the decreased body weight that is observed in patients with PD is due to an imbalance between energy expenditure and energy intake. There are many factors involved in this complicated equation including nausea, reduced appetite, anosmia, altered taste, dysphagia, early satiety, altered absorption, and increased energy expenditure from a plethora of causes including neuroendocrine dysregulation. It is noteworthy that midlife adiposity is associated with an increased risk of developing PD later in life[28]; however, other studies refute this finding.[29] Several studies have shown that PD patients have lower body weight than controls,[30–32] although the reasons are probably multifactorial. The assessment of body weight in the clinic is a necessary part of the routine review of the patient with PD. Over time, clinically significant weight loss of >5% of baseline occurs in more than 50% of patients with PD,[33] with worsening of parkinsonism (as assessed by the motor UPDRS) the strongest predictor of weight loss, as well as older age, female gender, the presence of visual illusions/hallucinations, and cognitive impairment. Dyskinesia is commonly associated with weight loss although the literature is divided on whether dyskinesia is cause or effect.[34–37]

Pathology and Pathophysiology

Neural Control of Gastrointestinal Function and Body Weight

Gastrointestinal motility and secretion rely on the intrinsic enteric nervous system (ENS), which is modulated by extrinsic parasympathetic and sympathetic inputs (Figure 5B-1).[38]

In brief, the ENS is a complex structure derived from the neural crest and consists of two ganglionated plexuses supported by glial cells within the walls of the digestive tract: the myenteric plexus (of Auerbach) and the submucosal plexus (of Meissner) (Figure 5B-1). Mechanical or chemical stimuli in the gut activate intrinsic primary afferent neurons that trigger local reflexes mediating peristalsis and secretion. Although most enteric neurons

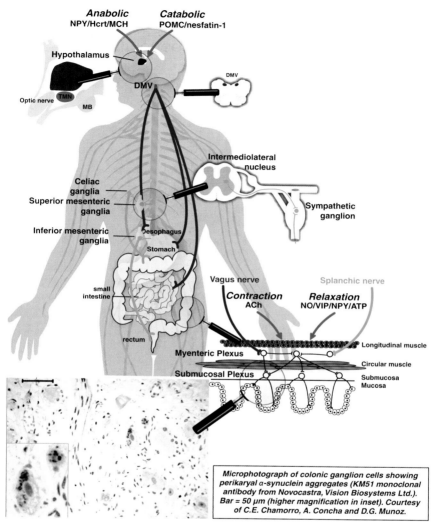

Figure 5B-1. Diagram of regions involved in the regulation of gut motility and function. The tuberal region (TMN) of the hypothalamus plays an important role in the neuroendocrine regulation of energy intake and expenditure. Parasympathetic regulation of the gut is largely via the dorsal motor nucleus of the vagus nerve (DMV) as well as the sacral parasympathetic neurons through peripheral ganglia relays. Sympathetic regulation of the gut is through the intermediolateral cell column of the spinal cord and paravertebral ganglia which give rise to the splanchnic nerves. All of these pathways impact on the enteric nervous system (myenteric and submucosal nerve plexuses) found within the gut wall that mediate gut motility and secretions. Photomicrograph of α-synuclein pathology found within the colonic ganglia of 1 of 3 out of 56 older patients undergoing colonic surgery who had yet to develop PD.

are cholinergic, chemical signaling is complex and includes other neurotransmitters such as vasoactive intestinal peptide (VIP), nitric oxide, and substance P, among others (Figure 5B-1). There is also a small proportion of intrinsic dopaminergic and serotonergic neurons.[39] Parasympathetic modulatory efferents, which promote gastrointestinal motility and secretion, originate in the dorsal motor nucleus of the vagus nerve (DMV) (supplying cholinergic neurons of ganglia adjacent to the esophagus, stomach, small intestine and proximal colon) (Figure 5B-1), and in the sacral parasympathetic nucleus (supplying ganglia close to the distal colon and rectum). On the other hand, motility-inhibitory sympathetic efferents that originate in the intermediolateral nucleus of the spinal cord supply, via the splanchnic nerves, catecholaminergic neurons in the prevertebral sympathetic ganglia (celiac, superior, and inferior mesenteric ganglia), innervating the upper, medium, and lower segments of the gut, respectively (Figure 5B-1).

Maintenance of body weight depends on energy intake (food intake and absorption) and expenditure (metabolism and physical activity) and is regulated by multiple factors with highly complex interactions. Neuroendocrine control of food intake comprises central and peripheral mechanisms (the latter include signals from the digestive system and adipose tissue) integrated in the hypothalamus, acting as a link between the nervous and endocrine systems. The tuberal hypothalamic area regulates feeding behavior and metabolism through the production of neuropeptides with anabolic (e.g., neuropeptide Y, hypocretin/orexin, or melanin-concentrating hormone) or catabolic effects (e.g., pro-opiomelanocortin or nesfatin-1) (Figure 5B-1).[40]

Pathological Substrate in PD and Incidental Lewy Body (LB) Disease

Post-mortem studies of patients with PD have consistently shown the occurrence of neuronal loss and LBs in CNS autonomic nuclei, peripheral sympathetic ganglia, the ENS, and the hypothalamus (Table 5-1). Additionally, a high proportion of incidental LB disease autopsies (neurologically unimpaired subjects who have PD-related pathology in the brain suggestive of presymptomatic PD) also show LB pathology in central and peripheral autonomic neurons, indicating an early involvement of the autonomic nervous system in the disease process (Table 5-1).

CNS Autonomic Nuclei

In the lower brainstem, the DMV is characteristically damaged in PD. Before the era of α-synuclein immunoreactivity, several studies identified reduced numbers of neurons and abundant LBs in this autonomic nucleus, but not in medullary motor neurons such as those in the nucleus ambiguus

Table 5b-1. Main Structures Involved in the Neural Control of Gastrointestinal Function and Body Weight with Indication of the Earliest Braak's Stage at Which Parkinson's Disease-related Pathology has Been Described (see text for further details).

			Stage 1	Stage 2	Stage 3	Stage 4	Stage 5	Stage 6
Brain	Diencephalon	Hypothalamic tuberomammillary nucleus						
	Mesencephalon	Substantia nigra						
	Rhombencephalon	Dorsal motor nucleus of the vagus nerve						
		Caudal raphe nuclei						
		Medullary catecholaminergic melanoneurons						
Spinal Cord	Thoracic	Sympathetic intermediolateral nucleus						
	Sacral	Parasympathetic nucleus						
Peripheral Autonomic Nervous System	Prevertebral plexuses	Sympathetic ganglia	?					
	Digestive tract	Enteric nervous system	?					

(which supply, via the vagus nerve, the striated musculature of the larynx and upper esophagus).[41,42] Later, α-synuclein immunoreactive inclusions were repeatedly described in the soma and axons of DMV unmyelinated projection neurons that connect the brainstem with the ENS. These inclusions are one of the earliest pathologic findings within the CNS and are characteristic of Braak Stage 1 in incidental LB disease cases.[43] Caudal raphe nuclei, implicated in the supraspinal control of defecation, are damaged at Stage 2, whereas catecholaminergic melanoneurons in the dorsal vagal area and in the intermediate reticular zone (with ascending projections) become involved at Stage 3.[43]

In the spinal cord, PD-related lesions are observable in several regions of the thoracic, lumbar, and sacral segments. The number of neurons in the sympathetic intermediolateral nucleus of the thoracic spinal cord was found to be reduced by up to 69% in PD patients versus controls, with occasional LBs in the remaining cells.[44] In the sacral segment of the spinal cord, LBs are consistently found in the parasympathetic nucleus, notably in the dorsal group of neurons innervating the internal anal sphincter.[42] Involvement of spinal cord autonomic nuclei appears to occur early in the disease process: α-synuclein pathology was detected by Bloch et al in 17 out of 17 cases of incidental LB disease staged as 2 or above (100%)[45] and by Klos et al in 9 out of 13 such cases (69%).[46]

Sympathetic Ganglia
LBs in the paravertebral and prevertebral (celiac) sympathetic ganglia were found in more than 90% of PD autopsy cases, mainly in the nerve cell processes, and in 5 out of 60 (8.3%) non-parkinsonian subjects aged over 60 yrs.[44] In the study by Bloch et al on incidental LD disease cases (stage 2 or above), 14 out of 17 (82%) showed PD-related pathology in the paravertebral chain, indicating early involvement of peripheral sympathetic neurons.[45]

Enteric Nervous System (ENS)
The presence of LBs in the ENS was first reported by Qualman et al in post-mortem studies [47] and later by Kupsky et al in the surgically-resected colon of a PD patient with acquired megacolon.[48] In 28 of 30 (93%) PD patients, Wakabayashi et al found LBs which were widely distributed in the myenteric and submucosal plexuses from the upper esophagus to the rectum, although they were more numerous in the myenteric plexus of the lower esophagus. The majority of LBs were observed in cell bodies and processes of intrinsic VIPergic neurons.[42] In the stomach, α-synuclein immunoreactive inclusions were present in the myenteric and submucosal plexuses of 3 PD patients and of 2 individuals with incidental LB disease

(Braak Stage 2 and 3).[49] Among 17 incidental LB disease cases in Braak Stage 2 or above, 14 (82%) exhibited inclusions in the esophageal myenteric plexus and only 3 (18%) in the submucosal plexus.[45] Hence, the ENS is also involved at an early stage in the disease process.

Hypothalamus

The hypothalamus is involved in PD pathology, with the tuberomammillary nucleus and lateral and posterior nuclei showing the highest LB counts.[42] Post-mortem studies staged for PD-related pathology reported involvement of the tuberomammillary nucleus from Braak stage 3.[49] Increasing loss of hypocretin/orexin and melanin-concentrating hormone cells and rising levels of glial fibrillary acidic protein throughout the hypothalamus have been associated with progression of the disease.[50]

Pathophysiology

The pathophysiological mechanisms of gastrointestinal manifestations of PD are complicated and multiple, although early degeneration of extrinsic and intrinsic autonomic innervation of the gut undoubtedly plays a pivotal role. Delayed gastric emptying appears to be largely related to the loss of vagal efferents to the stomach (DMV and cholinergic myenteric neurons), since parasympathetic influence is essential for adequate motility of the upper digestive tract.[51] Gastric emptying in PD patients is improved by domperidone, a peripherally-acting dopamine (D_2) receptor antagonist, or by 5-hydroxytryptamine ($5\text{-}HT_4$) receptor agonists such as mosapride and tegaserod, presumably by increasing local acetylcholine (ACh) release.[52] Helicobacter pylori gastroduodenitis may impair levodopa absorption in some PD patients and its eradication has been shown to improve motor fluctuations.[53]

Motility of the small bowel and colon is primarily controlled by local reflexes,[52] therefore slow intestinal transit in PD may be mainly related to degeneration of the ENS. Loss of excitatory cholinergic neurons, which also occurs in normal aging with an oral-to-anal gradient (distal tract more severely affected),[54] may result in bloating and constipation. In this regard, increasing local ACh release by $5\text{-}HT_4$ agonists improves constipation in patients with PD.[55–57] Loss of inhibitory VIPergic motor neurons of the myenteric plexus may restrict peristaltic movements by impairing the normal relaxation of distal segments.[52] A similar mechanism may come from the loss of dopaminergic myenteric neurons, which also inhibit intestinal motility,[58] although they constitute only a small proportion of the ENS.[39] These neurons are lost in PD patients [59] and in 1-methyl 4-phenyl 1,2,3,6-tetrahydropyridine (MPTP)-treated mice, who demonstrate a colonic relaxation defect.[60]

Additional factors may influence constipation in PD. In an epidemiological study, decreased water intake preceded and correlated with the
severity of constipation.[61] Many PD patients also suffer from defecatory
dysfunction due to impaired anorectal coordination.[14,21,62] The sacral defecation reflex is modulated by supraspinal mechanisms and involves reciprocal interactions between sacral parasympathetic and Onuf nucleus
neurons. In PD, paradoxical contraction of the puborectalis muscle during
attempted defecation, which prevents the normal opening of the anorectal
angle, probably results from impaired supraspinal modulatory efferences.[52]
Implication of central dopaminergic transmission seems probable since
apomorphine administration improves defecatory dysfunction,[63] although
other pathways have also been proposed, such as loss of efferents from
medullary raphe nuclei.[52]

The pathophysiology of unintended weight loss in PD is poorly understood and probably relies on multiple mechanisms. Some patients may
reduce their food intake due to impairment of olfaction and taste, depression, eating difficulties, dysphagia or side effects of medication such as
nausea and anorexia. On the other hand, energy expenditure may increase
due to severe rigidity, tremor, or dyskinesia and in relation to levodopa
treatment. However, these mechanisms do not seem to account for the
majority of cases, since weight loss appears to be a continuous process that
starts before the diagnosis and is not caused by reduced energy intake.[32]
In an epidemiological study, continuous weight loss since late adolescence
was identified as a risk factor for a diagnosis of PD later in life.[29] Although
speculative, these data suggest that weight loss may be related to the neurodegenerative process itself through early impairment of gastrointestinal
function (absorption, neuroendocrine signals) and/or CNS structures
implicated in feeding behavior and metabolism. In this regard, the loss of
hypothalamic neurons producing anabolic neuropeptides such as hypocre-
tin/orexin or melanin-concentrating hormone could play a role.[50]
Nevertheless, definitive evidence is lacking on specific absorptive or neuroendocrine dysfunction as a cause of weight loss in PD.

Early Gastrointestinal Dysfunction and the Pathogenesis of PD?

Clinical and epidemiological evidence indicates that gastrointestinal dysfunction precedes motor manifestations of PD. In a cohort study of 6,790
men with a 24-year follow-up, those with more severe constipation had at
least a 3-fold increased risk of being clinically diagnosed with PD a decade
after inclusion.[12] In an extension of this study, post-mortem examination
of the brain of 245 men without clinical PD revealed that 12% had incidental LB disease, with a higher prevalence (24%) among those with more

severe constipation.[13] These observations strongly suggest that LB pathology may affect neurons that regulate intestinal motility (largely myenteric neurons) years before the appearance of the typical extrapyramidal manifestations of PD.

Post-mortem studies of PD and incidental LB disease cases also support the early pathologic involvement of autonomic neurons controlling gastrointestinal function. Whereas clinically diagnosed PD patients are commonly assigned to Braak stages 4 to 6, PD-related pathology in the DMV is characteristic of Braak stage 1, and involvement of other central or peripheral autonomic neurons has been described as early as stage 2.[43] Hence, it is not clear from these studies whether LB pathology begins in the peripheral autonomic nervous system without prior or simultaneous involvement of the DMV. Using conventional stains, Wakabayashi et al found occasional LBs in the myenteric plexus of the esophagus or small intestine in 8 out of 24 (33%) non-parkinsonian subjects aged over 50 yrs without LBs in the CNS.[64] This finding suggests that myenteric neurons are especially vulnerable to LB formation. However, whether this is an age-related phenomenon or represents the earliest stage of an ongoing process such as PD remains to be elucidated. In this regard, new data have been obtained by means of a novel pathologic-clinical approach. Minguez-Castellanos et al found α-synuclein aggregation in abdominopelvic autonomic neurons in 9/100 (9%) of an apparently neurologically normal patient population undergoing surgical procedures.[65] Concerning gut specimens, α-synuclein aggregates were found in the perikarya of colonic ganglion cells (Figure 5B-1 micrographs) in 3 out of 56 specimens but were not detected in gastric (n = 12) or small bowel (n = 9) specimens. Follow-up of patients with α-synuclein aggregation versus controls disclosed increasing subclinical sympathetic cardiovascular dysfunction and a trend to progressive motor impairment. These results strongly suggest that, rather than being an incidental finding, α-synuclein aggregation in peripheral autonomic neurons reflects early events in the development of LB disorders.

Bearing in mind the early involvement of the ENS and the DMV and assuming a predictable caudo-rostral progression of PD pathology, Braak's group hypothesized that an environmental agent in the gut might induce the pathologic process locally and subsequently reach the DMV via retrograde axonal transport.[49] In this regard, the stomach might be the entry point since it is innervated by a disproportionately large segment of the DMV. Taking into account that all vulnerable nerve cells in PD are closely interconnected projection neurons with a long and sparingly myelinated axon, this putative pathogen (presumably prion-like or a neurotoxin) might further spread to rostral CNS structures by axonal transport and trans-synaptic transmission.

This intriguing hypothesis is supported by the demonstration of a stomach-DMV pathogenic connection in rats, since intragastric injections of a selective proteasome inhibitor induced α-synuclein inclusions and activated microglia in the DMV; however, the procedure was insufficient to cause cell death.[66]

Nevertheless, the above hypothesis does not clarify the widespread peripheral autonomic involvement that seems to occur from early stages, which might rather suggest a multicentric process. In asymptomatic subjects, the prevalence and severity of incidental α-synuclein aggregation in autonomic neurons was higher in vesicoprostatic (26%) versus digestive tract (4%) specimens and was associated with diffuse cardiac sympathetic denervation observed by [123-I]metaiodobenzylguanidine scintigraphy.[65] As inferred from incidental LB disease autopsies, α-synuclein aggregation in the cardiac sympathetic system appears to occur first in distal axons, followed by centripetal degeneration, and later involvement of the neuronal somata in the paravertebral ganglia.[67] Certainly, this dying-back type of degeneration of vulnerable neurons is more suggestive of a systemic pathogenic mechanism. At any rate, large prospective full-body autopsy studies and the development of appropriate animal models are required to further address these issues.

Therapy

As might be predicted from the above discourse, the therapies for disturbances of the gastrointestinal tract in PD are diverse. The therapy of gastrointestinal dysfunction in PD begins with a problem-specific history and examination, medication review, and consideration of alternative causes. It is not sufficient to assume that abdominal symptoms and weight loss are due to PD alone. Directed questioning for 'alarm' symptoms are required, including blood in the stool, as well as features of other local and systemic disease. Physical examination is required, including digital rectal examination. If the treating neurologist is uncomfortable or unfamiliar with these facets of the physical exam, then the assistance and advice of a general physician or gastroenterologist should be sought. Stool diaries are uncommonly employed in the evaluation of constipation in patients with PD, even though PD patients often underestimate the number of stools, highlighting the differences in understanding the term constipation. It is important to remember that symptoms alone are often unable to distinguish between various intestinal conditions including constipation due to prolonged colonic transit time, constipation from anorectal dysfunction, and intestinal pseudo-obstruction. General investigations with biochemistry, hematology and endocrinology tests are helpful to evaluate possible inter-current systemic disease that might cause gastrointestinal dysfunction such as hypothyroidism and hypercalcemia. These tests may also help to identify the consequences of significant intercurrent disease such as anemia secondary to colonic carcinoma. Specific tests of the gastrointestinal tract such as endoscopy should be undertaken with the assistance of a specialist physician such as a gastroenterologist. Tests of colonic transit time and anorectal physiology including manometry and neurophysiology are seldom undertaken, but should be considered if anorectal dysfunction is a possibility. Significant and continued weight loss despite adequate caloric intake should be investigated thoroughly, as an underlying cause is often identified. Specialist dietary advice is required for some patients.

The medical management of constipation in PD includes hydration, exercise, increasing dietary fiber (psyllium et al), laxatives (stimulant and osmotic), dopamine replacement therapy, dopamine antagonists, serotiner-gic agents, and other drugs (including erythromycin, colchicine and botu-linum toxin). General recommendations for the treatment of constipation begin with dietary modification including adequate hydration and a high fiber diet.[2] Empiric therapy with a high fiber diet is inexpensive and effec-tive in patients with chronic constipation from any cause, with the addition of 25g of dietary fiber (typically psyllium) a day increasing stool frequency, together with adequate hydration of 1.5 to 2 liters a day. PD patients often have reduced water intake, which has an impact on the consistency of the stool.[61] Trials of the use of fiber in the therapy on constipation in PD support its use.[15,18,19,68] Increased physical exercise is also helpful in the therapy of constipation of any cause,[69] but no trials exist to address this issue in PD subjects. There is scant or no literature to support the use of common stimulant laxatives such as bicosadyl, senna, or other agents in the therapy of constipation in PD. A meta-analysis of 11 large studies on the use of these agents in chronic constipation does not support their use.[70] Furthermore, the prolonged usage of stimulant laxatives can result in the development of a cathartic colon, which worsens constipation.

Osmotic laxatives such as lactulose and polyethylene glycol are also used in the therapy of constipation. These agents work solely by osmotic action, increasing the water content and volume of the stool, and as a result, stool frequency. While there are no trial data to support the use of lactulose in constipation in patients with PD, there are several reports of the efficacy of macrogol, which is polyethylene glycol with a molecular weight of 3350. It is used in combination with electrolytes to produce an isotonic solution, marketed in most countries as Movicol®. Eichorn and Oertel first demonstrated the efficacy of macrogol in the constipation of PD, an observation later confirmed by Zanaglia and coworkers.[20,71]

In routine clinical practice, the majority of PD patients with symptomatic constipation respond to daily macrogol therapy that is easily titrated according to response.

Pharmacological therapy of constipation in PD is sometimes of use. The effect of dopamine on the intestine is complicated.[9] Endogenous dopamine is thought to inhibit intestinal motility, whereas exogenous dopamine has variable effects on intestinal motility. Intravenous dopamine in the intensive care setting reduces intestinal motility,[72] probably by action on an intact ENS. Levodopa, in contrast to dopamine, crosses the blood brain barrier via active transport, and acts on both the central and enteric nervous systems. There are no conclusive data regarding the exacerbation of constipation by levodopa/dopa decarboxylase combination therapy, although experience from the clinic is that some patients may unpredictably develop worsening constipation with either Sinemet® (levodopa/carbidopa) or Madopar® (levodopa/benserazide), prompting a switch from one to the other. Dopamine agonists, including pramipexole, cabergoline, pergolide, pramipexole and apomorphine can either produce diarrhea and/or constipation, and although these adverse effects might be a reason to cease the agonist therapy, rarely are they employed to counter constipation specifically.[21,63,73,74] Inhibitors of catechol-o-methyltransferase, such as tolcapone[75,76] and entacapone,[77,78] can produce diarrhea, possibly by different mechanisms. In the occasional patient in the clinic these adverse effects can be used to advantage, particularly in compound preparations such as Stalevo®.

Blockade of peripheral D2 receptors can enhance intestinal motility, although domperidone is more useful in the therapy of gastroparesis and delayed gastric emptying.[79] There are no data to support the use of maintenance domperidone for constipation in PD, as the effect is minimal. Domperidone is effective in relieving symptoms of gastroparesis, and may help levodopa absorption,[80] as well as minimize nausea via blockade of D2 receptors in the chemoreceptor trigger zone.

Other pro-motility agents have been used in the treatment of constipation in PD. These include serotinergic agents, erythromycin, colchicine, and botulinum toxin. 5-HT agents include cisapride, which, although shown to be effective in the therapy of constipation in PD,[55,81] is now not available in many countries due to cardiac toxicity.[82] Newer agents include mosapride[56,83] and tegaserod,[57] although their place in PD therapy of gastroparesis and constipation is yet to be determined. The macrolide antibiotic erythromycin is often trialed in the therapy of gastroparesis,[84] but no trials of this therapy exist specifically in the PD population. Caution is required regarding drug interactions, particularly via macrolide inhibition of cytochrome P450 and other PD medications.[85] This interaction is particularly important if helicobacter therapy containing clarythromycin (another macrolide) is used in PD patients, as inhibition of cabergoline metabolism may produce significant adverse effect. Colchicine is reported to be useful in the therapy of constipation in PD in one small trial.[86] Other physical methods including enemas and colonic irrigation are also used clinically, with no trials to support their use. If constipation is due to ano-rectal dysfunction, and overactivity of the striated muscles of the anus, injection of botulinum toxin is effective.[87]

The therapy of weight loss begins with the monitoring of weight on clinical review. Keeping a weight record, and emphasizing the importance of weight maintenance is a critical factor. Immobility is a risk factor for weight loss, but there are no trials yet to determine whether regular exercise is important in the maintenance of weight in PD. No convincing trials exist to guide recommendations regarding specific dietary changes in patients with significant weight loss. From a practical point of view, ensuring that PD patients recognize their weight as an important parameter to monitor, together with the maintenance of a high energy diet will often suffice. Sometimes it is useful to obtain the advice of a dietitian. Severe weight loss secondary to dysphagia sometimes requires the insertion of a percutaneous gastrostomy feeding tube in order to preserve life, although this is almost never reported in the literature.[88] Interestingly, there are many reports of increased weight gain following functional surgery in PD, either pallidotomy[89] or the insertion of stimulators into the subthalamic nucleus or globus pallidus.[90–94] The mechanism behind this weight gain is the subject of considerable conjecture, but little convincing data to date.

Conclusion

Gastrointestinal dysfunction in PD is very common, and underscores the widespread involvement that occurs as a result of the disease. There is widespread pathological and therefore clinical involvement that requires careful evaluation of the patient with PD, and even more considered research into the processes that are involved. Intriguingly, it is possible that gastrointestinal dysfunction is critical in the evolution of PD.

References

1. Parkinson J. An Essay on the Shaking Palsy. 1817, London: Whittingham and Rowland.
2. Ternent CA, et al. Practice parameters for the evaluation and management of constipation. *Dis Colon Rectum*. 2007;50(12): 2013–22.

3. Longstreth GF et al. Functional bowel disorders. *Gastroenterology*. 2006;130(5): 1480–91.

4. Bachmann CG, Trenkwalder C. Body weight in patients with Parkinson's disease. *Mov Disord*. 2006;21(11): 1824–30.

5. Edwards LL, et al. Gastrointestinal symptoms in Parkinson's disease. *Mov Disord*. 1991;6(2): 151–6.

6. Edwards L, et al. Gastrointestinal symptoms in Parkinson disease: 18-month follow-up study. *Mov Disord*. 1993;8(1): 83–6.

7. Jost WH, Schimrigk K. Constipation in Parkinson's disease. *Klin Wochenschr*. 1991;69(20): 906–9.

8. Magerkurth C, Schnitzer R, Braune S. Symptoms of autonomic failure in Parkinson's disease: prevalence and impact on daily life. *Clin Auton Res*. 2005;15(2): 76–82.

9. Sakakibara R, et al. Bladder and bowel dysfunction in Parkinson's disease. *J Neural Transm*. 2008;115(3): 443–60.

10. Wiley JW. Aging and neural control of the GI tract: III. Senescent enteric nervous system: lessons from extraintestinal sites and nonmammalian species. *Am J Physiol Gastrointest Liver Physiol*. 2002;283(5): G1020–6.

11. Siddiqui MF, et al. Autonomic dysfunction in Parkinson's disease: a comprehensive symptom survey. *Parkinsonism Relat Disord*. 2002;8(4): 277–84.

12. Abbott RD, et al. Frequency of bowel movements and the future risk of Parkinson's disease. *Neurology*. 2001;57(3): 456–62.

13. Abbott RD, et al. Bowel movement frequency in late-life and incidental Lewy bodies. *Mov Disord*. 2007;22(11): 1581–6.

14. Sakakibara R. et al. Colonic transit time and rectoanal videomanometry in Parkinson's disease. *J Neurol Neurosurg Psychiatry*. 2003;74(2): 268–72.

15. Jost WH, Eckardt VF. Constipation in idiopathic Parkinson's disease. *Scand J Gastroenterol*. 2003;38(7): 681–6.

16. Rosenthal MJ, Marshall CE. Sigmoid volvulus in association with parkinsonism. Report of four cases. *J Am Geriatr Soc*. 1987;35(7): 683–4.

17. Bassotti G, et al. Normal aspects of colorectal motility and abnormalities in slow transit constipation. *World J Gastroenterol*. 2005;11(18): 2691–6.

18. Jost WH, Schrank B. Defecatory disorders in de novo Parkinsonians–colonic transit and electromyogram of the external anal sphincter. *Wien Klin Wochenschr*. 1998;110(15): 535–7.

19. Ashraf W, et al. Constipation in Parkinson's disease: objective assessment and response to psyllium. *Mov Disord*. 1997;12(6): 946–51.

20. Zangaglia R, et al. Macrogol for the treatment of constipation in Parkinson's disease. A randomized placebo-controlled study. *Mov Disord*. 2007;22(9): 1239–44.

21. Mathers SE, et al. Anal sphincter dysfunction in Parkinson's disease. *Arch Neurol*. 1989;46(10): 1061–4.

22. Mathers SE, et al. Constipation and paradoxical puborectalis contraction in animus and Parkinson's disease: a dystonic phenomenon? *J Neurol Neurosurg Psychiatry*. 1988;51(12): 1503–7.

23. Ashraf W, Pfeiffer RF, Quigley EM. Anorectal manometry in the assessment of anorectal function in Parkinson's disease: a comparison with chronic idiopathic constipation. *Mov Disord*. 1994;9(6): 655–63.

24. Goetze O, et al. Predictors of gastric emptying in Parkinson's disease. *Neurogastroenterol Motil.* 2006;18(5): 369–75.
25. Hardoff R, et al. Gastric emptying time and gastric motility in patients with Parkinson's disease. *Mov Disord.* 2001;16(6): 1041–7.
26. Pfeiffer RF. Gastrointestinal dysfunction in Parkinson's disease. *Lancet Neurol.* 2003;2(2): 107–16.
27. Hermanowicz N. Fatal gastroparesis in a patient with Parkinson's disease. *Mov Disord.* 2008;23(1): 152–3.
28. Abbott RD, et al. Midlife adiposity and the future risk of Parkinson's disease. *Neurology.* 2002;59(7): 1051–7.
29. Logroscino G, et al. Body mass index and risk of Parkinson's disease: a prospective cohort study. *Am J Epidemiol.* 2007;166(10): 1186–90.
30. Abbott RA, et al. Diet, body size and micronutrient status in Parkinson's disease. *Eur J Clin Nutr.* 1992;46(12): 879–84.
31. Beyer PL, et al. Weight change and body composition in patients with Parkinson's disease. *J Am Diet Assoc.* 1995;95(9): 979–83.
32. Chen H, et al. Weight loss in Parkinson's disease. *Ann Neurol.* 2003;53(5): 676–9.
33. Uc EY, et al. Predictors of weight loss in Parkinson's disease. *Mov Disord.* 2006;21(7): 930–6.
34. Zappia M, et al. Body weight influences pharmacokinetics of levodopa in Parkinson's disease. *Clin Neuropharmacol.* 2002;25(2): 79–82.
35. Sharma JC, et al. Cascade of levodopa dose and weight-related dyskinesia in Parkinson's disease (LD-WD-PD cascade). *Parkinsonism Relat Disord.* 2006;12(8):499–505.
36. Arabia G, et al. Body weight, levodopa pharmacokinetics and dyskinesia in Parkinson's disease. *Neurol Sci.* 2002;23 Suppl 2: S53–4.
37. Sharma JC. Body weight in patients with Parkinson's disease. *Mov Disord.* 2007;22(9): 1365; author reply 1365–6.
38. Benarroch EE. Enteric nervous system: functional organization and neurologic implications. *Neurology.* 2007;69(20): 1953–7.
39. Anlauf M, et al. Chemical coding of the human gastrointestinal nervous system: cholinergic, VIPergic, and catecholaminergic phenotypes. *J Comp Neurol.* 2003;459(1): 90–111.
40. Fort P, et al. The satiety molecule nesfatin-1 is co-expressed with melanin concentrating hormone in tuberal hypothalamic neurons of the rat. *Neuroscience.* 2008;155(1): 174–81.
41. Gai WP, et al. Age-related loss of dorsal vagal neurons in Parkinson's disease. *Neurology.* 1992;42(11): 2106–11.
42. Wakabayashi K, Takahashi H. Neuropathology of autonomic nervous system in Parkinson's disease. *Eur Neurol.* 1997;38 Suppl 2: 2–7.
43. Braak H, Del Tredici K. Invited Article: Nervous system pathology in sporadic Parkinson disease. *Neurology.* 2008;70(20): 1916–25.
44. Wakabayashi K, Takahashi H. The intermediolateral nucleus and Clarke's column in Parkinson's disease. *Acta Neuropathol.* 1997;94(3): 287–9.
45. Bloch A, et al. Alpha-synuclein pathology of the spinal and peripheral autonomic nervous system in neurologically unimpaired elderly subjects. *Neuropathol Appl Neurobiol.* 2006;32(3):284–95.

46. Klos KJ, et al. Alpha-synuclein pathology in the spinal cords of neurologically asymptomatic aged individuals. *Neurology*. 2006;66(7): 1100–2.
47. Qualman SJ, et al. Esophageal Lewy bodies associated with ganglion cell loss in achalasia. Similarity to Parkinson's disease. *Gastroenterology*. 1984;87(4): 848–56.
48. Kupsky WJ, et al. Parkinson's disease and megacolon: concentric hyaline inclusions (Lewy bodies) in enteric ganglion cells. *Neurology*. 1987;37(7):1253–5.
49. Braak H, et al. Gastric alpha-synuclein immunoreactive inclusions in Meissner's and Auerbach's plexuses in cases staged for Parkinson's disease-related brain pathology. *Neurosci Lett*. 2006;396(1):67–72.
50. Thannickal TC, Lai YY, Siegel JM. Hypocretin (orexin) cell loss in Parkinson's disease. *Brain*. 2007;130(Pt 6):1586–95.
51. Travagli RA, et al. Brainstem circuits regulating gastric function. *Annu Rev Physiol*. 2006;68: 279–305.
52. Cersosimo MG, Benarroch EE. Neural control of the gastrointestinal tract: implications for Parkinson disease. *Mov Disord*. 2008;23(8): 1065–75.
53. Pierantozzi M, et al. Helicobacter pylori eradication and l-dopa absorption in patients with PD and motor fluctuations. *Neurology*. 2006;66(12): 1824–9.
54. Phillips RJ, Powley TL. Innervation of the gastrointestinal tract: patterns of aging. *Auton Neurosci*, 2007;136(1-2):1–19.
55. Jost WH, Schimrigk K. Long-term results with cisapride in Parkinson's disease. *Mov Disord*. 1997;12(3):423–5.
56. Liu Z, et al. Mosapride citrate, a novel 5-HT4 agonist and partial 5-HT3 antagonist, ameliorates constipation in parkinsonian patients. *Mov Disord*. 2005;20(6):680–6.
57. Sullivan KL, et al. Tegaserod (Zelnorm) for the treatment of constipation in Parkinson's disease. *Mov Disord*. 2006;21(1): 115–6.
58. Li ZS, et al. Physiological modulation of intestinal motility by enteric dopaminergic neurons and the D2 receptor: analysis of dopamine receptor expression, location, development, and function in wild-type and knock-out mice. *J Neurosci*. 2006;26(10): 2798–807.
59. Singaram C, et al. Dopaminergic defect of enteric nervous system in Parkinson's disease patients with chronic constipation. *Lancet*. 1995;346(8979): 861–4.
60. Anderson G, et al. Loss of enteric dopaminergic neurons and associated changes in colon motility in an MPTP mouse model of Parkinson's disease. *Exp Neurol*. 2007;207(1): 4–12.
61. Ueki A, Otsuka M. Life style risks of Parkinson's disease: association between decreased water intake and constipation. *J Neurol*. 2004;251 Suppl 7: vII18–23.
62. Stocchi F, et al. Anorectal function in multiple system atrophy and Parkinson's disease. *Mov Disord*. 2000;15(1):71–6.
63. Edwards LL, et al. Defecatory function in Parkinson's disease: response to apomorphine. *Ann Neurol*. 1993;33(5): 490–3.
64. Wakabayashi K, et al. Parkinson's disease: the presence of Lewy bodies in Auerbach's and Meissner's plexuses. *Acta Neuropathol*. 1988;76(3): 217–221.
65. Minguez-Castellanos A, et al. Do alpha-synuclein aggregates in autonomic plexuses predate Lewy body disorders?: a cohort study. *Neurology*. 2007;68(23): 2012–8.

66. Miwa H, et al. Intragastric proteasome inhibition induces alpha-synuclein-immunopositive aggregations in neurons in the dorsal motor nucleus of the vagus in rats. *Neurosci Lett.* 2006;401(1-2): 146–9.

67. Orimo S, et al. Axonal alpha-synuclein aggregates herald centripetal degeneration of cardiac sympathetic nerve in Parkinson's disease. *Brain.* 2008;131(Pt 3): 642–50.

68. Astarloa R, et al. Clinical and pharmacokinetic effects of a diet rich in insoluble fiber on Parkinson disease. *Clin Neuropharmacol.* 1992;15(5): 375–80.

69. De Schryver AM, et al. Effects of regular physical activity on defecation pattern in middle-aged patients complaining of chronic constipation. *Scand J Gastroenterol.* 2005;40(4): 422–9.

70. Ramkumar D, Rao SS. Efficacy and safety of traditional medical therapies for chronic constipation: systematic review. *Am J Gastroenterol.* 2005;100(4):936–71.

71. Eichhorn TE, Oertel WH. Macrogol 3350/electrolyte improves constipation in Parkinson's disease and multiple system atrophy. *Mov Disord.* 2001;16(6):1176–7.

72. Dive A, et al. Effect of dopamine on gastrointestinal motility during critical illness. *Intensive Care Med.* 2000;26(7): 901–7.

73. Kempster PA, Iansek R, Larmour I. Intermittent subcutaneous apomorphine injection treatment for parkinsonian motor oscillations. *Aust N Z J Med.* 1991;21(3): 314–8.

74. Navan P, et al. Double-blind, single-dose, cross-over study of the effects of pramipexole, pergolide, and placebo on rest tremor and UPDRS part III in Parkinson's disease. *Mov Disord.* 2003;18(2): 176–80.

75. Brooks DJ. Safety and tolerability of COMT inhibitors. *Neurology.* 2004;62(1 Suppl 1): S39–46.

76. Gerlach M, et al. Different modes of action of catecholamine-O-methyltransferase inhibitors entacapone and tolcapone on adenylyl cyclase activity in vitro. *J Neural Transm.* 2002;109(5-6): 789–95.

77. Brooks DJ. Optimizing levodopa therapy for Parkinson's disease with levodopa/carbidopa/entacapone: implications from a clinical and patient perspective. *Neuropsychiatr Dis Treat.* 2008;4(1): 39–47.

78. Parashos SA, Wielinski CL, Kern JA. Frequency, reasons, and risk factors of entacapone discontinuation in Parkinson disease. *Clin Neuropharmacol.* 2004;27(3): 119–23.

79. Soykan I, et al. Effect of chronic oral domperidone therapy on gastrointestinal symptoms and gastric emptying in patients with Parkinson's disease. *Mov Disord.* 1997;12(6): 952–7.

80. Langdon N, Malcolm PN, Parkes JD. Comparison of levodopa with carbidopa, and levodopa with domperidone in Parkinson's disease. *Clin Neuropharmacol.* 1986;9(5): 440–7.

81. Jost WH, Schimrigk K. Cisapride treatment of constipation in Parkinson's disease. *Mov Disord.* 1993;8(3):339–43.

82. Hennessy S, et al. Cisapride and ventricular arrhythmia. *Br J Clin Pharmacol.* 2008;66(3): 375–85.

83. Asai H, et al. Increased gastric motility during 5-HT4 agonist therapy reduces response fluctuations in Parkinson's disease. *Parkinsonism Relat Disord.* 2005;11(8):499–502.

84. Friedenberg FK, Parkman HP. Delayed gastric emptying: whom to test, how to test, and what to do. *Curr Treat Options Gastroenterol.* 2006;9(4): 295–304.

85. Nakatsuka A, et al. Effect of clarithromycin on the pharmacokinetics of cabergoline in healthy controls and in patients with Parkinson's disease. *J Pharmacol Sci.* 2006;100(1): 59–64.

86. Sandyk R, Gillman MA. Colchicine ameliorates constipation in Parkinson's disease. *J R Soc Med.* 1984;77(12): 1066.

87. Albanese A, et al. Severe constipation in Parkinson's disease relieved by botulinum toxin. *Mov Disord.* 1997;12(5): 764–6.

88. Lieberman AN, et al. Dysphagia in Parkinson's disease. *Am J Gastroenterol.* 1980;74(2): 157–60.

89. Ondo WG, et al. Weight gain following unilateral pallidotomy in Parkinson's disease. *Acta Neurol Scand.* 2000;101(2): 79–84.

90. Barichella M, et al. Body weight gain rate in patients with Parkinson's disease and deep brain stimulation. *Mov Disord.* 2003;18(11):1337–40.

91. Macia F, et al. Parkinson's disease patients with bilateral subthalamic deep brain stimulation gain weight. *Mov Disord.* 2004;19(2): 206–12.

92. Montaurier C. et al. Mechanisms of body weight gain in patients with Parkinson's disease after subthalamic stimulation. *Brain.* 2007;130(Pt 7):1808–18.

93. Novakova L, et al. Increase in body weight is a non-motor side effect of deep brain stimulation of the subthalamic nucleus in Parkinson's disease. *Neuro Endocrinol Lett.* 2007;28(1):21–5.

94. Tuite PJ, et al. Weight and body mass index in Parkinson's disease patients after deep brain stimulation surgery. *Parkinsonism Relat Disord.* 2005;11(4): 247–52.

Chapter 5C

Lesions Associated with Autonomic Dysfunction: Orthostatic Hypotension

Kathryn K. Post and Spiridon Papapetropoulos

Introduction

Although Parkinson's disease (PD) is classically thought of in terms of motor dysfunction, it was evident even at the time of this disorder's original description in 1817 that features of autonomic dysfunction are often present.[1] Documented abnormalities in the gastrointestinal, urogenital, cardiovascular, sexual, and thermoregulatory systems illustrate the widespread impact of dysautonomia on patients' clinical condition.[2,3] The relevance of this topic in terms of patients' morbidity is underscored by one report that estimates that a PD patient has a 1 in 3 lifetime risk of developing a significant autonomic dysfunction.[4] Orthostatic hypotension (OH), in particular, has been a focus of recent study. While its exact prevalence has been subject to debate, a thorough review of the literature by one study found the average prevalence of OH in PD patients to be 41%.[5] OH poses a significant problem to the PD patient as it markedly increases the risk of falling in this already susceptible population, adding to the impact this disorder exerts on a patient's quality of life.[6,7] The focus of this chapter will thus be the origins of OH and the possible screening applications associated with this clinical sign. We will first explore where OH of PD fits in the classification scheme of syncope. Subsequent analysis will delve into the question of whether OH is central or peripheral in nature through

a detailed comparison with multiple system atrophy (MSA) and pure autonomic failure (PAF). Finally, this chapter will end with a discussion of the
potential screening techniques for pre-motor diagnosis of PD associated
with the clinical sign of OH, as well as an assessment of other possible
techniques.

Syncope

The Consensus Committee of the American Autonomic Society and the
American Academy of Neurology define OH as: a reduction of systolic
blood pressure of at least 20 mmHg or diastolic blood pressure of at least
10 mmHg within 3 minutes of standing.[8] Since OH is a clinical sign and
not a symptom, care must be taken to read the presenting features of the
patient that may indicate a subsequent need for dysautonomia evaluation.[8]
Symptoms associated with OH range from a feeling of lightheadedness to
outright syncope. Physicians must recognize such symptoms upon clinical
encounter and evaluate their basis.

Syncope (fainting) is due to a disturbance in the autonomic system that
results in inadequate cerebral perfusion to maintain consciousness.[9,10] Its
causes are varied and, at times, quite difficult to discern.[11,12] Blood pressure maintenance requires the functioning of an elaborate autonomic
system evolutionarily designed upon man's transition to upright posture to
maintain cerebral perfusion.[13,14] A peripheral or central insult within this
complex system can often upset the balance. An effort to classify the
resulting mix of conditions known to elicit syncope has led to a classification schema consisting of three general headings:

- neurally mediated syncope (reflex syncope)
- postural orthostatic tachycardia syncope (POTS)
- autonomic failure (see Figure 5C-1) [10]

This system of classification is dependent upon an understanding of how
the autonomic system maintains blood pressure normally in the human
body.

Upon standing, approximately 500–800mL of blood drops to the abdomen and lower limbs.[13] As a result, venous return to the heart decreases
and there is a 40% decline in stroke volume.[10] The corresponding drop in
blood pressure is corrected within the first minute of adopting an upright
posture in a normal person by autonomic compensatory mechanisms.[13]
The baroreflex arc contains both peripheral and central components.
A drop in blood pressure is detected peripherally by high pressure receptors in the aortic arch and carotid sinus, as well as low pressure receptors

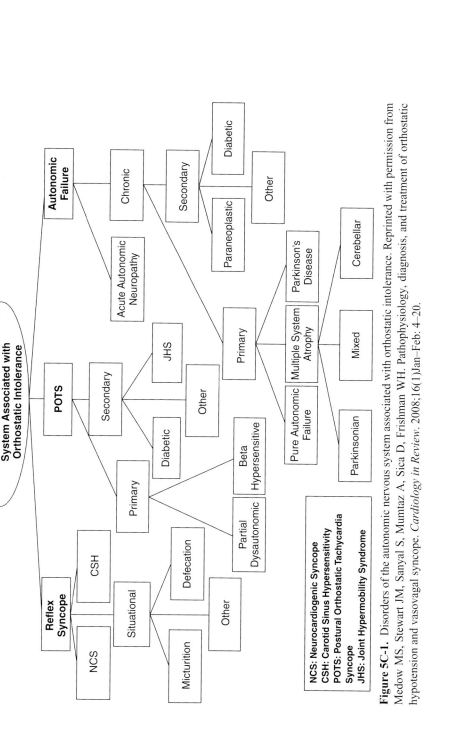

Figure 5C-1. Disorders of the autonomic nervous system associated with orthostatic intolerance. Reprinted with permission from Medow MS, Stewart JM, Sanyal S, Mumtaz A, Sica D, Frishman WH. Pathophysiology, diagnosis, and treatment of orthostatic hypotension and vasovagal syncope. *Cardiology in Review.* 2008;16(1)Jan–Feb: 4–20.

in the heart and lungs.[10] A decrease in blood pressure causes the barore-ceptors to decrease their firing rate.[13] This afferent signal then travels to the medullary cardiovascular center, discussed subsequently, wherein there is a corresponding decrease in parasympathetic outflow and an increase in sympathetic outflow.[13] Sympathetic activation will, through various mechanisms, work to increase blood pressure and heart rate.[13] For example, it will increase venous and arteriolar constriction as well act on the heart to increase contractility and heart rate.[15] In addition, sympathetic activity may cause the hypothalamus to release vasopressin (AVP) from the posterior pituitary.[16–18] Muscle contraction of the legs upon standing, also known as the skeletal muscle pump system, will aid in the return of venous blood to the heart and recovery of blood pressure.[10] If a person remains upright for an extended period of time (20–30 minutes), plasma volume loss will occur, triggering the activation of long term compensa-tory mechanisms such as the renin-angiotensin-aldosterone system.[10,19]

The medullary cardiovascular system relies upon afferent input from peripheral baroreceptors. The signal travels via the glossopharyngeal and vagus nerves to the nucleus tractus solitarius (NTS) where the first steps of integration occur.[10,20] The NTS likewise receives signals from higher brain centers.[20] Cortical and limbic structures which influence the hypo-thalamus as well as the insular cortex have all been implicated as possible sources of central autonomic control.[13,20–22] Much is still unknown about the integration of peripheral and central signals within the medulla.[15] Neurohormonal influences may also affect this process due to this region's proximity to the area postrema, a site where the blood brain barrier may be weak.[20] Once integration has occurred, efferent sympathetic and parasym-pathetic information travels out, respectively, through the ventrolateral medulla (VLM) and nucleus ambiguous.[15]

Appropriate diagnosis is important, as improved understanding of the pathophysiological mechanisms behind syncopal disorders has led to better treatment options.[10,13] The two most common categories, neurally medi-ated syncope and autonomic failure, differ as to whether an intact auto-nomic system is present and whether the condition is acute or chronic in nature.[10,21] Neurally mediated syncope represents an acute episode of an abnormal reflex within an intact autonomic system.[21] Episodes are elicited in response to a specific trigger, whether known or unknown, and ulti-mately result in bradycardia and vasodilation.[20,21] This is due to a reversal of the normal autonomic outflow that maintains blood pressure while stand-ing, causing an increased parasympathetic and decreased sympathetic outflow.[20,21] Neurally mediated syncope can in turn be divided, based on central or peripheral origin.[21] Recall that both sources of input can affect the output of the medullary cardiovascular center. Vasovagal syncope (fainting spell) is an example of neurally mediated syncope of central origin and is the most common cause of syncope.[10,20] In this situation, triggers such as emotional or painful stimuli cause, through an incompletely understood mechanism, regions of the brain such as the limbic system to influence the hypothalamus and thereby the medullary cardiovascular center.[21] Carotid sinus hypersensitivity, micturation, and defecation syncope are all examples of neurally mediated syncope of peripheral origin.[21] The culprits in this scenario are highly sensitive peripheral receptors that upon stimulation, for example in the case of a tight shirt collar, signal the medullary cardiovascular center to invert the normal relationship between parasympathetic and sympathetic outflow.[21] In contrast to the episodic nature of neurally mediated syncope, recurring syncopal incidents upon orthostasis point to a disorder of autonomic failure.[10,13,21] Numerous conditions fall under this category and so autonomic failure is divided into primary and secondary forms.[10,21] PD with OH (PD + OH), MSA with OH (MSA + OH), and PAF are all considered to be primary chronic autonomic disorders.[10,23] Lesions in the autonomic pathway are reported to occur centrally in MSA and peripherally in PAF.[21] As yet, however, it is unclear whether central, peripheral, or perhaps both types of lesions are involved in PD + OH patients. Various studies have implicated higher brain centers, the medullary portion of the brainstem, and post-ganglionic sympathetic neurons as all possible sites of damage along the autonomic pathway.[22,24–35] The upcoming section will focus on these reports. Lastly, POTS is a disorder with syncopal manifestations that has been characterized rather recently.[10] Considered a variant of autonomic failure as a result of a likely problem with peripheral vasoconstriction, these patients possess a rather unique pattern of expression. While displaying symptoms of lightheadedness, dizziness, or syncope upon upright posture, patients experience an increase in heart rate of more than 30 beats per minute or obtain a heart rate of more than 120 beats per minute.[9,10] This singular pattern makes POTS the easiest to rule out of the three categories of syncopal disorders.

To clinically differentiate neurally mediated syncope from syncope of autonomic failure, a thorough history and physical exam should be performed, noting the setting in which the symptoms occur and whether the patient cites a particular triggering factor.[11] Associated symptoms can also provide clues.[10,13,20] Nausea, pallor, vomiting, diaphoresis, loss of peripheral vision, and diminished hearing have all been recorded as possible accompanying symptoms of neurally mediated syncope.[10,13,20] In contrast, autonomic dysfunction incurred by multiple organ systems is the usual hallmark of patients who present with the latter.[13] Symptoms may include urinary and fecal incontinence, constipation or diarrhea, hypohidrosis, and impotence.[10,13] After taking a full history from the patient, an orthostatic blood pressure check should be performed.[11] It is important to recognize that even if symptoms of OH are present, patients may fail to meet the criteria for OH upon measurement, in which case repeated measurements may be needed.[8] Repeated measurements are encouraged in such cases.[8] In conjunction with a patient's history and physical exam, an electrocardiogram should be ordered.[11]

Despite our best efforts, though, only approximately 45% of syncopal episodes are diagnosed by careful history and physical exam.[11,12] Thus, syncope remains unexplained in half of patients after initial work up and in these cases further testing strategies should be considered although there is no diagnostic gold standard.[11,12] As well, there is no assurance that further testing may reveal definitive answers. Syncope is a complex problem and although some progress has been made in understanding the science behind its causes, a battery of negative tests may at times yield only more questions.[12]

One test often discussed in the literature is the head-up tilt test (HUTT), which elicits different responses from patients with neurally mediated syncope compared to those with autonomic failure.[21] This procedure involves a passive maneuver and therefore the skeletal muscle pump that normally functions upon standing is inactive.[21] Thus, the test exaggerates the decrease in venous return to the heart that would normally occur upon assuming an upright posture.[21] A disturbance in the autonomic system created by this hemodynamic trigger may occur and cause patients with neurally mediated syncope to experience symptoms during the HUTT.[21] Symptoms would appear after an extended period (40 to 50 minutes for example).[21] In contrast, symptoms would appear shortly (within minutes) after onset of the HUTT in patients with autonomic failure.[21] This is because the autonomic system that governs blood pressure maintenance is simply not intact in the latter group of patients and thus no trigger, other than assuming an upright posture, is necessary to elicit symptoms. If symptoms are not elicited during passive HUTT, a reattempt is often made with isoproterenol infusion.[12] Reports on the sensitivity and specificity of such tests are inconsistent.[12,36]

Orthostatic Hypotension in Parkinson's Disease

OH is commonly encountered in PD patients, yet its pathophysiological mechanism remains uncertain. Evidence suggests a resemblance to mechanisms thought to play a role in the development of OH in both PAF and MSA. However, these disorders sit on opposite ends of the spectrum; autonomic dysfunction in the former is thought to be dominated by peripheral lesions, while the latter is considered to be a centrally mediated disturbance. Investigators are charged with the task of resolving this paradox.

Loss of peripheral vasoconstrictor ability may be the most important factor in determining whether a patient becomes susceptible to hypotension upon standing. This is certainly true in PAF. This disorder, originally described by Bradbury and Eggleston in 1925, involves a generalized loss of peripheral postganglionic sympathetic neurons.[10,13,14] Onset of PAF usually occurs after the age of 60 years and its progression is characterized by a decline in the body's ability to manage functions dependent on the autonomic system such as bladder control, sexual ability, and prolonged standing, with symptoms of lightheadedness and syncope being the typical presenting features.[4,10] Unlike PD and MSA, no robust signs and symptoms of central neurodegeneration have been reported.[27] Ultimately, the most disabling component of this disorder is OH, imposing severe restrictions on patients' movements.[4] Although MSA patients may express similar symptoms of lightheadedness and syncope, the pathophysiological mechanism behind OH in this disorder is thought to be more centrally located.[10] Lesions have been noted in the brainstem, cerebellum, and spinal cord of MSA patients.[10,27] MSA presents with both parkinsonian and cerebellar signs and symptoms, although different levels of combination are possible.[4] Patients may either be parkinsonian predominant (MSA-P) or cerebellar predominant (MSA-C).[4]

Despite these differences, both disorders share much in common with each other and with PD. PD, MSA, and PAF are all synucleinopathic (α-synuclein inclusion bodies noted in either neuronal or glial cells) neurodegenerative disorders frequently associated with the clinical sign of OH.[4,27] PD + OH, MSA + OH and PAF are all considered to be forms of primary chronic autonomic failure.[10,23] It is well known that the mechanisms behind OH in MSA and PAF differ greatly, and it may be possible to infer how the PD + OH mechanism relates to the other two by comparing and contrasting the respective patient groups.

Many view PD + OH as more akin to PAF and thus argue that the autonomic dysfunction involved in the former is more peripheral in nature. Presently, there is no direct method by which to examine the integrity of peripheral postganglionic sympathetic neurons, though denervation can be inferred through multiple techniques. Neurochemical evidence has suggested that there is a generalized loss of postganglionic sympathetic neurons in PAF.[37] Upon activation of peripheral sympathetic neurons, the neurotransmitter norepinephrine (NE) is released and mediates vasoconstriction through interaction with $\alpha 1$ adrenergic receptors. Supine plasma NE levels in PAF patients are significantly lower than normal, and multiple studies have looked into the question of whether the same finding might be apparent in PD + OH patients.[8,37] Lower levels of plasma NE in PD + OH patients have been reported compared to normal controls and PD

patients without OH.[3,38–40] However, other studies have not found significant differences.[1,26,27] These inconsistencies may be due to the effects of
levodopa, which acts as a precursor in the synthesis of dopamine and subsequently of catecholamines.[26] Peripheral conversion of this medication,
despite co-administration of carbidopa, may be responsible for artificially
increasing plasma NE levels in patients.[26] Support for this hypothesis is
derived from one study which compared PD + OH patients on and off
levodopa. The resultant findings demonstrated that PD + OH patients who
were off levodopa had lower levels of supine plasma NE than did PD
patients without OH.[26] These results, however, did not hold true for PD +
OH patients being treated with levodopa.[26] Both sets of patients had similar and normal plasma NE levels.[26] Within the same study, a comparison
was also made between non-treated PD + OH patients and PAF patients.[26]
PAF patients displayed even lower levels of plasma NE, illustrating that
the groups differ but by degree of peripheral noradrenergic nerve loss.[26]
MSA patients, however, displayed normal levels of plasma NE.[26] This
outcome is expected of a disorder thought to be centrally mediated.[26]

Since levodopa may serve as a confounding factor in experiments that
attempt to utilize supine plasma NE levels to judge the general integrity of
peripheral sympathetic nerves, an alternative approach based on neuropharmacology was devised. Appropriate drug response signifies an intact
underlying mechanism that functions in predicted manners. Sharabi and
colleagues used medications to examine the autonomic vasoconstrictor
abilities of MSA, PAF, and PD + OH patients.[27] Yohimbine (pressor) is an
α2 selective antagonist that promotes NE release and subsequent blood
pressure elevation via blockade of the sympathetic negative feedback system.[41] Trimethaphan (depressor), on the other hand, works by inhibiting
sympathetic neurotransmission via ganglionic blockade, thereby hinder-
ing NE release and lowering blood pressure.[42] Previous studies have
reported that blood pressure changes (in either direction) upon administration of these peripherally acting drugs were diminished in PAF patients
owing to postganglionic lesions present in this disorder.[43] Thus the drugs
were not able to perform their designed function. However, because MSA
does not involve a postganglionic lesion, the drugs' ability to act is not
hindered and thus demonstrable changes in blood pressure have been
reported.[44,45] To discover which group PD + OH patients most resemble,
Sharabi and colleagues performed neuropharmacological testing on all
three patient populations.[27] In accordance with a pathophysiological
mechanism of OH thought to be more centrally located, MSA patients
responded appropriately to the peripherally acting drugs.[27] Upon administration of yohimbine and subsequently of trimethaphan, these patients displayed marked increases and decreases, respectively, in blood pressure,

indicating an intact peripheral autonomic system.[27] PD + OH and PAF patients, however, did not respond well to either drug.[27] Little change in blood pressure was noted among the patients.[27] This inappropriate response signifies a damaged sympathetic system in the periphery which suggests a closer resemblance of PD + OH to PAF than to MSA.[27]

Neuroimaging techniques, such as ^{123}I-metaiodobenzylguanidine (MIBG) and 6-[^{18}F]fluorodopamine (6F-DA) PET scans, provide additional evidence of peripheral autonomic impairment. These scans can be used to visualize sympathetic innervation of multiple organs, and it has become apparent that cardiac denervation is present in both PD + OH and PAF patients.[27] It is the loss of postganglionic sympathetic neurons that causes cardiac denervation.[46] Catecholamine neurotransmitters are released by postganglionic neurons and bind to cardiac adrenergic receptors.[46] MIBG is a norepinephrine analog that uses the re-uptake transporter system to accumulate in postganglionic sympathetic neurons.[29,46] PET scans utilizing 6F-DA work similarly as this radioisotope is another catecholamine analog.[31,34,35] In both PD + OH and PAF patients it has been shown that myocardial MIBG uptake is decreased, implying some degree of cardiac sympathetic denervation.[27,29–33, 46] Similar results are obtained from 6F-DA PET scans, while analogous scans in MSA patients revealed autonomic cardiac innervation to be intact.[27,28,31,34,35] One study has explored this further to see whether similarities between PD + OH and PAF patients extend to involve extracardiac noradrenergic denervation.[28] 6F-DA PET scans revealed that both groups exhibited decreased uptake in the renal cortex.[28] This may be of particular significance owing to its known role in the regulation of blood pressure.[28] PD + OH patients additionally displayed decreased radioactivity in the thyroid gland.[28] No MSA patients were tested so results cannot be compared.[28] To summarize, evidence of cardiac, extracardiac, and generalized sympathetic postganglionic denervation has been presented.

Others believe central mechanisms may be involved in the manifestation of OH in PD and point to similarities between these patients and those suffering from MSA. The VLM is the site of sympathetic outflow from the medullary cardiovascular center and consists of different neuronal subpopulations.[15–17] Adrenergic C1 neurons are located in the rostral VLM.[16,17] Upon standing, afferent signals are relayed to the NTS and subsequently VLM neurons are signaled to increase sympathetic outflow.[15–17] C1 neurons provide excitatory input to preganglionic sympathetic neurons of the intermediolateral column (IML).[16,17] The result is an increase in vasomotor tone and consequently, blood pressure.[16,17] The caudal VLM houses noradrenergic A1 neurons and they are responsible for signaling hypothalamic cells (magnocellular neurons) to produce vasopressin (AVP) that will subsequently be released from the posterior pituitary.[16,17] Multiple studies have documented decreases in both C1 and A1 catecholaminergic neurons in MSA + OH patients via immunohistochemical staining techniques.[17,47] Similar decreases in C1 neurons were observed by Gai and colleagues in PD patients.[24] In this early study, investigators utilized the presence of phenylethanolamine N-methyltransferase (PNMT) as a marker of adrenergic neurons (this enzyme is responsible for the final conversion of norepinephrine to epinephrine).[24] This immunohistochemical stain is more selective for adrenergic neurons, such as C1, than stains utilizing tyrosine hydroxylase (TH) (this enzyme catalyzes an earlier step in the pathway and is present in all catecholaminergic neurons).[24] Results from this study indicated that PNMT + C1 adrenergic neurons in PD patients were reduced to 47% of control levels.[24] Unfortunately, the authors did not specify whether PD patients experienced OH during their lifetime.[24] Soon after, Kato and colleagues published a study that placed additional emphasis on OH.[25] In this case, investigators chose to perform immunohistochemical staining with TH antibodies and studied medullary regions of both MSA + OH and PD + OH patients.[25] Significant decreases of TH immunoreactive neurons in C1 and A2 regions (A2 region represents noradrenergic neurons of the NTS) were seen in autopsy samples from both groups.[25] While decreases were consistently observed in MSA + OH patients, not all PD + OH patients displayed reduced levels.[25] Some PD patients without OH were observed to have neuronal decreases in either the C1 or A2 region.[25] This raises the question of whether we are simply looking at background noise. Decreases in medullary neuronal populations may be unspecific to the pathophysiological mechanism of OH. Rather, they may be a byproduct of the neurodegenerative process in PD. Additional evidence of a central mechanism is provided by studies looking at other brain regions linked to the normal control of the autonomic nervous system. The insular cortex is thought to be involved in the autonomic regulation of blood pressure.[22] One study looked at Lewy body density as a quantifiable measure of neurodegeneration in PD.[22] A post-mortem comparison of the insular cortex in PD and PD+OH patients revealed that patients with OH had a significantly higher Lewy body density.[22] In contrast, other areas of the brain did not show comparable differences.[22]

Signals travelling from the NTS to VLM are relayed to sympathetic preganglionic neurons of the IML.[25,47] This information is then passed on to sympathetic postganglionic neurons that directly mediate peripheral vasoconstriction. The IML column, and its function as an intermediate relay station in this pathway, may also be involved in autonomic impairment. MSA + OH patients experience significant losses of sympathetic preganglionic neurons of the IML and this may be the most important contributing factor to the development of OH in MSA patients.[25,47] Braak and colleagues demonstrated the presence of α-synuclein aggregates in these preganglionic neurons and suggested the IML's involvement in PD.[48] While OH status was not documented in this study, previous case reports in PD + OH patients have indicated IML involvement.[48–50] With the addition of this evidence, both components of the CNS (brain and spinal cord) have been implicated in the pathophysiological mechanism of OH in PD. A centrally mediated mechanism is plausible given the argued parallel between PD + OH and MSA + OH patients.

The question as to the degree of similarity between these two disorders, though, is still debated. The results of recent reports are inconsistent, with respect to the previous studies, as to which medullary neuronal populations are most involved.[51–53] Benarroch and colleagues conducted an immunohistochemical comparison study between MSA + OH, PD + OH, and a control group of patients.[51] MSA + OH patients consistently displayed marked decreases in TH immunoreactive neurons in the rostral VLM, but results varied widely among PD + OH patients and overall the mean number of TH immunoreactive neurons in the rostral VLM did not significantly differ from that of controls.[51] As well, TH number could not be predicted by the severity of the PD patient's OH.[51] This lack of correlation seems to suggest an alternative autonomic mechanism is behind OH in the PD patient.

Figure 5C-2 displays all the areas cited to date as possible locations of autonomic impairment in the PD + OH patient. The reader will note that for every major step in the autonomic pathway responsible for blood pressure maintenance upon standing, evidence of some type of lesion has been put forth. However, a definite conclusion as to whether a particular lesion causes OH in PD cannot be made by simple virtue of its location within the autonomic pathway. We suggest accurate assessment can only be made when the following two conditions are met. First, studies should include a comparison between PD + OH and PD patients. If similar abnormalities are noted in PD patients without OH, then it stands to reason that such lesions are more suggestive of background noise than indicative of a pathophysiological process causing OH despite any presence noted in PD + OH patients. For example, a study which only compares PD + OH patients to MSA or PAF patients would not allow for this check. Second, a proven correlation should be seen between severity of damage and severity of OH. Most studies have lacked either one or both of these conditions. This is a possible reason for both the discrepancy among reports and the lack of consensus upon whether OH is peripheral or central in nature. Apart from methodology, individual variation among patients may be partially responsible for inconsistent results. It is plausible that in lieu of one

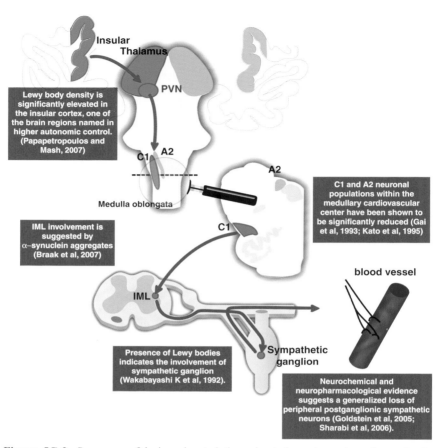

Figure 5C-2. Summary of lesions located throughout the autonomic pathway in the Parkinson's patient. The anatomic structures depicted in this diagram (cortex, medulla, intermediolateral column of the spinal cord, sympathetic ganglion, postganglionic sympathetic neurons) are each important relay stations in the sequence of information regulating the autonomic control of blood pressure. Researchers have described lesions in each region and suggest they may play a role in the development of OH.

pathophysiological mechanism governing the appearance of OH in PD patients, we are in fact dealing with multiple possible mechanisms. Whether that mechanism is central or peripheral could depend largely on the insult(s) suffered by the patient. This could explain both the inconsistencies in plasma NE level reports and the marked individual variations seen in the Benarroch study.[1,26,27,51] A heterogeneous PD + OH patient population would also explain the vastly differing accounts of which medullary neuronal populations are affected. However, the notoriously small sample sizes of post-mortem studies may also have been a contributing factor. It is also possible that one pathophysiological mechanism of OH may dominate in PD. Whether that mechanism is peripheral or central in nature is still up for debate.

Potential Screening Applications Associated with OH

PD + OH patients tend to display abnormal results on tests thought to indicate cardiovascular autonomic dysfunction at higher rates than PD patients without OH. The Valsalva maneuver is one type of experimental manipulation thought to evaluate underlying cardiovascular autonomic dysfunction. Over a period of 8 years, one group of studies showed that all PD + OH patients displayed abnormal Valsalva patterns, whereas only 25% of PD patients without OH did so.[3] Abnormalities occurred in phase II_L and phase IV of the Valsalva pattern.[3] Phase II_L represents a failure to initiate a blood pressure climb back towards normal, while phase IV represents a failure to overshoot.[3] These 2 phases are thought to indicate both peripheral (Phase II_L) and cardiac adrenergic impairment (Phase II_L, Phase IV).[54] Increased blood pressure recovery time (time taken for blood pressure to recover from the phase III drop) and decreased baroreflex-cardiovagal gain are quantitative measurements that are also commonly seen in the PD + OH patient during the Valsalva maneuver.[3,55] Plasma NE level is another test often reported as abnormal in PD + OH patients (although some reports are inconsistent).[1,3,26,27,38–40] Low circulatory levels of catecholamines have been cited as a theoretical cause of denervation supersensitivity.[56,57] Administration of an adrenoceptor agonist is one method to test for this phenomenon.[3,56] For example, the dose required to elicit a 25 mmHg increase in systolic blood pressure in PD + OH patients was significantly less than that necessary in PD patients and controls.[56]

Manifestations of cardiovascular dysautonomia are important because of recent evidence that points to cardiac sympathetic denervation early on in PD.[29,30,58] Both MIBG and PET (6F-DA) scans demonstrate reduced catecholamine analog reuptake, indicating sympathetic postganglionic loss.[29–33,35] Denervation has been observed in both early stage (Hoehn and Yahr I, II) and newly diagnosed PD patients.[29,30,58] Evidence such as this raises the question of whether cardiac denervation may serve as a pre-motor marker of PD. Identifying PD at an earlier stage may aid in the development of more effective/neuroprotective treatment strategies. A cardiovascular premotor marker may be plausible given that Goldstein and colleagues recently published a case report describing a patient with cardiac sympathetic denervation that preceded the symptoms and diagnosis of PD by 4 years.[59]

However, MIBG and PET (6F-DA) scans cannot be performed on the general population. Additional research into the development of simpler sensitive and predictive autonomic tests is warranted.

Other Potential Premotor Screening Techniques

The drawback of many potential screening techniques is that they are not uniformly sensitive to the entire PD population. Current methods to identify undiagnosed PD patients based upon cardiovascular autonomic dysfunction recognize mostly those with OH. This leaves many PD patients undiagnosed. Yet both types of patients reportedly suffer from early cardiac sympathetic denervation (imaging studies have revealed denervation to be independent of OH).[3] The problem may be that tests which involve measurements reliant upon blood pressure, such as blood pressure recovery time or baroreflex-cardiovagal gain, are confounded by the exceptional ability of the cardiovascular system to compensate. For example, there are many ways that variables within the blood pressure equation could interact to mask the pathological loss of direct autonomic neuronal connections to the heart in PD, as blood pressure = cardiac output x total peripheral resistance.[46] Patients with OH may have suffered a severe enough insult to the system that compensation is not possible, and thus are positively identified by these screening techniques.

Heart rate (HR) may serve as a purer marker of changes in cardiac autonomic innervation, and thus screening techniques based upon this variable may be able to identify undiagnosed PD patients with and without OH. Studies have revealed that PD patients as a group exhibit decreased HR variability, a finding which is even apparent in de novo patients.[60–62] It is not yet possible to make conclusions on an individual scale, though, as HR variability is only functional for group assessment at the present time.[60] However, HR may still serve as a vital marker for recognizing the early onset of cardiac dysautonomia; heart transplant patients, whom also suffer from cardiac autonomic denervation, may provide insight into how.[46] Postoperatively, these patients must undergo extensive "warm up" and "cool down" periods before and after engaging in exercise.[46,63] This is due to the absence of direct autonomic connection to the heart.[46,63–65] Instead of rapid adjustments in HR, changes occur slowly over time due to the necessity of plasma catecholamine build up.[46,63–65] Time to reach peak HR in a heart transplant patient upon continuous exercise is reported to be prolonged (approximately 10 min).[46,63] This may prove to be an informative measurement of autonomic integrity in our patients as well. It is our hypothesis that time to reach peak HR will be prolonged in the PD and undiagnosed PD patient due to early cardiac sympathetic denervation.[46] If future studies reveal this hypothesis to be correct, screening could be accomplished by monitoring time to peak HR during cardiac stress tests, a procedure which is normally performed on patients of a similar age bracket as those with new onset PD.[46] Positive screens could then be referred for MIBG or PET (6FDA) imaging studies in a cost-effective manner.[46]

References

1. Micieli G, Tosi P, Marcheselli S, Cavallini A. Autonomic dysfunction in Parkinson's disease. *Neurol Sci.* 2003;24 Suppl 1:S32–4.

2. Mathias CJ. Cardiovascular autonomic dysfunction in Parkinson's disease and parkinsonian syndromes. In *Parkinson's disease*, ed Ebadi, Manuchair, and Ronald F. Pfeiffer, 295–317. 2005. Boca Raton, FL: CRC Press.

3. Goldstein, D.S. Cardiovascular autonomic dysfunction. In *Parkinson's disease and nonmotor dysfunction.* Pfeiffer Ronald F., and Bodis-Wollner I, eds. 149–157. 2005. Totowa, NJ: Humana Press.

4. Walter BL. Cardiovascular autonomic dysfunction in patients with movement disorders. *Cleve Clin J Med.* 2008;75 Suppl 2:S54–8.

5. Goldstein DS. Orthostatic hypotension as an early finding in Parkinson's disease. *Clin Auton Res.* 2006;16:46–54.

6. Michalowska M, Fiszer U, Krygowska-Wajs A, Owczarek K. Falls in Parkinson's disease: Causes and impact on patients' quality of life. *Funct Neurol.* 2005;20:163–168.

7. Martignoni E, Tassorelli C, Nappi G. Cardiovascular dysautonomia as a cause of falls in Parkinson's disease. *Parkinsonism Relat Disord.* 2006;12:195–204.

8. Consensus Committee of the American Autonomic Society and the American Academy of Neurology. Consensus statement on the definition of orthostatic hypotension, pure autonomic failure, and multiple system atrophy. *Neurology.* 1996;46:1470.

9. McLeod KA. Dysautonomia and neurocardiogenic syncope. *Curr Opin Cardiol.* 2001;16:92–96.

10. Medow MS, Stewart JM, Sanyal S, Mumtaz A, Sica D, Frishman WH. Pathophysiology, diagnosis, and treatment of orthostatic hypotension and vasovagal syncope. *Cardiol Rev.* 2008;16:4–20.

11. Linzer M, Yang EH, Estes NA III, Wang P, Vorperian VR, Kapoor WN. Diagnosing syncope. Part 1. Value of history, physical examination, and electrocardiography. Clinical efficacy assessment project of the American College of Physicians. *Ann Intern Med.* 1997;126:989–996.

12. Linzer M, Yang EH, Estes NA III, Wang P, Vorperian VR, Kapoor WN. Diagnosing syncope. Part 2: Unexplained syncope. Clinical efficacy assessment project of the American College of Physicians. *Ann Intern Med.* 1997;127:76–86.

13. Rocha EA. Neurally mediated syndromes. *Arq Bras Cardiol.* 2006;87:e34–44.

14. Grubb BP, Kosinski D. Dysautonomic and reflex syncope syndromes. *Cardiol Clin.* 1997;15:257–268.

15. Mohrman DE, Heller LJ. *Cardiovascular Physiology.* 6th ed. New York: McGraw-Hill Companies, Inc. 2006.

16. Saper CB. "All fall down": The mechanism of orthostatic hypotension in multiple systems atrophy and Parkinson's disease. *Ann Neurol.* 1998;43:149–151.

17. Benarroch EE. New findings on the neuropathology of multiple system atrophy. *Auton Neurosci.* 2002;96:59–62.

18. Kaufmann H, Oribe E, Miller M, Knott P, Wiltshire-Clement M, Yahr MD. Hypotension-induced vasopressin release distinguishes between pure autonomic failure and multiple system atrophy with autonomic failure. *Neurology.* 1992;42: 590–593.

19. Robertson D. The pathophysiology and diagnosis of orthostatic hypotension. *Clin Auton Res.* 2008;18 Suppl 1:2–7.

20. Benditt DG. Neurally mediated syncopal syndromes: Pathophysiological concepts and clinical evaluation. *Pacing Clin Electrophysiol.* 1997;20:572–584.

21. Kaufmann H. Neurally mediated syncope and syncope due to autonomic failure: Differences and similarities. *J Clin Neurophysiol.* 1997;14:183–196.

22. Papapetropoulos S, Mash DC. Insular pathology in Parkinson's disease patients with orthostatic hypotension. *Parkinsonism Relat Disord.* 2007;13:308–311.

23. Goldstein DS, Holmes C, Sharabi Y, Brentzel S, Eisenhofer G. Plasma levels of catechols and metanephrines in neurogenic orthostatic hypotension. *Neurology.* 2003;60:1327–1332.

24. Gai WP, Geffen LB, Denoroy L, Blessing WW. Loss of C1 and C3 epinephrine-synthesizing neurons in the medulla oblongata in Parkinson's disease. *Ann Neurol.* 1993;33:357–367.

25. Kato S, Oda M, Hayashi H, et al. Decrease of medullary catecholaminergic neurons in multiple system atrophy and Parkinson's disease and their preservation in amyotrophic lateral sclerosis. *J Neurol Sci.* 1995;132:216–221.

26. Goldstein DS, Eldadah BA, Holmes C, et al. Neurocirculatory abnormalities in Parkinson's disease with orthostatic hypotension: Independence from levodopa treatment. *Hypertension.* 2005;46:1333–1339.

27. Sharabi Y, Eldadah B, Li ST, et al. Neuropharmacologic distinction of neurogenic orthostatic hypotension syndromes. *Clin Neuropharmacol.* 2006;29:97–105.

28. Tipre DN, Goldstein DS. Cardiac and extracardiac sympathetic denervation in Parkinson's disease with orthostatic hypotension and in pure autonomic failure. *J Nucl Med.* 2005;46:1775–1781.

29. Takatsu H, Nishida H, Matsuo H, et al. Cardiac sympathetic denervation from the early stage of Parkinson's disease: Clinical and experimental studies with radiolabeled MIBG. *J Nucl Med.* 2000;41:71–77.

30. Courbon F, Brefel-Courbon C, Thalamas C, et al. Cardiac MIBG scintigraphy is a sensitive tool for detecting cardiac sympathetic denervation in Parkinson's disease. *Mov Disord.* 2003;18:890–897.

31. Goldstein DS, Holmes C, Li ST, Bruce S, Metman LV, Cannon RO III. Cardiac sympathetic denervation in Parkinson's disease. *Ann Intern Med.* 2000;133:338–347.

32. Orimo S, Ozawa E, Nakade S, Sugimoto T, Mizusawa H. (123)I-metaiodobenzylguanidine myocardial scintigraphy in Parkinson's disease. *J Neurol Neurosurg Psychiatry.* 1999;67:189–194.

33. Yoshita M, Hayashi M, Hirai S. Decreased myocardial accumulation of 123I-meta-iodobenzyl guanidine in Parkinson's disease. *Nucl Med Commun.* 1998;19:137–142.

34. Amino T, Orimo S, Itoh Y, Takahashi A, Uchihara T, Mizusawa H. Profound cardiac sympathetic denervation occurs in Parkinson's disease. *Brain Pathol.* 2005;15:29–34.

35. Li ST, Dendi R, Holmes C, Goldstein DS. Progressive loss of cardiac sympathetic innervation in Parkinson's disease. *Ann Neurol.* 2002;52:220–223.

36. Parry SW, Kenny RA. Tilt table testing in the diagnosis of unexplained syncope. *QJM.* 1999;92:623–629.

37. Polinsky RJ. Clinical autonomic neuropharmacology. *Neurol Clin.* 1990;8:77–92.

38. Senard JM, Rascol O, Durrieu G, et al. Effects of yohimbine on plasma catecholamine levels in orthostatic hypotension related to Parkinson's disease or multiple system atrophy. *Clin Neuropharmacol.* 1993;16:70–76.

39. Galinier M, Senard JM, Valet P, et al. Relationship between arterial blood pressure disturbances and alpha adrenoceptor density. *Clin Exp Hypertens.* 1994;16:373–389.

40. Barbic F, Perego F, Canesi M, et al. Early abnormalities of vascular and cardiac autonomic control in Parkinson's disease without orthostatic hypotension. *Hypertension.* 2007;49:120–126.

41. Hoffman BB. Adrenoceptor antagonist drugs. In: Katzung BG, ed. *Basic & Clinical Pharmacology.* 9th ed. New York: McGraw-Hill Companies, Inc. 2004:142.

42. Pappano AJ, Katzung BG. Cholinoceptor-blocking drugs. In: Katzung BG, ed. *Basic & Clinical Pharmacology.* 9th ed. New York: McGraw-Hill Companies, Inc.; 2004:109.

43. Polinsky RJ, Kopin IJ, Ebert MH, Weise V. Pharmacologic distinction of different orthostatic hypotension syndromes. *Neurology.* 1981;31:1–7.

44. Jordan J, Shannon JR, Biaggioni I, Norman R, Black BK, Robertson D. Contrasting actions of pressor agents in severe autonomic failure. *Am J Med.* 1998;105:116–124.

45. Shannon J, Jordan J, Costa F, Robertson RM, Biaggioni I. The hypertension of autonomic failure and its treatment. *Hypertension.* 1997;30:1062–1067.

46. Post KK, Singer C, Papapetropoulos S. Cardiac denervation and dysautonomia in Parkinson's disease: A review of screening techniques. *Parkinsonism Relat Disord.* 2008.

47. Benarroch EE, Smithson IL, Low PA, Parisi JE. Depletion of catecholaminergic neurons of the rostral ventrolateral medulla in multiple systems atrophy with autonomic failure. *Ann Neurol.* 1998;43:156–163.

48. Braak H, Sastre M, Bohl JR, de Vos RA, Del Tredici K. Parkinson's disease: Lesions in dorsal horn layer I, involvement of parasympathetic and sympathetic pre- and post-ganglionic neurons. *Acta Neuropathol (Berl).* 2007;113:421–429.

49. Johnson RH, Lee Gde J, Oppenheimer DR, Spalding JM. Autonomic failure with orthostatic hypotension due to intermediolateral column degeneration. A report of two cases with autopsies. *Q J Med.* 1966;35:276–292.

50. Bannister R, Oppenheimer DR. Degenerative diseases of the nervous system associated with autonomic failure. *Brain.* 1972;95:457–474.

51. Benarroch EE, Schmeichel AM, Parisi JE. Involvement of the ventrolateral medulla in parkinsonism with autonomic failure. *Neurology.* 2000;54:963–968.

52. Malessa S, Hirsch EC, Cervera P, Duyckaerts C, Agid Y. Catecholaminergic systems in the medulla oblongata in parkinsonian syndromes: A quantitative immunohistochemical

study in Parkinson's disease, progressive supranuclear palsy, and striatonigral degeneration. *Neurology.* 1990;40:1739–1743.

53. Saper CB, Sorrentino DM, German DC, de Lacalle S. Medullary catecholaminergic neurons in the normal human brain and in Parkinson's disease. *Ann Neurol.* 1991;29:577–584.

54. Vogel ER, Sandroni P, Low PA. Blood pressure recovery from Valsalva maneuver in patients with autonomic failure. *Neurology.* 2005;65:1533–1537.

55. Oka H, Yoshioka M, Onouchi K, et al. Characteristics of orthostatic hypotension in Parkinson's disease. *Brain.* 2007;130:2425–2432.

56. Senard JM, Valet P, Durrieu G, et al. Adrenergic supersensitivity in parkinsonians with orthostatic hypotension. *Eur J Clin Invest.* 1990;20:613–619.

57. Niimi Y, Ieda T, Hirayama M, et al. Clinical and physiological characteristics of autonomic failure with Parkinson's disease. *Clin Auton Res.* 1999;9:139–144.

58. Oka H, Mochio S, Onouchi K, Morita M, Yoshioka M, Inoue K. Cardiovascular dysautonomia in de novo Parkinson's disease. *J Neurol Sci.* 2006;241:59–65.

59. Goldstein DS, Sharabi Y, Karp BI, et al. Cardiac sympathetic denervation preceding motor signs in Parkinson's disease. *Clin Auton Res.* 2007;17:118–121.

60. Haapaniemi TH, Pursiainen V, Korpelainen JT, Huikuri HV, Sotaniemi KA, Myllyla VV. Ambulatory ECG and analysis of heart rate variability in Parkinson's disease. *J Neurol Neurosurg Psychiatry.* 2001;70:305–310.

61. Devos D, Kroumova M, Bordet R, et al. Heart rate variability and Parkinson's disease severity. *J Neural Transm.* 2003;110:997–1011.

62. Pursiainen V, Haapaniemi TH, Korpelainen JT, Huikuri HV, Sotaniemi KA, Myllyla VV. Circadian heart rate variability in Parkinson's disease. *J Neurol.* 2002;249:1535–1540.

63. Thompson CJ. Denervation of the transplanted heart: Nursing implications for patient care. *Crit Care Nurs Q.* 1995;17:1–14.

64. Shephard RJ. Responses of the cardiac transplant patient to exercise and training. *Exerc Sport Sci Rev.* 1992;20:297–320.

65. Cooper DKC, Lanza RP, eds. Heart Transplantation: The Present Status of Orthotopic and Heterotopic Heart Transplantation. Lancaster, MA: MTP Press Limited; 1984.

Chapter 6

Lesions Associated with Pain and Sensory Abnormalities

Andreas Hartmann and Glenda M. Halliday

Introduction

Intuitively, we consider Parkinson's disease (PD) as a motor disorder (similarly to amyotrophic lateral sclerosis as a 'pure' motorneuron disorder) and thus, the 'opposite' of a sensory disorder. However, as with many non-motor and non-dopaminergic signs in PD (which are not necessarily equivalent!), sensory dysfunction in PD is gaining renewed attention, although it probably remains the most under-recognized and under-treated of the parkinsonian non-motor symptoms.

Pain Receptors and Pathways

The perception of pain differs from other sensory perceptions in that it is both a discriminative sensation and a behavioral drive,[1] with both of these influenced by memories, and emotional, pathological, genetic and cognitive factors. This complexity has lead to the concept of central pain processing through a 'pain matrix' where cortical and subcortical structures influence critical brainstem regions to modify peripheral sensations, ensuring that any painful experience is appropriate for the circumstance.[2]

This top-down integration can be disrupted via both bottom-up and top-down influences to contribute to the generation and maintenance of a heightened pain experience.

Nociceptors are free nerve endings of pseudo-unipolar neurons located in dorsal root or trigemenal ganglia that can detect mechanical, thermal or chemical tissue changes above certain thresholds. Two types of nociceptor fibers (fast myelinated Aδ fibers and slow unmyelinated C fibers) transmit peripheral information on the physiological status of tissues (both damaging and innocuous) directly to their nearest spinal trigeminal or spinal cord segment level.[1] Aδ fibers directly transfer peripheral information somatotopically, but only the summated activity of C nociceptors causes conscious pain perception in humans, as many C fibers relay information on ongoing tissue metabolic status.[1] The peripheral information includes temperature, local metabolism (acidic pH, hypoxia, hypoglycemia, hypoosmolarity, lactic acid), cell rupture (potassium, ATP, glutamate), parasite penetration (histamines, proteinases), mast cell activation (serotonin, bradykinin, eicosanoids), and immune and hormonal activity (cytokines, somatostatin). Within the spinal cord and brainstem two types of nociceptive neurons collect information for relay to higher centers—one specific for the type of information (lamina 1 nociceptor-specific neurons) and one collecting multimodal information from the same region (lamina V polymodal neurons).[1] This second type of neuron can be viewed as integrating the convergent intensity of the stimulus.

This nociceptor information ascends to the thalamus through the spinothalamic tract and to the medulla and brainstem through spinoreticular and spinomesencephalic tracts (Figure 6-1). The thalamus is a major center for pain processing, with ongoing projections to critical forebrain and spinal regions (Figure 6-1). Brainstem regions are now thought to be the critical integration center for nociception with homeostatic, arousal, and autonomic processes, as well as to convey processed information back to the spinal cord and to forebrain regions (Figure 6-1).[2]

A variety of other brain regions can also influence pain perception. A meta-analysis of human data identified primary and secondary somatosensory, insular, anterior cingulate, and prefrontal cortices as commonly active during acute pain (Figure 6-1).[3] Other regions such as the basal ganglia, cerebellum, amygdala, hippocampus and areas within parietal and temporal cortices can also be active depending on the set of circumstances. These brain regions modulate pain perception through a descending system which includes the frontal lobe, anterior cingulate cortex, insula, amygdala, hypothalamus, periaqueductal grey, cuneiformis nucleus, and rostral ventromedial medulla (Figure 6-1).[2] Brain activation to pain can be modified by endogenous opioids and dopamine pathways.[2]

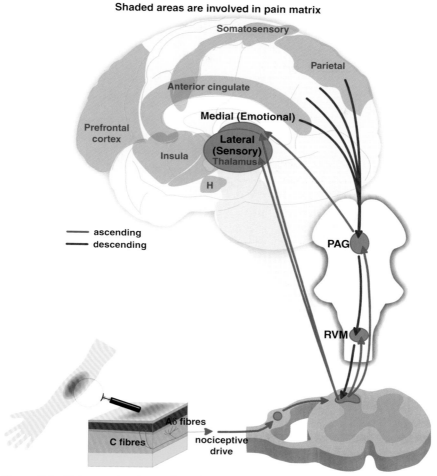

Figure 6-1. Main neural pathways for pain perception. Peripheral nociceptor fiber endings in the skin transmit painful stimuli to the dorsal horn of the spinal cord. This nociceptor information ascends to the thalamus through the spinothalamic tract and to the medulla and brainstem through spinoreticular and spinomesencephalic tracts. The thalamus is a major center for processing the sensory and emotional aspects of painful stimuli, with ongoing projections to critical forebrain and spinal regions that form the pain matrix of cortical and subcortical structures which influence the critical brainstem regions to modify peripheral sensations and ensure that any painful experience is appropriate for the circumstance. These regions include the primary and secondary somatosensory, insular, anterior cingulate, prefrontal, parietal and hippocampal cortices. H = hippocampus, PAG = periaqueductal grey area, RVM = rostral ventromedial medulla.

Recent data suggest that in chronic pain syndromes there is more substantive structural remodeling of the brain. A meta-analysis identified decreased grey matter in the cingulate, orbitofrontal and insular cortices, and ventral midbrain as common to a variety of pain syndromes.[4] These regions are associated with pain surpression, and whether this neural plasticity is a cause or consequence, or can be considered degenerative, needs further evaluation.

Sensory Abnormalities in PD

Sensory abnormalities in PD are multiple. Prominently, there is kinaesthesia, which refers to the conscious awareness of limb position and plays an important role in planning and controlling voluntary movement. It is both dependent on proprioception[5] and central integration of proprioceptive signals; this integration likely occurs at the basal ganglia level.[6] Impaired kinaesthesia may have several deleterious consequences for PD patients but these are rather motor than non-motor, i.e. impaired fine-tuning of movement, postural instability, falls, or dyskinesia.

Peripheral sensory abnormalities in parkinsonian patients have been reported, namely a possible association between PARK2 (parkin) mutations and peripheral neuropathy.[7-9] Possibly, similar associations will be detected in other forms of familial PD. In a recent intriguing study, skin biopsies were obtained from 18 PD patients, 3 with paresthesia and 3 with burning feet, the remaining 12 being symptom-free on the sensory level.[10] Compared to 30 controls, the PD patients had a significant increase in tactile and thermal thresholds and a significant reduction in mechanical pain perception. Accordingly, on the anatomical level, PD patients had less nociceptors than controls.[10] These findings are intriguing because they suggest both a peripheral deafferentation in PD and a relative insensitivity to pain, contrasting with several other reports (see below).

A Brief History of Pain in PD

In this chapter we will focus on pain, which is likely the most debilitating sensory abnormality in PD. Pain as a prominent feature of PD had already been recognized by James Parkinson in his original 1817 essay, where the term 'pain' appears 21 times.[11] In 1877 Charcot, who renamed the 'shaking palsy' after its describer, reported neuropathic and rheumatologic pains in PD patients.[12] A similar observation was made in 1888 by Gowers who commented on aching pains in the limbs, 'rheumatic' in character.[13]

In 1911, Mendel observed a multitude of paraesthetic sensations in PD patients.[14] In 1921 Souques was the first to suggest that parkinsonian pain might be of central origin in some cases, caused by alterations in the connections between the striatum and suboptic region within the thalamus.[15]

Yet, as with many other non-motor symptoms, pain was somewhat referred backstage with the advent of pharmacological and surgical therapies in the late 1940s and 1950s. A notable exception was the study by Sigwald and Solignac (1960), who described painful sensations in 108 out of 213 PD patients.[16] Painful manifestations were subdivided into paresthesias (cramps and restlessness) and pain symptoms, which were catalogued according to affected body regions (legs, arms, neck, lumbar region, epigastrium, abdomen), but not to the type of pain (burning pain, cold numbness, cramping or 'arthritic' pain).

The introduction of levodopa in the late 1960s was a double-edged sword with regard to pain in PD: levodopa was both able to alleviate certain types of PD-related pain, mainly those related to off-conditions; but it also caused, in the middle and long term, pain syndromes related to motor complications, i.e., fluctuations.

Between 1976 and 1986, five seminal papers looked into pain in PD. Snider et al reported that 43 out of 101 PD patients described spontaneus abnormal sensations, e.g. either burning or pain, which preceded the onset of motor symptoms in 9% of the total population studied.[17] The latter was often described as poorly localized, albeit more frequent in the affected limb(s). Importantly, patients with arthritis and diabetes were excluded from this study. Painful muscle cramps or spasms were discarded as secondary to the motor symptoms; all other painful symptoms were considered as primary parkinsonian sensations. Thus, the authors suggested that parkinsonian pain was directly related to central nervous system (CNS) dysfunction and not to the peripheral motor symptoms of the disease.

In 1984 Koller studied 50 PD patients, out of whom 19 had sensory complaints.[18] Similarly to Snider et al,[17] patients with arthritis, musculoskeletal disease, or diabetes were excluded from the study and all abnormal sensations were considered 'primary'. He further showed that nerve conduction velocities and sensory-evoked potentials were normal in his PD patient cohort, thus indicating a central rather than peripheral (neuropathic or other) origin of these symptoms. Koller speculated that these pains might be related to the nigrostriatal pathology and/or treatment of pain signals in the striatum or the insula.[18]

The possible existence of a 'central' parkinsonian pain was also raised by Schott in 1985 based on the examination of 3 PD patients and discussed with regard to the role of dopaminergic pathways on pain modulation.[19] Schott also underlined that pain may be a symptom *preceding* motor abnormalities in PD, often localized to the shoulder or affected arm.[19] Recent reports suggest that up to 11% of patients with PD have significant shoulder pain, with 20% of these patients presenting with significant shoulder pain prior to the onset of PD.[20]

In 1986 Goetz et al surveyed 95 PD patients and asked them to describe the frequency, duration, character, location, and temporal qualities of pain.[21] Pain was classified into musculoskeletal, dystonic, and 'thalamic', i.e., central. Of the patients surveyed, 46% (43/95) indeed suffered from pain: muscle cramps or tightness (74%), painful dysonia (28%), joint pains (14%), radicular or neuritic pain (14%), and diffuse generalized pain considered akathitic (2%). Pain symptoms reminiscent of a central, 'thalamic' origin were not observed in this study. Since pain was associated with the worsening of PD motor symptoms in 89% of cases, Goetz et al concluded that parkinsonian pain is mainly controllable by dopaminergic medication.[21]

Quinn et al[22] proposed a classification of parkinsonian pain clearly related to motor status and medication intake, into 4 types: (1) presymptomatic, (2) non-dystonic off, (3) dystonic off, and (4) peak-dose-related. Thus, similar to Goetz et al,[21] these authors rather dismissed the idea of central pain in PD, since in almost all of their cases (44 outpatients) pain fluctuated in parallel with the motor changes associated with levodopa treatment.

Epidemiology of Pain in PD

The frequency of pain syndromes in PD has been estimated between 40–75%,[23] although more recent studies have estimated the prevalence as even higher.[24] Out of these, 10–30% of pain syndromes cannot be explained by motor status and medication intake and are therefore considered 'central'. A recent retrospective study on 388 consecutive patients assessed in Lausanne, Switzerland, indicated that two-thirds of PD patients (68.8%) suffered from some form of pain.[25] Patients received an auto-questionnaire on which they were asked to categorize pain as follows: muscular (94%), rheumatologic (51%), neurogenic (16%) or others (akathisia, restless legs syndrome – 10%). The results showed that 90% of painful sensation appeared in the off phase, with maximum intensity always on the most affected body side. Also, 26% of patients experienced pain in early disease stages. There were no correlations of pain with age, gender, disease duration, disease stage, levodopa equivalent doses, dysautonomic symptoms, sleep disturbances, or depression. A recent comparison of 450 PD patients and 98 patients with other chronic disorders showed that chronic pain was twice as frequent in PD after adjusting for osteo-articular comorbidities.[26]

In this comparison, 25% of PD patients had acute pain, 26% had chronic pain unrelated to PD (mainly oesteoarthritis), and 40% had chronic pain related to PD. Those with chronic PD pain were younger at PD onset, had more motor complications and severe depressive symptoms than those without.[26,27] They less frequently reported their pain to doctors so were less likely to receive analgesic medication.[26]

Categories of Pain in PD

Categorizing pain in PD can be done according to different criteria:

- Type of pain[23]: (1) dystonic (associated with movements and posture); (2) musculoskeletal/rheumatic (aching, cramping, arthraltic joint); (3) neuritic/radicular (pain in the territory of a nerve/root); (4) akathitic discomfort; (5) primary/central (burning, tingling, formication, bizarre quality) (Table 6-1).
- Kinetics of pain: preceding and/or occuring with the initial motor signs; in the intermediate stages and late stages. Pain in PD is associated with the degree of motor complications[28]; this applies both to dystonic and non-dystonic pain. Therefore, pain can be expected to increase with disease duration, as indeed shown by regression analysis.[28] Off dystonia and biphasic dyskinesia can both cause significant pain, whereas peak-dose dykinesias are usually (but not always) less painful.[29]

For practical purposes (management, see below), the relation of pain syndromes to dopaminergic 'state', as initially proposed by Quinn,[22] is helpful. From a pathophysiological point of view, the classification by Ford[23] into peripheral mechanical pain (types 1-4) and central neurological pain (type 5) (Table 6-1) remains the most practical to date. In the present chapter, we will focus on central neurological pain or primary parkinsonian pain (PPP) as the most elusive and under-recognized pain syndrome in PD. Also, PPP, in contrast to peripheral mechanical pain, is both dopaminergic and non-dopaminergic in origin (Figure 6-2).

Primary Parkinsonian Pain (PPP)

PPP is difficult to clearly characterize clinically; it includes bizarre unexplained sensations of stabbing, burning, scalding, and formication, all quite similar to neuropathic pain originating from the periphery.[23] Although these pains occur typically in the more affected body sides, their location

Table 6-1. Classification of Painful Sensations in PD

Pain Category	Clinical Description	Etiology	Comments
Musculoskeletal	Aching, cramping, arthralgic, myalgic sensations. May be associated with muscle tenderness, arthritic changes, skeletal deformities and limited joint mobility. May be exacerbated by rigidity, stiffness, immobility. May improve with dopaminergic medication and exercise. May fluctuate with medication status.	Parkinsonian rigidity. Associated rheumatologic disease or skeletal deformity.	Frozen shoulder as presenting PD symptom.
Radicular-neuropathic	Pain in the territory of a root or nerve or in a neuropathic distribution.	Associated with root lesion, focal or peripheral neuropathy.	
Dystonic	Associated with dystonic movements and postures. May fluctuate with medication status.	Off period dystonia (includes early morning dystonia). Diphasic (beginning and end of dose) dyskynesia. Peak dose dyskinesia.	Dystonic foot as presenting PD symptom.
Akathisia	Subjective sensation of restlessness or intolerance of remaining still. Objective signs of restless behavior. May fluctuate with medication status. May improve with dopaminergic medication.	Off period ('parkinsonian') related. Drug-induced (neuroleptics).	Shares some phenomenological similarities with RLS.
Central ('primary') pain	Burning, tingling, formication. Relentless, bizarre quality. Location not confined to root or nerve territory. Not explained by rigidity or dystonia. May fluctuate with medication status.	Unknown.	

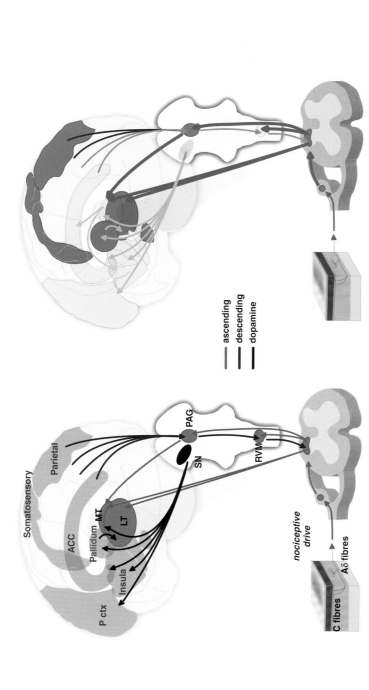

Figure 6-2. Pain pathways in PD. Left side = normal pathways, right side = PD. The peripheral nerve fibers in PD patients have abnormal α-synuclein accumulations and this intraneural pathology appears to trigger an increase in central signaling from dorsal root ganglia neurons. This, in association with an early loss of dopamine regulation of the pain matrix and a loss of the medullary pain relay centers, heightens ascending spinal pain signaling in PD. Over the disease course, these changes impact on the pain matrix itself, further diminishing its ability to modulate an intact lateral pain system (LT). ACC=anterior cingulate cortex, LT=lateral sensory thalamic relay, MT=medial emotional thalamic relay, P ctx=prefrontal cortex, PAG=periaqueductal grey area, RVM=rostral ventromedial medulla, SN=dopaminergic substantia nigra.

149

is unusual insofar as they involve areas in which painful dystonia or musculoskeletal conditions are unlikely or implausible, i.e., the face, head, epigastrium, abdomen, pelvis, rectum, and genitalia.[23] Oral pain syndromes remiscent of the 'burning mouth syndrome' have also been described; they tend to correlate with off periods but are not necessarily abolished by dopaminergic therapy.[30] Moreover, these pains are not abolished by peripheral nerve blocks, supporting a CNS origin.[31]

An initial report described that levodopa administration in PD increased heat pain thresholds and tolerance.[32] Three decades later, Djaldetti et al compared heat pain thresholds in 36 PD patients with predominantly unilateral disease to 28 controls.[33] In the PD group, 28 patients experienced spontaneous pain, whereas the remaining 8 did not. The initial hypothesis was that parkinsonian pain is similar to post-stroke central pain which is caused by lesions of the thalamus or spinothalamocortical pathways and is associated with elevation of heat pain thresholds. Suprisingly, however, the researchers found an increase in thermal pain sensitivity in PD patients, especially in those suffering from spontaneous pain. Also, heat pain thresholds were lower in the affected compared to the non-affected limbs. However, no correlation of heat pain thresholds with on/off states was observed in patients with response fluctuations (n=15); the authors therefore concluded that heat pain thresholds were insensitive to levodopa. A further study of 50 PD patients who had a stable levodopa response (n=12) or were fluctuators (n=15) or dyskinetic (n=23), used cold water immersion and levodopa challenge to show that all PD patients off medication have low cold pain thresholds and tolerance, but following levodopa adminstration this is ameliorated only in dyskinetic patients.[34] This supports a role for dopamine modulation of pain pathways in patients with advanced disease.

Brefel-Courbon et al[35] examined 9 PD patients and 9 controls with regard to their pain thresholds after thermal stimulation, which consisted of the cold pressor test, thus differing from the heat pain paradigm used by Djaldetti et al.[33] Also, they only included patients who did not complain of spontaneous pain. Thermal stimulation was done in off and on conditions (after levodopa administration) and combined with $H_2^{15}O$ positron emission tomography (PET). They found decreased pain thresholds in PD patients compared to controls, as had Djaldetti et al.[33] However, in contrast to the previous study, they observed that levodopa administration increased pain thresholds. In addition, they administered levodopa to control subjects, where it had no effect on pain thresholds, suggesting that a certain degree of nigrostriatal denervation is necessary to produce an analgetic effect by central dopamine. Finally, they measured a significant increase in pain-induced activation in the ipsilateral insula and ipsilateral prefrontal cortex, as well as in the contralateral anterior cingulate cortex in PD patients compared to controls. Levodopa was effective in decreasing activation in the insula and the anterior cingulate cortex. These areas are strongly connected with the basal ganglia and also receive direct dopaminergic projections from the midbrain, thus lending support to a central dopaminergic mediation of pain.[36] A dopamine receptor 2 (D2) PET activation study by Scott et al demonstrates increased basal ganglia dopamine transmission in response to pain, and also increased mesolimbic dopamine transmission with increased emotion and fear in response to pain. In agreement with the clinical observation by Djaldetti et al,[33] Brefel-Courbon et al[35] did not detect any thalamic activation in their PET aquisitions.

In an extension of this initial study, Slaoui et al included heat threshold testing, albeit without nuclear imaging.[37] Next, Gerdelat-Mas et al[38] demonstrated that the *objective* pain threshold (assessed by the nociceptive flexion reflex – RIII) was decreased in 13 PD patients compared to 10 controls, since previous studies[33,35] had relied on measuring subjective pain thresholds. As previously shown using the the cold pressor test,[35] levodopa was able to increase pain thresholds in the PD but not in the control group. Using another kind of objective pain measurement—scalp CO_2 laser evoked potentials to hand skin stimulation—Tinazzi et al found, in 18 pain-free PD patients compared to 18 controls, that the N2/P2 peak-to-peak amplitude was reduced in the PD group, regardless of affected body side or medication state (on/off; but only 7 patients tested).[39] They concluded that there exists an abnormal nociceptive input in PD patients compared to controls. Interestingly, the N2/P2 potentials are thought to originate from the cingulate gyrus and insula, cortical structures indentified previously by Brefel-Courbon et al[35] in their $H_2{}^{15}O$ PET study, and regions known to influence pain perception (see above).

Is Every Type of Pain Disabling and Thus Worthy of Treatment?

In recent years, it has been recognized that dyskinesias, especially peak-dose dykinesias, do not necessarily affect health-related quality of life (HRQOL) in PD patients; thus, we now speak of 'disabling' vs. 'non-disabling' dyskinesia.[40] Concerning sensory abnormalities in PD, the same perspective probably applies: not every tingling or paraesthesia requires special attention and treatment. However, most would agree that pain is a symptom that is not easily dismissed. Accordingly, Rahman et al, in a series of 130 consecutive PD patients, using the PDQ-39 questionnaire, confirmed that HRQOL is significantly diminished in PD patients affected by pain.[41] Quittenbaum and Grahn submitted auto-questionaires (SF-36, visual analogue pain scales, pain drawing and pain-specific questions) to 57 PD patients and 95 controls.[42] About two-thirds of PD patients complained of pain, and HRQOL was significantly decreased in the PD group due to pain. A case-control study shows that the overall frequency of pain is significantly greater in PD due to dystonic pain, but there is a significant association between PD and non-dystonic pain, beginning after the onset of symptoms.[43]

As a general rule, it appears that pain overtakes motor or other non-motor symptoms (especially depression) as a distressing factor only in a minority of patients. Moreover, since most painful parkinsonian states are related to motor status and/or medication intake, pain therapy in PD parallels therapy of motor disturbances (see below). However, patients presenting with PPP are likely an under-recognized and under-served community. Therefore, careful history taking and examination is crucial in these patients; and therapy, for now, based mostly on a case-to-case approach (see below).

Is Pain Necessarily Deleterious as Long as Akinesia/Bradykinesia Persists?

From a conceptual point of view, we must ask whether decreased pain thresholds in PD are not useful as long as satisfactory motor functions have not been re-established. In other words, prolonged reaction times due to akinesia/bradykinesia may favor a decreased pain threshold to effectively counter noxious/dangerous stimuli. Therefore, levodopa's ability to raise pain thresholds and improve motor function may not be co-incidental.[44]

Pathology in Pain Pathways in Parkinson's Disease

As described earlier, peripheral neuropathy occurs in parkinsonian patients, particularly those with PARK2 (parkin) mutations,[7–9] but also in sporadic PD patients with peripheral sensory abnormalities and a reduction in the numbers of peripheral nociceptors.[10] In a recent study of 142 autopsied cases, the accumulation of phosphorylated α-synuclein in peripheral nerves from skin biopsies has been reported in 70% of patients with PD and not in patients with multiple system atrophy, progressive supranuclear palsy or corticobasal degeneration, so-called 'parkinson plus' syndromes.[45] The use of phosphorylated α-synuclein deposition in skin biopsies has been suggested as a highly specific and useful biomarker for PD, based on the frequency of this pathology in PD. It also suggests that remaining peripheral nerve endings contain significant abnormalities.[45]

In patients with PD, abnormal accumulation of α-synuclein occurs in a proportion of one of the 3 types of projection neurons found in lamina 1 of the spinal cord with significant deposition in the terminal arbors of peripheral spinal nerves innervating this region of the spinal cord.[46,47] Although only limited PD specimens have been assessed, this pathology is in general greater at caudal compared with rostral spinal segments.[47] Lamina 1 neurons are not affected in patients with preclinical disease and lamina 5 neurons are largely unaffected at any disease stage.[46,47] These studies suggest that over the course of PD, degenerative changes occur in a selective population of centrally-projecting spinal neurons integrating peripheral pain, particularly from the lower body.

A few critical brainstem regions modify peripheral sensations, ensuring that any painful experience is appropriate for the circumstance.[2] Lamina 1 neurons in the spinal cord rapidly excite two brainstem regions—the parabrachial area and periaqueductal gray (PAG). The parabrachial area coordinates appropriate changes in breathing through various pathways.[48] Projections from the PAG to the nucleus raphe magnus and adjacent structures of the rostral ventromedial medulla (RVM) and then onto the spinal dorsal horn, constitute the descending control of the pain matrix.[2] No significant pathology has been described in the parabrachial area or PAG of patients with PD (apart from the involvement of nearby catecholamine neurons), but substantial pathology occurs in the medullary raphe and RVM. In addition to significant α-synuclein deposition in these medullary regions, there is a significant loss of neurons in the medullary raphe.[49–51] Neurodegeneration in this region occurs early in the preclinical phase,[49] suggesting an early loss of decending control over painful stimuli.

Rapid integration of painful stimuli also occurs in the thalamus with information processed in two systems—a lateral (ventral posterior thalamus with somatosensory and parietal relays) and a medial (midline and intralaminar thalamus with prefrontal and anterior cingulate relays) system. The lateral pain system is thought to be responsible for the sensory aspects of pain such as its location and duration,[52] and this system shows no substantial α-synuclein pathology or neurodegeneration at either the thalamic or cortical levels in PD.[53] The medial pain system is thought to be responsible for the more emotional aspects of pain, such as how unpleasant the pain feels,[51] and by end stage PD there is significant deposition of α-synuclein mainly in Lewy neurites in most of the midline and intralaminar thalamic nuclei,[53] although only the parafascicular nucleus has any loss of neurons (~50% loss[54]). Additionally, the anterior cingulate and insular cortices and amygdala are predeliction sites for intraneuronal Lewy body formation,[50] suggesting abnormalities in higher order neurons in the medial pain system. These changes occur following the onset of motor symptoms in PD[50] and are not accompanied by major neuronal loss.[55] This indicates that degenerative changes are restricted to the emotional medial pain system with substantial pathology in higher order processing centers which appear to impact on midline and intralaminar thalamic neurons integrating pain.

Pathophysiology

As stated above, there is considerable pathology in only certain brain regions integrating painful stimuli. While peripheral deafferentation may suggest less sensitivity to pain, the peripheral nerve fibers with abnormal α-synuclein accumulations are still *in situ* and this intraneural pathology may itself trigger abnormal central signaling from dorsal root ganglia neurons. This is consistent with normal conduction velocities along peripheral and central pain pathways in PD patients with or without PPP.[56] Degenerative changes of peripheral nerve endings prior to abnormalities in the neuronal cell bodies within peripheral ganglia occurs in cardiac nerves in PD[57] as well as being a hallmark of the degenerative changes centrally (dopaminergic terminal degeneration in the basal ganglia causing the symptoms of PD occurs prior to degeneration of their neuronal cell bodies[58,59]). In this latter senario of distal-dominant degeneration, PD patients would have constant stimulation of their peripheral nociceptors. This in association with an early loss of descending analgesic control due to the degeneration of medullary relay centers suggests a heightened spinal pain signaling in PD. Over the disease course, these changes appear to impact on pathways in the pain matrix mediating the emotional context of pain, regions identified in human imaging studies as more highly active in people with pathological tissue damage[60] and regions that undergo significant atrophy in all forms of chronic pain syndromes.[4] Thus with time it appears that PD patients have less ability to modulate this heightened sense of pain within the pain matrix with an intact and unchecked lateral pain system clearly able to identify the site and intensity of peripheral pain signals (Figure 6-2).

In addition to this impact on primary pain pathways, over time neuronal degeneration in PD affects noradrenergic, serotoninergic, cholinergic, and peptidergic neurons. The locus ceruleus (LC) contains the largest group of noradrenergic neurons in the CNS. Noradrenergic fibers from the LC and A5/A7 groups of noradrenergic neurons in the pontine tegmentum innervate the medullary RVM and the dorsal horn of the spinal cord where they inhibit the ascending nociceptive pathways. Overall, these changes in PD would amplify further heightened spinal pain.

Management of Pain in PD

A careful history taking and examination should reveal whether pain is related to the cardinal PD symptoms and whether antiparkinsonian medications induce, relieve or exarcerbate pain. Clearly, the first step is to treat PD, i.e., to optimize treatment with dopaminergic agents, for two reasons. First, to avoid pain related to motor fluctuations (both high and low levodopa-associated states). Second, in case of low dopaminergic innervation, to raise thresholds for central basal ganglia pain.[35] Unfortunately, there are very few studies that systematically investigate treatment either of peripheral mechanical pain in PD or of PPP. A crucial question remains as to whether levodopa and dopamine agonists are equivalent in controlling PPP. Theroretically, dopamine is also converted into noradrenaline, which probably plays a role in pain generation: therefore, levodopa (and subsequently dopamine in the CNS) may be superior to dopamine agonists in PPP control. However, the special role played by basal ganglia D2 receptors[61] suggests that dopamine agonists with special affinity for these receptors may be a better choice. Controlled clinical trials are warranted to answer this question.

For the treatment of PD-related motor fluctuations and dyskinesia, we refer to the review by Pahwa et al.[62] An overview of pharmacological interventions related to dopaminergic state in non-PPP are summarized in Tables 6-2a and 6-2b.

PPP Management

As stated, PPP can respond to dopaminergic medication. However, if pain persists despite optimal dopaminergic therapy, the following options need to be considered.

First, is the patient depressed? Depression can significantly augment the subjective feeling of pain; and conversely, chronic pain can favor depression, ultimately engaging a vicious cycle. Cantello et al reported that IV methylphenidate may improve primary sensory symptoms in PD.[63] Since the effects of methylphenidate could be blocked by adrenergic and serotonergic antagonists, these findings suggest a role for noradrenaline and serotonin in PPP, apart from their role in the pathogenesis of depression. In addition, degeneration of brainstem noradrenergic and

Table 6-2a. Treatment of Pain Related to Low Dopaminergic State

	Comments	Pharmacotherapy	Surgery	Others
Off period dystonia	Correlates with dopaminergic deficiency states. Often the first PD symptom (frozen shoulder, dystonic foot). After therapy initiation, occurs often in the morning before first medication intake; or as part of wearing off phenomena during the day. Writer's cramp as an initial complaint in PD.[77]	*Optimize (increase) dopaminergic treatment.* Levodopa Dopamine agonists: pramipexole, ropinirole, rotigotine, apomorphine COMT inhibitors: entacapone, tolcapone MAO-B inhibitors: Selegiline, rasagiline. In advanced cases: continuous dopaminergic stimulation; either by apomorphine infusions[78] s.c. or duodenal levodopa infusions.[79] *Others :* Lithium[80] Baclofen[31, 81]	*Reserved for advanced cases:* Abolition of dystonia and pain 12/24 PD patients after pallidotomy (radiosurgery).[82] Major reduction in pain and discomfort scores in 9/12 PD patients after pallidotomy.[83] Major relief from off period dystonia in 5/9 PD patients after GPi DBS.[84] Complete relief in 12/16 PD patients and decrease in 4/16 PD patients from off period dystonia after STN DBS.[85] Improvement of dystonia (-90%) and pain (-66%) in 8 PD patients after STN DBS.[86] 16 PD patients with advanced PD treated by GPi DBS. Improvement at 1 year post-surgery for contralateral off period dystonia in 100%, cramps by 74% and dysaesthesia in 100%.[72]	Activity partly relieves early morning dystonia. Rehabilitation/physical therapy. NSAIDs/analgesics Botulinum toxin: pain relief in 67% of patients for 3-4 months post-injection.[87]

Diphasic dyskinesia	Painful dystonia occurs at the beginning and/or the end of efficacy of dopaminergic treatment (threshold between on and off states).	Mantain patient above off threshold. In practice increase individual doses of dopaminergic treatment and maintain these levels (COMT inhibitors; long acting dopamine agonists).	Effective on diphasic dyskinesias by virtue of a continuous, levodopa-mimicking effect.	In advanced cases: continuous dopaminergic stimulation; either by apomorphine infusions s.c. or levodopa infusions (duodenal).
Pseudoradicul-opathy	Radicular pain distribution. Often (but not always) associated with severe limb rigidity.	If associated with rigidity, optimize (increase) dopaminergic treatment. In refractory cases, consider NSAIDs, gabapentin and tricyclic antidepressants.		In severe refractory cases: spinal analgesia for levodopa-associated leg pain.[88]
Trigeminal-neuralgia-like pain	Associated with off periods.[89]	Optimize (increase) dopaminergic treatment.		
Akathisia	Patient feels that he/she will not be able to take another breath. Sometimes accompanied by anxiety. Usually observed during off periods.	Optimize (increase) dopaminergic treatment. Clozapine.[90]		Check for 'hidden' neuroleptics, i.e. some anti-emetics.
Sensory dyspnea		Optimize (increase) dopaminergic treatment.		
Abdominal pain	Associated with abdominal spasms or dystonia.	Optimize (increase) dopaminergic treatment.		

Table 6-2b. Treatment of Pain Related to High Dopaminergic State

	Comments	Pharmacotherapy	Surgery	Others
Peak dose dyskinesia	Choreatic in nature. Becomes painful ('disabling') when excessive range of motion cause muscular and/or joint pains. Radicular and neuritic pain exacerbations.[21]	*Optimize (decrease) dopaminergic treatment.* In practice, dopaminergic treatment needs to be fractioned into smaller individual doses. Care must be taken to avoid biphasic dyskinesias by lowering dopaminergic medication below the off threshold. Amantadine.[91] Clozapine.[92] Tricyclic antidepressants and/or gabapentin for neuropathic pain.	Both GPi and STN DBS are effective in reducing peak dose dyskinesia; first, through a reduction in concomittant levodopa dosage and second, through a 'direct' antidyskinetic effect (GPi DBS).[93]	
Peak dose dystonia	Usually associated with neck and facial dystonia but may spread to the limbs.[22, 94]	Optimize (decrease) dopaminergic treatment.		
Abdominal symptoms	Levodopa and dopamine agonists may cause abdominal cramping, bloating and nausea.	Optimize (decrease) dopaminergic treatment.		

serotonergic systems is an early event in the progression of parkinsonian neurodegeneration.[50] Therefore, clinical trials with norepinephrine reuptake blockers (e.g., desipramine and venlafaxine) may reduce pain in early cases in which some neurons are preserved, in addition to managing the depression that is common in these patients. In patients with advanced disease in which few descending noradrenergic neurons may remain, adrenergic agonists such as epidural or systemic clonidine might be considered [64] although they may potentiate orthostasis.

The potential involvement of the cholinergic system in PPP is less clear. In one study, Sandyk reported that benzhexol, an anticholinergic, relieved pain in PD patients refractory to oral narcotics, NSAIDs, and levodopa.[65] However, care must be taken when using anticholinergics in PD patients: they may, as a positive side (or primary) effect alleviate tremor, but may also cause cognitive impairment and confusion, especially in elderly patients.

'Neuropathic' types of pain may respond well to tricyclic antidepressants [66] with the additional advantage of relieving any concomittant depression. However, this class of drugs offers a side effect profile that is inferior to serotonin and noradrenaline reuptake inhibitors. Other medications that have proven efficient in treating neuropathic pain, most prominently gabapentin and pregabalin, may prove helpful.[67]

Oral/genital pain syndromes in PD have responded to atypical neuroleptics, e.g., clozapine.[31] The fact that these drugs act preferentially on D_3/D_4 receptors underlines the selectivity of certain pain syndromes to dopaminergic subtypes involved.[36] However, clozapine is known to exert effects on other receptor types as well, such as 5-HT2a receptors.[68]

In a high number of PD patients, abdominal discomfort/pain is due to constipation; although not strictly corresponding to PPP, these pain syndromes may be exacerbated by enhanced pain perception. In these patients, the use of laxatives[69] should be considered in addition to other interventions focused on reducing pain perception. Also, non-pharmacologic interventions (relaxation techniques etc.) should not be disregarded, especially when coupled with physiotherapy to improve movement range and precision.[70]

Pain is not an indication for lesioning procedures or deep brain stimulation (DBS) in advanced PD patients. However, some studies have indicated that DBS may exert pain-relieving effects which seem to be independent from the improvement of motor status. Honey et al reported on 21 PD patients treated by unilateral pallidotomy and observed a decrease in pain in 40% of patients, although the type of pain was unspecified.[71] Loher et al treated 16 advanced PD patients with GPi DBS.[72] Interestingly, they reported an improvement at 1 year post-surgery for dysaesthesia in 100% of their patients. Witjas et al focused on the effects of subthalamic nucleus (STN) DBS on non-motor fluctuations, to which pain and sensory fluctuations (i.e. *not* associated with dystonia) belong.[73] Of PD patients who underwent STN DBS, 84.2% were improved for pain and sensory fluctuations and thus showed the best response of all non-motor fluctuations to surgery. In this regard, a recent paper demonstrating the integration of motor, sensory, and/or limbic functions in the STN[74] suggests that the STN may be a prime target for patients suffering from PPP, although this assumption remains theoretic at present.

Finally, pain management in PD may rely on classical analgesics, such as NSAIDs and opioids. Concerning the latter, care must be taken not to increase akinesia[75] and/or constipation. We suggest that in difficult cases, a specialized pain service may be contacted and pain treated according to World Health Organization guidelines for cancer pain management based on a 3-step analgesic ladder,[76] with which most movement disorder specialists may not be familiar (Figure 6-3).

Perspectives/Outlook

As has become apparent, PPP remains an understudied entity. It is very likely a consequence of peripheral nerve pathology in association with

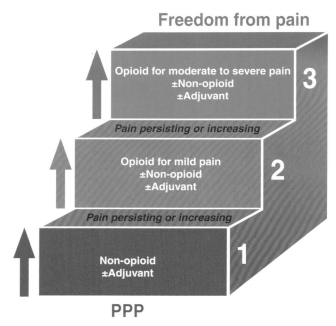

Figure 6-3. Analgesic ladder for PPP (Adapted from the World Health Organization, 1990).

degeneration of part of the central pain matrix in PD. To improve our understanding of PPP, it will first be necessary to establish rigorous clinical criteria to diagnose this syndrome. Also, instruments to assess and quantify PPP should be developed. This will enable practitioners and researchers to identify concerned patients and, to begin with, assess the impact of PPP on HRQOL. In addition, there will be a need for imaging and postmortem studies in PPP to better understand its pathophysiology and the timing of the changes observed. Based on these finding, rational therapeutic interventions can be designed and tested in controlled clinical trials.

References

1. Craig AD. Pain mechanisms: labeled lines versus convergence in central processing. *Annu Rev Neurosci.* 2003;26:1–30.
2. Tracey I, Mantyh PW. The cerebral signature for pain perception and its modulation. *Neuron.* 2007;55:377–391.
3. Apkarian AV, Bushnell MC, Treede RD, Zubieta JK. Human brain mechanisms of pain percpetion and regulation in health and disease. *Eur J Pain.* 2005(4);9:463–484.
4. May A. Chronic pain may change the structure of the brain. *Pain.* 2008;137(1):7–15.
5. Jobst EE, Melnick ME, Byl NN, Dowling GA, Aminoff MJ. Sensory perception in Parkinson disease. *Arch Neurol.* 1997;54(4):450–454.
6. Maschke M, Gomez CM, Tuite PJ, Konczak J. Dysfunction of the basal ganglia, but not the cerebellum, impairs kinaesthesia. *Brain.* 2003;126(Pt 10):2312–2222.
7. Okuma Y, Hattori N, Mizuno Y. Sensory neuropathy in autosomal recessive juvenile parkinsonism (PARK2). *Parkinsonism Relat Disord.* 2003;9(5):313–314.
8. Abbruzzese G, Pigullo S, Schenone A, et al. Does parkin play a role in the peripheral nervous system? A family report. *Mov Disord.* 2004;19(8):978–981.
9. Ohsawa Y, Kurokawa K, Sonoo M, et al. Reduced amplitude of the sural nerve sensory action potential in PARK2 patients. *Neurology.* 2005;65(3):459–462.
10. Nolano M, Provitera V, Estraneo A, et al. Sensory deficit in Parkinson's disease: evidence of a cutaneous denervation. *Brain.* 2008;131(7):1903–1911.
11. Parkinson J. An essay on the shaking palsy (1817). London: Sherwood, Neely, and Jones.
12. Charcot JM. Lectures sur les maladies du système nerveux central. Paris, Delahaye (1877) pp. 155–188.
13. Gowers WR. *Manual of diseases of the nervous system* (1888). Philadelphia: Blakiston.
14. Mendel K. *Die paralysis agitans. Berlin*, Karger (1911), pp. 39–42.
15. Souques MA. Des douleurs dans la paralysie agitante. *Rev Neurol (Paris).* 1921;37: 629–633.
16. Sigwald J, Solignac J. Manifestations douloureuses de la maladie de Parkinson et paréthesies provoquées par les neuroléptiques. *Sem Hosp Paris.* 1960;41: 2222–2225.

17. Snider SR, Fahn S, Isgreen WP, Cote LJ. Primary sensory symptoms in parkinsonism. *Neurology.* 1976;26(5):423–429.
18. Koller WC. Sensory symptoms in Parkinson's disease. *Neurology.* 1984;34(7): 957–959.
19. Schott GD. Pain in Parkinson's disease. *Pain.* 1985;22(4):407–411.
20. Stamey W, Davidson A, Jankovic J. Shoulder pain: a presenting symptom of Parkinson disease. *J Clin Rheumatol.* 2008;14(4):253–254.
21. Goetz CG, Tanner CM, Levy M, Wilson RS, Garron DC. Pain in Parkinson's disease. *Mov Disord.* 1986;1(1):45–49.
22. Quinn NP, Koller WC, Lang AE, Marsden CD. Painful Parkinson's disease. *Lancet.* 1986;1(8494):1366–1369.
23. Ford B. Pain in Parkinson's disease. *Clin Neurosci.* 1998;5(2):63–72.
24. Beiske AG, Loge JH, R nningen A, Svensson E. Pain in Parkinson's disease: Prevalence and characteristics. *Pain.* 2009;141(1–2):173–177.
25. Giuffrida R, Vingerhoets FJ, Bogousslavsky J, Ghika J. [Pain in Parkinson's disease] *Rev Neurol (Paris).* 2005;161(4):407–418.
26. Nègre-Pagès L, Regragui W, Bouhassira D, Grandjean H, Rascol O; DoPaMiP Study Group. Chronic pain in Parkinson's disease: the cross-sectional French DoPaMiP survey. *Mov Disord.* 2008;23(10):1361–1369.
27. Roh JH, Kim BJ, Jang JH, et al. The relationship of pain and health-related quality of life in Korean patients with Parkinson's disease. *Acta Neurol Scand.* 2009;119(6): 397–403.
28. Tinazzi M, Del Vesco C, Defazio G, et al. Abnormal processing of the nociceptive input in Parkinson's disease: A study with CO_2 laser evoked potentials. *Pain.* 2008;136(1–2):117–124.
29. Ilson J, Fahn S, Côté L. Painful dystonic spasms in Parkinson's disease. *Adv Neurol.* 1984;40:395–398.
30. Grushka M, Sessle BJ. Burning mouth syndrome. *Dent Clin North Am.* 1991;35(1): 171–184.
31. Ford B, Louis ED, Greene P, Fahn S. Oral and genital pain syndromes in Parkinson's disease. *Mov Disord.* 1996;11(4):421–426.
32. Battista AF, Wolff BB. Levodopa and induced-pain response. A study of patients with Parkinsonian and pain syndromes. *Arch Intern Med.* 1973;132(1):70–74.
33. Djaldetti R, Shifrin A, Rogowski Z, Sprecher E, Melamed E, Yarnitsky D. Quantitative measurement of pain sensation in patients with Parkinson disease. *Neurology.* 2004;62(12):2171–2175.
34. Lim SY, Farrell MJ, Gibson SJ, Helme RD, Lang AE, Evans AH. Do dyskinesia and pain share common pathophysiological mechanisms in Parkinson's disease? *Mov Disord.* 2008;23(12):1689–1695.
35. Brefel-Courbon C, Payoux P, Thalamas C, et al. Effect of levodopa on pain threshold in Parkinson's disease: a clinical and positron emission tomography study. *Mov Disord.* 2005;20(12):1557–1563.
36. Scott DJ, Heitzeg MM, Koeppe RA, Stohler CS, Zubieta J-K. Variations in the human pain stress experience mediated by ventral and dorsal basal ganglia dopamine activity. *J Neurosci.* 2006 Oct;26(42):10789–10795.

37. Slaoui T, Mas-Gerdelat A, Ory-Magne F, Rascol O, Brefel-Courbon C. [Levodopa modifies pain thresholds in Parkinson's disease patients] *Rev Neurol (Paris)*. 2007;163(1):66–71.
38. Gerdelat-Mas A, Simonetta-Moreau M, Thalamas C, et al. Levodopa raises objective pain threshold in Parkinson's disease: a RIII reflex study. *J Neurol Neurosurg Psychiatry*. 2007;78(10):1140–1142.
39. Tinazzi M, Del Vesco C, Fincati E, et al. Pain and motor complications in Parkinson's disease. *J Neurol Neurosurg Psychiatry*. 2006;77(7):822–825.
40. Marras C, Lang A, Krahn M, Tomlinson G, Naglie G; Parkinson Study Group. Quality of life in early Parkinson's disease: impact of dyskinesias and motor fluctuations. *Mov Disord*. 2004;19(1):22–28.
41. Rahman S, Griffin HJ, Quinn NP, Jahanshahi M. Quality of life in Parkinson's disease: The relative importance of the symptoms. *Mov Disord*. 2008;23(10):1428–1434.
42. Quittenbaum BH, Grahn B. Quality of life and pain in Parkinson's disease: a controlled cross-sectional study. *Parkinsonism Relat Disord*. 2004;10(3):129–136.
43. Defazio G, Berardelli A, Fabbrini G, et al. Pain as a nonmotor symptom of Parkinson disease: evidence from a case-control study. *Arch Neurol*. 2008;65(9):1191–1194.
44. Tison F. [Pain in Parkinson's disease]. *Rev Neurol (Paris)*. 2007;163(1):15–16.
45. Ikemura M, Saito Y, Sengoku R, et al. Lewy body pathology involves cutaneous nerves. *J Neuropathol Exp Neurol*. 2008;67(10):945–953.
46. Bloch A, Probst A, Bissig H, Adams H, Tolnay M. Alpha-synuclein pathology of the spinal and peripheral autonomic nervous system in neurologically unimpaired elderly subjects. *Neuropathol Appl Neurobiol*. 2006;32(3):284–295.
47. Braak H, Sastre M, Bohl JR, de Vos RA, Del Tredici K. Parkinson's disease: lesions in dorsal horn layer I, involvement of parasympathetic and sympathetic pre- and postganglionic neurons. *Acta Neuropathol*. 2007;113(4):421–429.
48. Jiang M, Alheid GF, Calandriello T, McCrimmon DR. Parabrachial-lateral pontine neurons link nociception and breathing. *Respir Physiol Neurobiol*. 2004;143(2–3):215–233.
49. Braak H, Rüb U, Sandmann-Keil D, et al. Parkinson's disease: affection of brain stem nuclei controlling premotor and motor neurons of the somatomotor system. *Acta Neuropathol*. 2000;99(5):489–495.
50. Braak H, Del Tredici K, Rüb U, de Vos RA, Jansen Steur EN, Braak E. Staging of brain pathology related to sporadic Parkinson's disease. *Neurobiol Aging*. 2003;24(2):197–211.
51. Benarroch EE, Schmeichel AM, Low PA, Boeve BF, Sandroni P, Parisi JE. Involvement of medullary regions controlling sympathetic output in Lewy body disease. *Brain*. 2005;128(Pt 2):338–344.
52. Vogt BA. Pain and emotion interactions in subregions of the cingulate gyrus. *Nat Rev Neurosci*. 2005;6(7):533–544.
53. Rüb U, Del Tredici K, Schultz C, et al. Parkinson's disease: the thalamic components of the limbic loop are severely impaired by alpha-synuclein immunopositive inclusion body pathology. *Neurobiol Aging*. 2002;23(2):245–254.
54. Brooks D, Halliday GM. Intralaminar nuclei of the thalamus in Lewy body diseases. *Brain Res Bull*. 2009;78(2–3):97–104.

55. Harding AJ, Stimson E, Henderson JM, Halliday GM. Clinical correlates of selective pathology in the amygdala of patients with Parkinson's disease. *Brain*. 2002;125 (Pt 11):2431–2445.
56. Schestatsky P, Kumru H, Valls-Solé J, et al. Neurophysiologic study of central pain in patients with Parkinson disease. *Neurology*. 2007;69(23):2162–2169.
57. Orimo S, Uchihara T, Nakamura A, et al. Axonal alpha-synuclein aggregates herald centripetal degeneration of cardiac sympathetic nerve in Parkinson's disease. *Brain*. 2008;131:642–650.
58. Greffard S, Verny M, Bonnet AM, et al. Motor score of the Unified Parkinson Disease Rating Scale as a good predictor of Lewy body-associated neuronal loss in the substantia nigra. *Arch Neurol*. 2006;63(4):584–548.
59. Lee J, Zhu WM, Stanic D, et al. Sprouting of dopamine terminals and altered dopamine release and uptake in Parkinsonian dyskinaesia. *Brain*. 2008;131(Pt 6):1574–1587.
60. Lorenz J, Casey KL. Imaging of acute versus pathological pain in humans. *Eur J Pain*. 2005;9(2):163–165.
61. Hagelberg N, Jääskeläinen SK, Martikainen IK, et al. Striatal dopamine D2 receptors in modulation of pain in humans: a review. *Eur J Pharmacol*. 2004;500(1–3): 187–192.
62. Pahwa R, Factor SA, Lyons KE, et al.; Quality Standards Subcommittee of the American Academy of Neurology. Practice Parameter: treatment of Parkinson disease with motor fluctuations and dyskinesia (an evidence-based review): report of the Quality Standards Subcommittee of the American Academy of Neurology. *Neurology*. 2006;66(7):983–995.
63. Cantello R, Aguggia M, Gilli M, Delsedime M, Riccio A, Rainero I, Mutani R. Analgesic action of methylphenidate on parkinsonian sensory symptoms. Mechanisms and pathophysiological implications. *Arch Neurol*. 1988;45(9):973–976.
64. Schug SA, Saunders D, Kurowski I, Paech MJ. Neuraxial drug administration: a review of treatment options for anaesthesia and analgesia. *CNS Drugs*. 2006;20(11): 917–933.
65. Sandyk R. Anticholinergic-induced analgesia: possible role for the cholinergic system in abnormal sensory symptoms in Parkinson's disease. *Postgrad Med J*. 1986; 62(730):749–751.
66. Jann MW, Slade JH. Antidepressant agents for the treatment of chronic pain and depression. *Pharmacotherapy*. 2007;27(11):1571–1587.
67. Eisenberg E, River Y, Shifrin A, Krivoy N. Antiepileptic drugs in the treatment of neuropathic pain. *Drugs*. 2007;67(9):1265–1289.
68. Meltzer HY. The role of serotonin in antipsychotic drug action. *Neuropsychopharmacology*. 1999;21(2 Suppl):106S-115S.
69. Eichhorn TE, Oertel WH. Macrogol 3350/electrolyte improves constipation in Parkinson's disease and multiple system atrophy. *Mov Disord*. 2001;16(6):1176–1177.
70. Keefer L, Blanchard EB.The effects of relaxation response meditation on the symptoms of irritable bowel syndrome: results of a controlled treatment study. *Behav Res Ther*. 2001;39(7):801–811.
71. Honey CR, Stoessl AJ, Tsui JK, Schulzer M, Calne DB. Unilateral pallidotomy for reduction of parkinsonian pain. *J Neurosurg*. 1999;91(2):198–201.

72. Loher TJ, Burgunder JM, Weber S, Sommerhalder R, Krauss JK. Effect of chronic pallidal deep brain stimulation on off period dystonia and sensory symptoms in advanced Parkinson's disease. *J Neurol Neurosurg Psychiatry*. 2002;73(4):395–399.

73. Witjas T, Kaphan E, Régis J, et al. Effects of chronic subthalamic stimulation on non-motor fluctuations in Parkinson's disease. *Mov Disord*. 2007;22(12):1729–1734.

74. Mallet L, Schüpbach M, N'Diaye K, et al. Stimulation of subterritories of the subthalamic nucleus reveals its role in the integration of the emotional and motor aspects of behavior. *Proc Natl Acad Sci U S A*. 2007;104(25):10661–10666.

75. Berg D, Becker G, Reiners K. Reduction of dyskinesia and induction of akinesia induced by morphine in two parkinsonian patients with severe sciatica. *J Neural Transm*. 1999;106(7–8):725–728.

76. World Health Organization. Cancer pain relief and palliative care. Report of a WHO Expert Committee. *World Health Organ Tech Rep Ser*. 1990;804:1–75.

77. Poewe WH, Lees AJ, Stern GM. Dystonia in Parkinson's disease: clinical and pharmacological features. *Ann Neurol*. 1988;23(1):73–78.

78. Reuter I, Ellis CM, Ray Chaudhuri K. Nocturnal subcutaneous apomorphine infusion in Parkinson's disease and restless legs syndrome. *Acta Neurol Scand*. 1999;100(3):163–167.

79. Nyholm D. Enteral levodopa/carbidopa gel infusion for the treatment of motor fluctuations and dyskinesias in advanced Parkinson's disease. *Expert Rev Neurother*. 2006;6(10):1403–1411.

80. Quinn N, Marsden CD. Lithium for painful dystonia in Parkinson's disease. *Lancet*. 1986;1(8494):1377.

81. Lees AJ, Shaw KM, Stern GM. Baclofen in Parkinson's disease. *J Neurol Neurosurg Psychiatry*. 1978;41(8):707–708.

82. Laitinen LV, Bergenheim AT, Hariz MI. Leksell's posteroventral pallidotomy in the treatment of Parkinson's disease. *J Neurosurg*. 1992;76(1):53–61.

83. Baron MS, Vitek JL, Bakay RA, et al. Treatment of advanced Parkinson's disease by posterior GPi pallidotomy: 1-year results of a pilot study. *Ann Neurol*. 1996;40(3):355–366.

84. Volkmann J, Sturm V, Weiss P, et al. Bilateral high-frequency stimulation of the internal globus pallidus in advanced Parkinson's disease. *Ann Neurol*. 1998;44(6):953–961.

85. Limousin P, Krack P, Pollak P, et al. Electrical stimulation of the subthalamic nucleus in advanced Parkinson's disease. *N Engl J Med*. 1998;339(16):1105–1111.

86. Krack P, Pollak P, Limousin P, Benazzouz A, Deuschl G, Benabid AL. From off-period dystonia to peak-dose chorea. The clinical spectrum of varying subthalamic nucleus activity. *Brain*. 1999;122 (Pt 6):1133–1146.

87. Pacchetti C, Albani G, Martignoni E, Godi L, Alfonsi E, Nappi G. "Off" painful dystonia in Parkinson's disease treated with botulinum toxin. *Mov Disord*. 1995;10(3):333–336.

88. Sage JI, Kortis HI, Sommer W. Evidence for the role of spinal cord systems in Parkinson's disease-associated pain. *Clin Neuropharmacol*. 1990;13(2):171–174.

89. Hillen ME, Sage JI. Nonmotor fluctuations in patients with Parkinson's disease. *Neurology*. 1996;47(5):1180–1183.

90. Factor SA, Friedman JH. The emerging role of clozapine in the treatment of movement disorders. *Mov Disord.* 1997;12(4):483–496.

91. Snow BJ, Macdonald L, Mcauley D, Wallis W. The effect of amantadine on levodopa-induced dyskinesias in Parkinson's disease: a double-blind, placebo-controlled study. *Clin Neuropharmacol.* 2000;23(2):82–85.

92. Durif F, Debilly B, Galitzky M, et al. Clozapine improves dyskinesias in Parkinson disease: a double-blind, placebo-controlled study. *Neurology.* 2004;62(3):381–388.

93. Vitek JL. Deep brain stimulation for Parkinson's disease. A critical re-evaluation of STN versus GPi DBS. *Stereotact Funct Neurosurg.* 2002;78(3–4):119–131.

94. Mark MH, Sage JI. Levodopa-associated hemifacial dystonia. *Mov Disord.* 1991;6(4):383.

Chapter 7

Lesions Associated with Sleep Disturbances

Marcus M. Unger, Wolfgang H. Oertel, Thomas C. Thannickal, Yuan-Yang Lai, and Jerome M. Siegel

Introduction

Sleep disturbances are frequently reported complaints in patients with Parkinson's disease (PD) and are seen throughout all stages of the illness. On the one hand, certain sleep disorders can emerge already at preclinical stages, heralding the emergence of PD. On the other hand, disease progression (as assessed by Hoehn and Yahr stage) has been shown to be associated with a worsening of sleep-related disturbances.[1] The relevance of sleep disturbances as a non-motor symptom for PD patients is illustrated by the fact that the subjective quality of sleep in PD patients is not only poorer compared to healthy subjects, but also compared to patients with other neurodegenerative disorders, e.g. Alzheimer's disease.[2]

The spectrum of sleep-related symptoms seen in PD patients comprises a variety of disorders, including disturbances that occur during daytime, like excessive daytime sleepiness (EDS) and sleep attacks (SA), as well as disturbances that occur at night, e.g. nocturnal recurrence of PD motor symptoms (akinesia, painful cramps), nocturia, vivid dreams, REM sleep behavior disorder (RBD), restless legs syndrome (RLS), periodic limb movements during sleep (PLMS), and others.

The etiology of sleep disturbances in PD is most likely multifactorial and in part due to the neurodegenerative process (affecting centers that regulate sleep and wakefulness), the pharmacological therapy, and the inter-individual susceptibility. The impact of drug intervention, especially dopaminergic therapy, on sleep disturbances in PD is debatable, as sleep disturbances are also seen in drug-naïve PD patients.[3]

The pathoanatomicial model of PD proposed by Braak and colleagues[4,5] provides a neuropathological correlate for the observation that sleep disturbances can already occur at preclinical stages of PD. According to Braak's scheme, the lower brainstem (pons and medulla)—involved in the regulation of sleep and wakefulness—is affected early by the neurodegenerative process, i.e. prior to degeneration at the midbrain level and the occurrence of motor impairments.

This chapter will give an overview of sleep-related disturbances in PD patients with respect to epidemiology, clinical presentation, therapeutic options and (where known) the respective underlying pathophysiology.

Sleep-related Disturbances in PD Occurring During Daytime

Excessive Daytime Sleepiness (EDS)

Excessive daytime sleepiness (EDS) as a recurrent compulsion to sleep during daytime is frequently seen in PD patients. A nationwide face-to-face survey on excessive daytime sleepiness (defined as an Epworth Sleepiness Scale (ESS) score ≥ 10) in 1625 PD patients (most of them treated with dopaminergic drugs) in France revealed a prevalence of 29% for EDS.[6] The etiology of EDS in PD remains unclear and disputed: involvement of brainstem structures that regulate sleep and wakefulness by the neurodegenerative process, untoward effects of the dopaminergic medication, as well as an interaction between the first and the latter are discussed. Daytime sleepiness in PD has been reported to be associated with nigrostriatal dopaminergic degeneration as visualized by presynaptic dopamine transporter imaging.[7] Yet these data do not allow conclusions as to whether the dopaminergic nigrostriatal degeneration represents the pathoanatomical correlate for EDS or is just an epiphenomenon.

The Honolulu-Asia aging study found that EDS in men aged 71 to 93 years without signs of PD or dementia was associated with a threefold excess in the risk of developing PD,[8] arguing that EDS might be a premotor feature of evolving PD rather than a medication-induced phenomenon. Yet, another study found that the prevalence for EDS does not differ between drug-naïve PD patients and age and sex-matched healthy controls.[9] In a follow-up of the same cohort one year post initiation of a dopaminergic therapy, Epworth Sleepiness Scale (ESS) scores significantly increased,[10] arguing for a pharmacological effect. Another study showed that frequency rates of EDS increase with time.[11]

A poor quality of sleep (sleep fragmentation, arousals, etc.) and sleep-disordered breathing may also account for EDS in PD patients. Yet, Arnulf and colleagues found that these factors did not correlate with sleepiness in PD patients [12] and that the dose of dopaminergic treatment did not contribute to sleepiness, but conversely showed vigilance-enhancing effects. This is in contrast to other studies which found that dopamine receptor agonists contribute to daytime sleepiness.[11,13]

In conclusion, the etiology of EDS in PD most likely is multifactorial and the contribution of (dopaminergic) drugs to EDS depends on an inter-individual susceptibility. Treatment of EDS in PD therefore includes (despite controversial data) reduction of dopamine receptor agonist treatment and screening for (treatable) nocturnal sleep disturbances (e.g. obstructive sleep apnea) that potentially can result in sleep fragmentation. If these measures are not sufficiently successful and the patient's quality of life is severely affected by EDS, stimulants like modafinil might be considered as a therapeutic option.[14–16]

A Narcolepsy-like Phenotype in PD?

EDS is also one of the chief complaints in another neurological disorder, i.e. narcolepsy. Arnulf and colleagues reported a narcolepsy-like phenotype (excessive daytime sleepiness, shortened sleep latency and sleep-onset REM periods) in PD patients with EDS.[12,17] In addition, daytime hallucinations in these patients showed a coincidence with short REM sleep intrusions during periods of wakefulness; also the presence of Lewy body pathology in the subcoeruleus nucleus (which is known to control REM sleep) in a PD patient with hallucinations suggests that visual hallucinations in PD might reflect a narcolepsy-like REM sleep disorder.[18] Other authors dispute a common pathophysiological basis for narcolepsy and PD [19] and refer to the conflicting data concerning hypocretin (orexin) CSF levels in PD.[20–23] Yet, recently published post-mortem data demonstrated hypocretin cell loss in PD: decreased hypocretin-1 tissue concentrations in the prefrontal cortex and a stage-dependent loss of hypothalamic hypocretin neurons were shown by Fronczek et al and Thannickal et al,[24,25] arguing again for some common pathological alterations in PD and narcolepsy.

Sleep Attacks (SA)

The issue of sleep attacks (SA) in PD has raised much attention because of the potential danger of falling asleep while driving.[26] Sleep attacks in PD are defined as an inappropriate sudden onset of an overwhelming, irresistible sleepiness occurring without warning and preventing the patient from taking appropriate measures to protect himself.[27] These SA are frequently associated with EDS, but can also occur in the absence of EDS.[28]

Sleep attacks have initially been described in PD patients on dopamine receptor agonist treatment,[29] but are also reported under levodopa monotherapy (showing a dose dependency),[30] and after initiation of entacapone.[31–33] These observations argue that SA are not exclusively due to dopamine receptor agonists but can be induced by any dopaminergic drug and that SA are related to the bioavailability of dopaminergic drugs and total dopaminergic load rather than to a single class of substances.

The absence of SA in patients treated with dopamine receptor agonists for restless legs syndrome, the fact that SA in PD can also occur at low doses of dopaminergic treatment in some patients (i.e. the lack of a clear dose effect correlation), and the lack of a clear temporal association with the introduction (specifically elevation of the dosage) of certain drugs argues for a susceptibility rather than a sole drug effect or disease-intrinsic mechanisms.[34] Genetic factors may also contribute to the occurrence of SA in PD patients: polymorphisms in the dopamine D2 and D4 receptor genes and polymorphisms in the preprohypocretin gene have been described.[35–37]

A cross-sectional study in 2952 PD patients revealed SA in 177 subjects (~6%). Sleep attacks occurred with all types of DA with no significant differences between ergot and non-ergot dopamine receptor agonists. Yet the risk for sleep attacks increased when comparing levodopa monotherapy to dopamine receptor agonist monotherapy and to a combination of levodopa *and* dopamine receptor agonist therapy,[38] arguing again that the total degree of dopaminergic stimulation contributes to SA. Another study in 6620 PD patients found that younger patients (below the age of 70 years) taking non-ergot dopamine receptor agonists are more susceptible to experience SA, yet medication was less effective in predicting SA than other factors (age, male gender, disease duration, etc.),[39] arguing for a multifactorial pathogenesis.

A cross-sectional case-control study in PD patients and healthy volunteers showed that the same proportion of PD patients and controls reported episodes of sleep attacks (approx. 1/3). Nevertheless, sleep attacks occurred more frequently in PD, especially during situations requiring attention. In this study, the most consistent factor associated with sleep attacks was the duration of levodopa therapy.[40]

In conclusion, PD patients should be routinely asked about the presence of SA and be informed about the potential risk of falling asleep at the wheel. It is disputed whether the Epworth Sleepiness Scale (ESS) is suitable to screen for SA (poor positive predictive value, but good negative predictive value).[40] If SA occur under dopamine receptor agonist treatment, a switch to another dopamine receptor agonist or a reduction of the dosage should be considered (if possible).

Sleep-related Disturbances Occurring at Night time

Sleep Apnea Syndrome (SAS)

Diederich et al found a frequency of sleep apnea syndrome (SAS) of 43% in an unselected sample of 49 PD patients.[41] Interestingly (in contrast to what is known for SAS in the general population), SAS in PD was not associated with obesity, and PD patients maintained a more favorable respiratory profile than non-PD SAS controls (matched in terms of age, gender and apnea/hypopnea index). In sum, in this study SAS was not a major cause for sleep fragmentation and SAS in PD seems to have a different profile in terms of polysomonographic and respiratory parameters. Thus, it is doubtful whether SAS in PD contributes to EDS. Continuous positive airway pressure (CPAP) treatment should be initiated if indicated by the respiratory profile seen in the cardio-respiratory polysomnography.

Insomnia, Vivid Dreams and (Nocturnal) Hallucinations

Stimulatory effect of drugs used to treat PD, especially amantadine and MAO-B-inhibitors (amphetamine metabolites), can induce insomnia. In addition, these drugs and also dopamine receptor agonists can cause vivid dreams and nocturnal hallucinations. Rescheduling, reduction, or (in more severe cases) discontinuation of these drugs should be considered to overcome these problems. In the case of severe (nocturnal) hallucinations that do not respond to the aforementioned measures, addition of atypical neuroleptic drugs (especially clozapine) is indicated. In order to treat insomnia, patients should also be informed about sleep hygiene, specifically how to maintain the circadian rhythm (bright light during the day, darkness during the night, use bedroom only for sleep, etc.). Any inappropriate aggressive nocturnal behavior in PD patients should also prompt checking for REM sleep behavior disorder (RBD).

REM Sleep Behavior Disorder (RBD)

REM sleep behavior disorder (RBD) is a male-predominant parasomnia that was scientifically described for the first time in 1986 by Schenck and colleagues. RBD presents with dream-enacting motor behaviors and speech during REM sleep.[42] Most patients with RBD seek medical help when their dream-enactments result in physical injury to themselves or their bed partner. A diagnosis of RBD is established by the typical history of dream enactments (including information from the patient's spouse/ caregiver about the sleep behavior) and loss of (the physiological) muscle atonia during REM sleep (documented by video-polysomnography).

In the absence of a concomitant neurological disorder, RBD is termed idiopathic RBD (iRBD), which has been shown to be a risk marker for subsequent development of neurodegenerative disorders, especially PD. In 1996, Schenck and colleagues reported that 11 out of 29 patients (i.e. 38%) initially diagnosed to suffer from iRBD eventually developed a parkinsonian syndrome, with a mean follow-up of 12.7 years.[43] On a second follow-up 7 years later, 19 of the initial 29 iRBD patients (i.e. 65%) presented with a parkinsonian syndrome, dementia or both diseases. Cross-sectional studies have shown that approximately one-third of PD patients exhibit RBD when examined by V-PSG.[44] Pachetti and colleagues also screened PD patients for RBD and found a similar prevalence of RBD (26.6%). Retrospectively, approximately one-third developed RBD before, and two-thirds after, diagnosis of PD.[45] The largest retrospective study investigating RBD and concomitant diseases has been published by Olsen and colleagues: among 93 patients with RBD 53 presented with a concomitant neurological disorder, 25 of these 53 patients had PD. With a closer look at the 25 patients with RBD and PD, it was found that RBD developed before PD in 13 patients, simultaneously in 2 patients and after diagnosis of PD in 10 patients.[46] It is unclear which mechanisms are responsible for the occurrence of RBD either before or after the manifestation of PD. One possible explanation for the divergent observations concerning the sequence of both diseases might be that in cases where RBD is reported and/or identified only in the course of PD there is a lack of sufficient investigation for subclinical stages at earlier time points. Interestingly, RBD (but also sleep disorders in general) constitute a predictor for emerging hallucinations in PD.[45,47,48]

The first post mortem studies in RBD patients described degeneration of monoaminergic (noradrenergic, dopaminergic, serotonergic) neurons and the presence of Lewy bodies in the brainstem and intracellular alpha-synuclein inclusions.[18,49] The pattern of lesions was very similar to the brainstem pathology seen in very early PD according to the neuropathologcial staging of PD proposed by Braak.[4] According to Braak's neuropathological staging, lesions in brainstem structures occur before the dopaminergic nigrostriatal pathway becomes affected. Braak's post mortem data support the assumption that RBD and PD are closely linked and even more, that from a neuroanatomical point of view, RBD should precede PD.

While routine imaging with magnetic resonance imaging (MRI) or computed tomography (CT) rarely detects or reveals brainstem pathology in RBD patients,[46] a reduced presynaptic striatal dopamine transporter uptake was shown using single photon emission computed tomography (SPECT) in RBD patients without motor symptoms of PD.[50] This finding and the proof of an olfactory dysfunction in RBD patients demonstrated by Stiasny-Kolster and colleagues[51] is in agreement with Braak's patho-anatomical staging.[4] According to Braak's model (Fig. 7-1), impaired olfactory function represents stage 1 of PD (Lewy body pathology in the olfactory bulb), the presence of PD stage 2 (Lewy body pathology is also seen in the medulla and pons), and the clinical manifestation of classical neurological signs such as akinesia, tremor or rigidity represents stage 3 PD (Lewy body pathology affects the midbrain level).

Hitherto, no causal therapeutical strategies for RBD have been available. Yet, the physical injuries that can result from the often violent behaviors during sleep and the morbidity associated with chronic sleep disruption, stress the need for a symptomatic therapy. Clonazepam (0.5 to 1 mg per night) is effective in most patients and is the drug of choice. In cases where the response to clonazepam is incomplete or when clonazepam is contraindicated, melatonin (0.5 to 12 mg per night) seems to be an alternative treatment option.[52–54] Boeve and colleagues have shown the effectiveness of melatonin specifically in patients with accompanying neurodegenerative disorders (n=14).[55] Improvement of RBD with oral administration of melatonin [52–55] as well as positive effects of melatonin on the subjective quality of sleep and even on motor function in PD patients[56] argue for involvement of the melatonin system. Melatonin has antioxidant properties that could modify the neurodegenerative process, but the short-term response directly after initiation of melatonin argues for a more direct action of melatonin. Interestingly, and in part controversial to the aforementioned, bright light therapy (melatonin antagonism) has also shown beneficial effects in PD.[57, 58] As RBD is often seen in the context of evolving PD, there have also been trials with levodopa and dopamine receptor agonists in a small group of patients. Tan and colleagues reported improvement of RBD symptoms when patients with early PD were treated with levodopa.[59] Ozekmekci and co-workers have shown that PD patients with RBD require higher levodopa doses to regain motor abilities compared to PD patients without RBD and that levodopa treatment cannot prevent the occurrence of RBD.[60] Pramipexole, a dopamine D2/D3-receptor agonist, has been shown to relieve RBD-related sleep disturbing symptoms.[61] However, pramipexole was not able to alter phasic EMG activity during REM sleep—when used as a possible quantitative marker of disease severity.[62] Also, cholinesterase inhibitors have been shown to relieve RBD symptoms in single patients. These drugs putatively modify the

BRAAK STAGE 1 PD

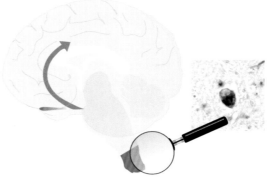

Non-motor symptoms
hyposmia
REM sleep behaviour disorder (RBD)
Excessive daytime sleepiness (EDS)
Sleep attacks (SA)

BRAAK STAGE 2 PD

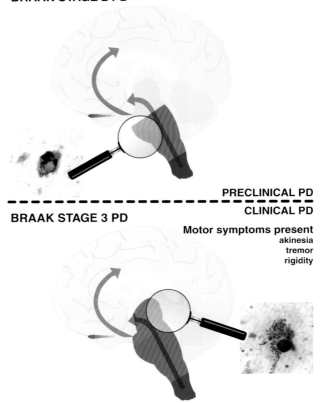

PRECLINICAL PD
CLINICAL PD

BRAAK STAGE 3 PD

Motor symptoms present
akinesia
tremor
rigidity

Figure 7-1. The distribution of Lewy body (LB) pathology in preclinical (premotor) and early clinical stages of PD according to Braak's pathoanatomical model. In preclinical stages (Braak stage 1 and 2) LB pathology in the brainstem (pons, medulla) and the olfactory bulb could explain the occurrence of sleep disorders and other non-motor symptoms (hyposmia, autonomic dysfunction, etc.). Upon involvement of the midbrain level with its nigrostriatal projections, the PD-typical motor symptoms occur and allow the clinical diagnosis of PD.

neuronal activity of the pedunculopontine nucleus.[63] Yet clinical trials that prove the effectiveness of any of the mentioned drugs in a double-blind placebo-controlled study remain to be initiated. Beside the pharmacological management, patients should be instructed about measures preventing physical injuries during RBD episodes (closing windows before sleep, removing sharp and dangerous objects from around the bed).

For experimental research, several animal models of RBD have been developed. Bilateral pontine tegmental lesions have been shown to provoke an RBD-like phenotype[64] and also circumscribed lesions in the ventral mesopontine junction (VMPJ) in cats resulted in a RBD-like phenotype.[65] There are a number of other animal models demonstrating that the lesion of brainstem structures can result in RBD.[66,67] Hence, brainstem nuclei in the pons and medulla are thought to be responsible for RBD.[66] This notion is supported by case reports of patients with defined structural brainstem lesions who developed RBD.[68,69] For example, even a minimal ischemic pontine lesion has been shown to be sufficient to cause RBD.[70] Mazza et al[71] also demonstrated abnormal cerebral blood flow in the pons in RBD patients, using 99mTc-ethylene cysteinate dimer SPECT technique. This observation strongly supports the assumption that the localization of a lesion, rather than its histological type is responsible for manifestation of RBD.

In PD, degeneration of cholinergic neurons in the pedunculopontine nucleus[72] as well as Lewy body pathology in the locus coeruleus[49] might be anatomical correlates of RBD. Post-mortem analysis of the brain of a patient with RBD who eventually developed cognitive decline and parkinsonism revealed marked neuronal loss in the locus coeruleus and substantia nigra—regions that may inhibit cholinergic neurons in the pedunculopontine nucleus (mediating atonia during REM sleep).[73]

In sum, RBD in (evolving) PD most likely reflects brainstem lesions in the medulla and pons. The presumed pathophysiology is that these lesions cause a net reduction in the inhibition of spinal motoneurons that are normally suppressed by a complex interaction of brainstem nuclei during REM sleep, thereby preventing motor activity during REM sleep.[74-76]

Sleepwalking

A sleep disorder that can clinically mimic RBD is sleepwalking. Adult-onset sleepwalking is seen in PD patients and can also present concomitant to RBD.[77] Its pathophysiology is unclear. Episodes with sleepwalking normally arise from non-REM sleep and can be distinguished from RBD episodes by a video-polysomnography. Coexistence of RBD and sleepwalking argue for a common pathophysiology of motor control during sleep.

Restless Legs Syndrome (RLS) and Periodic Leg Movements During Sleep (PLMS)

RLS is defined as an irresistible urge to move the legs, sometimes accompanied by uncomfortable, painful sensations. Typically, RLS symptoms emerge or become worse at rest, especially in bed at night, and are (partially) relieved by moving the legs or walking around. PLMS are periodic jerks of the lower extremity and can result in repeated awakenings and disruption of sleep. Restless legs syndrome (RLS) and periodic leg movements during sleep (PLMS) are seen as idiopathic entities, in the context of other sleep disorder, as well as in patients with PD. A recent study found a prevalence of 21.9% for RLS among 114 PD patients.[78]

The good clinical response to dopaminergic drugs and the association of PLMS with reduced striatal dopamine transporter binding suggests involvement of the dopaminergic system in PLMS.[79] The exact pathophysiology of PMLS and RLS in PD is still unclear. Disturbances in iron metabolism have been described for RLS. In RLS patients with a serum ferritin level below 50 µg/l, iron substitution can reduce RLS-related discomfort. Besides this, dopamine receptor agonists are the first line therapy for RLS; alternatively opioids and anticonvulsants can be used to treat RLS.

Lesions of the Arousal System in Parkinson's Disease

Altered sleep and vigilance are frequent symptoms in PD. As many as 60% of patients with PD experience insomnia, 15–59% show RBD, and 30% show excessive daytime sleepiness.[80] While PD is undoubtedly a disorder with a pathology of dopamine neuronal loss, most arousal systems including noradrenergic neurons in the locus coeruleus, serotonergic neurons in the raphe, cholinergic neurons in the basal forebrain, and orexin/hypocretin neurons in the hypothalamus, are affected by neuronal loss (Fig. 7-2). The loss of the neurotransmitter noradrenaline occurs consistently in PD and—according to Braak—earlier than in the dopaminergic neurons in the substantia nigra. This is thought to worsen with disease progression, either by increasing the vulnerability of dopamine-containing neurons or by reducing the recovery once they are damaged. There is 40–50% loss of noradrenergic neurons in the locus coeruleus and 20–40% loss of serotonergic neurons in the raphe median nucleus. In the basal forebrain, 32–93% of acetylcholine neurons are lost with disease progression.[81] However, loss of the dopaminergic neurons in the ventral periaqueducal gray region that contains "wake–active" dopaminergic neurons [82,83] is only 9% and histidine decarboxylase activity is reported to be normal in the brains of individuals with PD.[84]

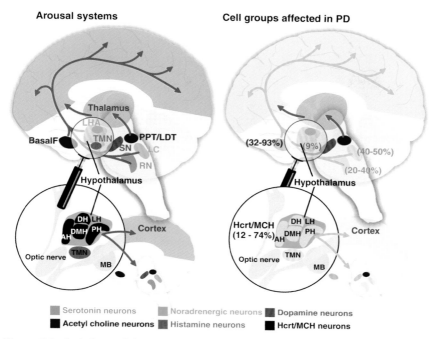

Figure 7-2. Pathology of the arousal system in Parkinson's disease. Left panel shows the cell groups involved in the arousal mechanism. The right panel shows the neuronal loss of the arousal system in PD. Arousal systems including noradrenergic neurons in the locus coeruleus; serotonergic neurons in the raphe; cholinergic neurons in the basal forebrain; Hcrt, MCH and histamine neurons in the hypothalamus are affected by neuronal loss.

Hypocretin/Orexin Cell Loss in Parkinson's Disease

The hypothalamic hypocretin (Hcrt or orexin) system plays a central role in the regulation of various functions, including sleep/wake regulation and metabolism. The two Hcrt peptides (Hcrt-1 and Hcrt-2), also known as orexins, are both encoded by the preprohypocretin gene, and the cell bodies are located in hypothalamus.[85,86] Two Hcrt receptors (Hcrtr-1 and Hcrtr-2) have been identified.[86] Hcrt fibers project widely throughout the brain, and generally have excitatory effects on their postsynaptic cells. Particularly notable are the projections of Hcrt cells to cholinergic and monoaminergic cells.[87] The similarity of the sleep disturbances of PD (discussed above) to narcolepsy suggest a common etiology. Narcolepsy is caused by loss of hypocretin-producing neurons, reflected in low cerebrospinal fluid (CSF) levels.[88–90]

Hcrt neurotransmission is affected in PD. Hcrt concentration in the prefrontal cortex was almost 40% lower in PD patients, while ventricular CSF levels were reduced by almost 25%.[24] Loss of hypocretin cells was found to correlate with disease progression [25] as measured by the Hoehn and Yahr rating scale, but not disease duration. The percentage loss of Hcrt cells was minimal in stage I (23%) and increased to a maximum of 62% in stage V (Fig. 7-3). Hcrt cells were lost throughout the A–P extent of their hypothalamic distributions (Fig. 7-3). Thus, the loss of Hcrt cells may be a cause of the narcolepsy-like symptoms of PD and may be ameliorated by treatments aimed at reversing the Hcrt deficit.[91,92]

Melanin Concentrating Hormone Cell Loss in PD

Melanin concentrating hormone (MCH) is a cyclic 19-amino-acid neuro-peptide that has been considered to play a key role in the regulation of feeding and energy homeostasis. Two receptors have been identified.[93] Hcrt and MCH neurons have a coextensive distribution in the hypothala-mus, but Hcrt and MCH are not co-localized within individual neurons.[94] MCH neurons have been suspected to play a role in arousal and modula-tion of memory. Expression of c-fos in these cells is particularly strong after sleep rebound, consequent to sleep deprivation.[95] Intracerebroventri-cular injections of low doses of MCH induce an increase of REM sleep and with lesser amounts of slow wave sleep, suggesting that MCH plays a role in the homeostatic regulation of REM sleep.[96]

MCH neurons are more abundant in the human hypothalamus and have a wider rostrocaudal distribution than hypocretin neurons. MCH neurons are relatively more numerous in the posterior hypothalamus (Fig. 7-3). In PD, MCH cells are lost throughout the anterior to posterior extent of their hypothalamic distributions. The percentage loss of MCH cells is correlated with clinical stages of PD, as is the case with hypocretin neurons, with the smallest loss in stage I (12%) and the highest in stage V (74%). MCH cell loss was not correlated with disease duration. There was a significant increase in the size of neuromelanin containing cells in PD patients, but no difference in the size of surviving MCH or Hcrt cells relative to controls.[25]

The cause and pathophysiological mechanisms for Hcrt and MCH cell death are currently unknown. Whether Hcrt and MCH neurons show some neuropathological signs of dysfunction before loss remains to be deter-mined. These issues need to be examined at the cellular and molecular level, but also in animal models. Dopamine replacement therapy has been the mainstay of antiparkinson treatment for the past three decades. Based on the new findings, detection of the loss of Hcrt and MCH cells and treat-ment of the deficits resulting from this loss may have a significant role in the diagnosis and treatment of Parkinson's disease.

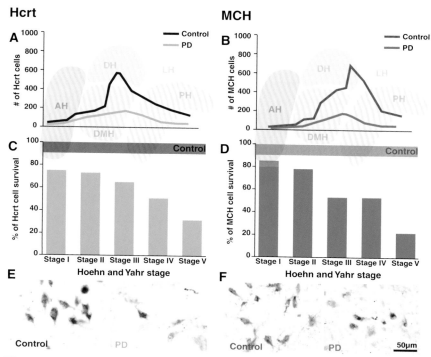

Figure 7-3. Hcrt and MCH pathology in Parkinson's disease. Hcrt cell loss (left panel) in different stages of PD (Hoehn and Yahr). The number of Hcrt cell was decreased with severity of the disease. The photomicrograph of Hcrt cells is from a control and a PD brain (stage V). Right panel shows MCH cell loss in different stages of PD. The number of MCH cells was decreased with severity of the disease. The photomicrograph of MCH cells is from a control and a PD brain (stage V). The loss of Hcrt and MCH cells was correlated with severity of the disease and not with duration. For cell count, a stereology program was used and for cell mapping a neurolucida program was used. The normal distribution of Hcrt and MCH cells in the hypothalamus is limited to AH, DH, DMH, LH and PH nulcei. AH=anterior hypothalamus, DH=dorsal hypothalamus, DMH=dorsomedial hypothalamus, LH=lateral hypothalamus, PH=posterior hypothalamus. Bar=50 μm.

Conclusions

In sum, sleep is frequently disturbed in PD patients. The spectrum of sleep-related disorders in PD patients comprises nocturnal troubles as well as symptoms that occur during daytime, like excessive daytime sleepiness and sleep attacks. Some of these disturbances (e.g. RBD and EDS) can emerge prior to the manifestation of PD-related motor symptoms and are potential markers that herald subsequent evolvement of PD. Pathophysiologically, degeneration of sleep-regulating centers in the brainstem (pons, medulla) that occurs early in the course of PD may account for the occurrence of these sleep disturbances.

The exact pathophysiology, specifically the patho-anatomic correlate, for most PD-related sleep disturbances is only marginally understood. A multifactorial pathogenesis with reciprocal interactions (drugs, genetic factors, neurodegeneration) is presumed. The existing data also indicate that not only dopaminergic, but different types of monoaminergic and cholinergic nuclei as well as the orexin/hypocretin system and perhaps also the melanin concentrating hormone are involved in the pathogenesis of the respective disorders.

Research focusing on the pathophysiological correlates of PD-associated sleep disorders is warranted as this research will largely contribute to our understanding of the neurodegenerative process in PD and might help to develop drugs for the treatment of sleep-related PD symptoms. These drugs could potentially have beneficial ("side") effects on other PD-associated symptoms as well.

Acknowledgments

Tissue specimens were obtained from the Human Brain and Spinal Fluid Resource Center, West Los Angeles Healthcare Center, Los Angeles, CA. Supported by grants to JMS (NS14610, HL41370 and MH64109) and to YYL (NS42566) and the Medical Research Service of the Department of Veterans Affairs and by grants to WHO from the German Federal Ministry of Education and Research (funding code: 01GI0401) and the Willy and Monika Pitzer Foundation.

References

1. Porter B, Macfarlane R, Walker R. The frequency and nature of sleep disorders in a community-based population of patients with Parkinson's disease. *Eur J Neurol*. 2008; 15(1):50–54.
2. Boddy F, Rowan EN, Lett D, O'Brien JT, McKeith IG, Burn DJ. Subjectively reported sleep quality and excessive daytime somnolence in Parkinson's disease with and without dementia, dementia with Lewy bodies and Alzheimer's disease. *Int J Geriatr Psychiatry*. 2007;22(6):529–535.
3. Dhawan V, Dhoat S, Williams AJ, et al. The range and nature of sleep dysfunction in untreated Parkinson's disease (PD). A comparative controlled clinical study using the Parkinson's disease sleep scale and selective polysomnography. *J Neurol Sci*. 2006; 248(1–2):158–162.

4. Braak H, Del Tredici K, Rub U, de Vos RA, Jansen Steur EN, Braak E. Staging of brain pathology related to sporadic Parkinson's disease. *Neurobiol Aging.* 2003;24(2): 197–211.

5. Braak H, Ghebremedhin E, Rub U, Bratzke H, Del Tredici K. Stages in the development of Parkinson's disease-related pathology. *Cell Tissue Res.* 2004;318(1):121–134.

6. Ghorayeb I, Loundou A, Auquier P, Dauvilliers Y, Bioulac B, Tison F. A nationwide survey of excessive daytime sleepiness in Parkinson's disease in France. *Mov Disord.* 2007;22(11):1567–1572.

7. Happe S, Baier PC, Helmschmied K, Meller J, Tatsch K, Paulus W. Association of daytime sleepiness with nigrostriatal dopaminergic degeneration in early Parkinson's disease. *J Neurol.* 2007;254(8):1037–1043.

8. Abbott RD, Ross GW, White LR, et al. Excessive daytime sleepiness and subsequent development of Parkinson disease. *Neurology.* 2005;65(9):1442–1446.

9. Fabbrini G, Barbanti P, Aurilia C, Vanacore N, Pauletti C, Meco G. Excessive daytime sleepiness in de novo and treated Parkinson's disease. *Mov Disord.* 2002;17(5): 1026–1030.

10. Fabbrini G, Barbanti P, Aurilia C, Pauletti C, Vanacore N, Meco G. Excessive daytime somnolence in Parkinson's disease. Follow-up after 1 year of treatment. *Neurol Sci.* 2003;24(3):178–179.

11. Gjerstad MD, Alves G, Wentzel-Larsen T, Aarsland D, Larsen JP. Excessive daytime sleepiness in Parkinson disease: is it the drugs or the disease?. *Neurology.* 2006;67(5);853–858.

12. Arnulf I, Konofal E, Merino-Andreu M, Houeto JL, Mesnage V, Welter ML, et al. Parkinson's disease and sleepiness: an integral part of PD. *Neurology.* 2002;58(7): 1019–1024.

13. Oved D, Ziv I, Treves TA, Paleacu D, Melamed E, Djaldetti R. Effect of dopamine agonists on fatigue and somnolence in Parkinson's disease. *Mov Disord.* 2006;21(8): 1257–1261.

14. Adler CH, Caviness JN, Hentz JG, Lind M, Tiede J. Randomized trial of modafinil for treating subjective daytime sleepiness in patients with Parkinson's disease. *Mov Disord.* 2003;18(3):287–293.

15. Hogl B, Saletu M, Brandauer E, et al. Modafinil for the treatment of daytime sleepiness in Parkinson's disease: a double-blind, randomized, crossover, placebo-controlled polygraphic trial. *Sleep.* 2002;25(8):905–909.

16. Ondo WG, Fayle R, Atassi F, Jankovic J. Modafinil for daytime somnolence in Parkinson's disease: double blind, placebo controlled parallel trial. *J Neurol Neurosurg Psychiatry.* 2005;76(12):1636–1639.

17. Rye DB, Johnston LH, Watts RL, Bliwise DL. Juvenile Parkinson's disease with REM sleep behavior disorder, sleepiness, and daytime REM onset. *Neurology.* 1999;53(8): 1868–1870.

18. Arnulf I, Bonnet AM, Damier P, et al. Hallucinations, REM sleep, and Parkinson's disease: a medical hypothesis. *Neurology.* 2000;55(2):281–288.

19. Baumann C, Ferini-Strambi L, Waldvogel D, Werth E, Bassetti CL. Parkinsonism with excessive daytime sleepiness—a narcolepsy-like disorder? *J Neurol.* 2005;252(2): 139–145.

20. Drouot X, Moutereau S, Nguyen JP, et al. Low levels of ventricular CSF orexin/hypo-cretin in advanced PD. *Neurology*. 2003;61(4):540–543.
21. Maeda T, Nagata K, Kondo H, Kanbayashi T. Parkinson's disease comorbid with narcolepsy presenting low CSF hypocretin/orexin level. *Sleep Med*. 2006;7(8):662.
22. Overeem S, van Hilten JJ, Ripley B, Mignot E, Nishino S, Lammers GJ. Normal hypocretin-1 levels in Parkinson's disease patients with excessive daytime sleepiness. *Neurology*. 2002;58(3):498–499.
23. Yasui K, Inoue Y, Kanbayashi T, Nomura T, Kusumi M, Nakashima K. CSF orexin levels of Parkinson's disease, dementia with Lewy bodies, progressive supranuclear palsy and corticobasal degeneration. *J Neurol Sci*. 2006;250(1-2):120–123.
24. Fronczek R, Overeem S, Lee SY, et al. Hypocretin (orexin) loss in Parkinson's dis-ease. *Brain*. 2007;130(6):1577–1585.
25. Thannickal TC, Lai YY, Siegel JM. Hypocretin (orexin) cell loss in Parkinson's dis-ease. *Brain*. 2007;130(6):1586–1595.
26. Meindorfner C, Körner Y, Möller JC, Stiasny-Kolster K, Oertel WH, Krüger HP. Driving in Parkinson's disease: mobility, accidents, and sudden onset of sleep at the wheel. *Mov Disord*. 2005;20(7):832–842.
27. Frucht SJ, Greene PE, Fahn S. Sleep episodes in Parkinson's disease: a wake-up call. *Mov Disord*. 2000;15(4):601–603.
28. Möller JC, Rethfeldt M, Körner Y, et al. Daytime sleep latency in medication-matched Parkinsonian patients with and without sudden onset of sleep. *Mov Disord*. 2005;20(12):1620–1622.
29. Frucht S, Rogers JD, Greene PE, Gordon MF, Fahn S. Falling asleep at the wheel: motor vehicle mishaps in persons taking pramipexole and ropinirole. *Neurology*. 1999;52(9): 1908–1910.
30. Ferreira JJ, Thalamas C, Montastruc JL, Castro-Caldas A, Rascol O. Levodopa monotherapy can induce "sleep attacks" in Parkinson's disease patients. *J Neurol*. 2001;248(5):426–427.
31. Bares M, Kanovsky P, Rektor I. Excessive daytime sleepiness and 'sleep attacks' induced by entacapone. *Fundam Clin Pharmacol*. 2003;17(1):113–116.
32. Santens P. Sleep attacks in Parkinson's disease induced by Entacapone, a COMT-inhibitor. *Fundam Clin Pharmacol*. 2003;17(1):121–123.
33. Tracik F, Ebersbach G. Sudden daytime sleep onset in Parkinson's disease: polysom-nographic recordings. *Mov Disord*. 2001;16(3):500–506.
34. Homann CN, Homann B, Ott E, Park KB. Sleep attacks may not be a side effect of dopaminergic medication. *Mov Disord*. 2003;18(12):1569–1570; author reply 1571.
35. Paus S, Seeger G, Brecht HM, et al. Association study of dopamine D2, D3, D4 recep-tor and serotonin transporter gene polymorphisms with sleep attacks in Parkinson's disease. *Mov Disord*. 2004;19(6):705–707.
36. Rissling I, Geller F, Bandmann O, et al. Dopamine receptor gene polymorphisms in Parkinson's disease patients reporting "sleep attacks". *Mov Disord*. 2004;19(11): 1279–1284.
37. Rissling I, Korner Y, Geller F, Stiasny-Kolster K, Oertel WH, Moller JC. Preprohypocretin polymorphisms in Parkinson disease patients reporting "sleep attacks". *Sleep*. 2005;28(7):871–875.

38. Paus S, Brecht HM, Koster J, Seeger G, Klockgether T, Wullner U. Sleep attacks, daytime sleepiness, and dopamine agonists in Parkinson's disease. *Mov Disord.* 2003;18(6): 659–667.

39. Korner Y, Meindorfner C, Moller JC, et al. Predictors of sudden onset of sleep in Parkinson's disease. *Mov Disord.* 2004;19(11):1298–1305.

40. Ferreira JJ, Desboeuf K, Galitzky M, et al. Sleep disruption, daytime somnolence and 'sleep attacks' in Parkinson's disease: a clinical survey in PD patients and age-matched healthy volunteers. *Eur J Neurol.* 2006;13(3):209–214.

41. Diederich NJ, Vaillant M, Leischen M, et al. Sleep apnea syndrome in Parkinson's disease. A case-control study in 49 patients. *Mov Disord.* 2005;20(11):1413–1418.

42. Schenck CH, Bundlie SR, Ettinger MG, Mahowald MW. Chronic behavioral disorders of human REM sleep: a new category of parasomnia. *Sleep.* 1986;9(2):293–308.

43. Schenck CH, Bundlie SR, Mahowald MW. Delayed emergence of a parkinsonian disorder in 38% of 29 older men initially diagnosed with idiopathic rapid eye movement sleep behaviour disorder. *Neurology.* 1996;46(2):388–393.

44. Gagnon JF, Bedard MA, Fantini ML, et al. REM sleep behavior disorder and REM sleep without atonia in Parkinson's disease. *Neurology.* 2002;59(4):585–589.

45. Pacchetti C, Manni R, Zangaglia R, et al. Relationship between hallucinations, delusions, and rapid eye movement sleep behavior disorder in Parkinson's disease. *Mov Disord.* 2005;20(11):1439–1448.

46. Olson EJ, Boeve BF, Silber MH. Rapid eye movement sleep behaviour disorder: demographic, clinical and laboratory findings in 93 cases. *Brain.* 2000;123(2): 331–339.

47. de Maindreville AD, Fenelon G, Mahieux F. Hallucinations in Parkinson's disease: a follow-up study. *Mov Disord.* 2005;20(2):212–217.

48. Onofrj M, Thomas A, D'Andreamatteo G, et al. Incidence of RBD and hallucination in patients affected by Parkinson's disease: 8-year follow-up. *Neurol Sci.* 2002; 23 Suppl 2: S91–4.

49. Uchiyama M, Isse K, Tanaka K, et al. Incidental Lewy body disease in a patient with REM sleep behavior disorder. *Neurology.* 1995;45(4):709–712.

50. Eisensehr I, Linke R, Noachtar S, Schwarz J, Gildehaus FJ, Tatsch K. Reduced striatal dopamine transporters in idiopathic rapid eye movement sleep behaviour disorder. Comparison with Parkinson's disease and controls. *Brain.* 2000;123(6):1155–1160.

51. Stiasny-Kolster K, Doerr Y, Moller JC, et al. Combination of 'idiopathic' REM sleep behaviour disorder and olfactory dysfunction as possible indicator for alpha-synucleinopathy demonstrated by dopamine transporter FP-CIT-SPECT. *Brain.* 2005; 128(1):126–137.

52. Kunz D, Bes F. Melatonin effects in a patient with severe REM sleep behavior disorder: case report and theoretical considerations. *Neuropsychobiology.* 1997;36(4): 211–214.

53. Kunz D, Bes F. Melatonin as a therapy in REM sleep behavior disorder patients: an open-labeled pilot study on the possible influence of melatonin on REM-sleep regulation. *Mov Disord.* 1999;14(3):507–511.

54. Takeuchi N, Uchimura N, Hashizume Y, et al. Melatonin therapy for REM sleep behavior disorder. *Psychiatry Clin Neurosci.* 2001;55(3):267–269.

55. Boeve BF, Silber MH, Ferman TJ. Melatonin for treatment of REM sleep behavior disorder in neurologic disorders: results in 14 patients. *Sleep Med.* 2003;4(4): 281–284.
56. Medeiros CA, Carvalhedo de Bruin PF, Lopes LA, Magalhaes MC, de Lourdes Seabra M, de Bruin VM. Effect of exogenous melatonin on sleep and motor dysfunction in Parkinson's disease. A randomized, double blind, placebo-controlled study. *J Neurol*;254(4):459–464.
57. Paus S, Schmitz-Hubsch T, Wullner U, Vogel A, Klockgether T, Abele M. Bright light therapy in Parkinson's disease: a pilot study. *Mov Disord.* 2007;22(10):1495–1498.
58. Willis GL, Turner EJ. Primary and secondary features of Parkinson's disease improve with strategic exposure to bright light: a case series study. *Chronobiol Int.* 2007;24(3):521–537.
59. Tan A, Salgado M, Fahn S. Rapid eye movement sleep behavior disorder preceding Parkinson's disease with therapeutic response to levodopa. *Mov Disord.* 1996;11(2): 214–216.
60. Ozekmekci S, Apaydin H, Kilic E. Clinical features of 35 patients with Parkinson's disease displaying REM behavior disorder. *Clin Neurol Neurosurg.* 2005;107(4): 306–309.
61. Schmidt MH, Koshal VB, Schmidt HS. Use of pramipexole in REM sleep behavior disorder: results from a case series. *Sleep Med.* 2006;7(5):418–423.
62. Fantini ML, Gagnon JF, Filipini D, Montplaisir J. The effects of pramipexole in REM sleep behavior disorder. *Neurology.* 2003;61(10):1418–1420.
63. Massironi G, Galluzzi S, Frisoni GB. Drug treatment of REM sleep behavior disorders in dementia with Lewy bodies. *Int Psychogeriatr.* 2003;15(4):377–383.
64. Hendricks JC, Morrison AR, Mann GL. Different behaviors during paradoxical sleep without atonia depend on pontine lesion site. *Brain Res.* 1982;239(1):81–105.
65. Lai YY, Hsieh KC, Nguyen D, Peever J, Siegel JM. Neurotoxic lesions at the ventral mesopontine junction change sleep time and muscle activity during sleep: An animal model of motor disorders in sleep. *Neuroscience.* 2008;154(2):431–443.
66. Lai YY, Siegel JM. Physiological and anatomical link between Parkinson-like disease and REM sleep behavior disorder. *Mol Neurobiol.* 2003;27(24):137–152.
67. Morrison AR. Paradoxical sleep without atonia. *Arch Ital Biol.* 1988;126(4): 275–289.
68. Plazzi G, Montagna P. Remitting REM sleep behavior disorder as the initial sign of multiple sclerosis. *Sleep Med.* 2002;3(5):437–439.
69. Xi Z, Luning W. REM sleep behavior disorder in a patient with pontine stroke. *Sleep Med.* 2009;10(1):143–146.
70. Kimura K, Tachibana N, Kohyama J, Otsuka Y, Fukazawa S, Waki R. A discrete pontine ischemic lesion could cause REM sleep behavior disorder. *Neurology.* 2000;55(6): 894–895.
71. Mazza S, Soucy J, Gravel P, et al. Assessing whole brain perfusion changes in patients with REM sleep behavior disorder. *Neurology.* 2006;67(9):1618–1622.
72. Hirsch EC, Graybiel AM, Duyckaerts C, Javoy-Agid F. Neuronal loss in the pedunculopontine tegmental nucleus in Parkinson disease and in progressive supranuclear palsy. *Proc Natl Acad Sci. U S A.* 1987;84(16):5976–5980.

73. Turner RS, D'Amato CJ, Chervin RD, Blaivas M. The pathology of REM sleep behavior disorder with comorbid Lewy body dementia. *Neurology*. 2000;55(11):1730–1732.

74. Boeve BF, Silber MH, Saper CB, et al. Pathophysiology of REM sleep behaviour disorder and relevance to neurodegenerative disease. *Brain*. 2007;130(11):2770–2788.

75. Lu J, Sherman D, Devor M, Saper CB. A putative flip-flop switch for control of REM sleep. *Nature*. 2006;441(7093):589–94.

76. Siegel,J.M. *REM sleep in Principles and Practice of Sleep Medicine* (eds. Kryger, M.H., Roth, T. & Dement, W.C. (Elsevier Saunders, Philadelphia). 2005;120–135.

77. Poryazova R, Waldvogel D, Bassetti CL. Sleepwalking in patients with Parkinson disease. *Arch Neurol*. 2007;64(10):1524–1527.

78. Gomez-Esteban JC, Zarranz JJ, Tijero B, et al. Restless legs syndrome in Parkinson's disease. *Mov Disord*. 2007;22(13):1912–1916.

79. Happe S, Pirker W, Klosch G, Sauter C, Zeitlhofer J. Periodic leg movements in patients with Parkinson's disease are associated with reduced striatal dopamine transporter binding. *J Neurol*. 2003;250(1):83–86.

80. De Cock VC, Vidailhet M, Arnulf I. Sleep disturbances in patients with parkinsonism. Nat. *Clin Pract Neurol*. 2008;4(5):254–66.

81. Jellinger KA. The pathology of Parkinson's disease. *Adv Neurol*. 2001;86:55–72.

82. Lu J, Jhou TC, Saper CD. Identification of wake-active dopaminergic neurons in the ventral periaqueductal gray matter. *J Neurosci*. 2006;26(1):193–202.

83. Damier P, Hirsch EC, Agid Y, Graybiel AM. The substantia nigra of the human brain. II. Patterns of loss of dopamine-containing neurons in Parkinson's disease. *Brain*. 1999; 122(8):1437–48.

84. Garbarg M, Javoy-Agid F, Schwartz JC, Agid Y. Brain histidine decarboxylase activity in Parkinson's disease. *Lancet*. 1983;1(8314-5):74–75.

85. de Lecea L, Kilduff TS, Peyron C, et al. The hypocretins: hypothalamus-specific peptides with neuroexcitatory activity. *Proc Natl Acad Sci U S A*. 1998;95(1):322–327.

86. Sakurai T, Amemiya A, Ishii M, et al. Orexins and orexin receptors: a family of hypothalamic neuropeptides and G protein-coupled receptors that regulate feeding behavior. *Cell*. 1998;92(4):573–85.

87. Siegel JM. Hypocretin (orexin): role in normal behavior and neuropathology. *Annu Rev Psychol*. 2004;55:125–48.

88. Peyron C, Faraco J, Rogers W, et al. A mutation in a case of early onset narcolepsy and a generalized absence of hypocretin peptides in human narcoleptic brains. *Nat Med*. 2000;6(9):991–997.

89. Thannickal TC, Moore RY, Nienhuis R, et al. Reduced number of hypocretin neurons in human narcolepsy. *Neuron*. 2000; 27(3):469–474.

90. Thannickal TC, Siegel JM, Nienhuis R, Moore RY. Pattern of hypocretin (orexin) soma and axon loss, and gliosis, in human narcolepsy. *Brain Pathol*. 2003;13(3):340–351.

91. Deadwyler SA, Porrino L, Siegel JM, Hampson RE. Systemic and nasal delivery of orexin-A (hypocretin-1) reduces the effects of sleep deprivation on cognitive performance in nonhuman primates. *Journal of Neuroscience*. 2007;27(52):14239–14247.

92. John J, Wu MF, Siegel JM. Systemic administration of hypocretin-1 reduces cataplexy and normalizes sleep and waking durations in narcoleptic dogs. *Sleep Res. Online*. 2000;3(1):23–28.

93. Shimazaki T, Yoshimizu T, Chaki S. Melanin-concentrating hormone MCH1 receptor antagonists: a potential new approach to the treatment of depression and anxiety disorders. *CNS Drugs.* 2006;20(10):801–811.

94. Broberger C, De Lecea L, Sutcliffe JG, Hökfelt T. Hypocretin/orexin- and melanin-concentrating hormone-expressing cells form distinct populations in the rodent lateral hypothalamus: relationship to the neuropeptide Y and agouti gene-related protein systems. *J Comp Neurol.* 1998;402(4): 60–74.

95. Modirrousta M, Mainville L, Jones BE. Orexin and MCH neurons express c-Fos differently after sleep deprivation vs. recovery and bear different adrenergic receptors. *Eur J Neurosci.* 2005;21(10):2807–2816.

96. Verret L, Goutagny R, Fort P, et al. A role of melanin-concentrating hormone producing neurons in the central regulation of paradoxical sleep. *BMC Neurosci.* 2003; 9:4:19.

Chapter 8

Lesions Associated with Depression and Apathy

Uwe Ehrt, Kenn F. Pedersen, and Dag Aarsland

Introduction

In this chapter, we aim to review and discuss the neuropathological and neurochemical basis of apathy and depression in Parkinson's disease (PD), two of the most common neuropsychiatric manifestations in PD. While it is likely that dopaminergic neurotransmitter systems are involved also in the pathophysiology of depression and apathy in PD, non-dopaminergic lesions probably play a key role in the etiology of these neuropsychiatric symptoms.

Depression

Depression is the most common psychiatric disorder diagnosed in patients with Parkinson's disease. It has a major impact on functional ability as well as on the quality of life of patients and their caregivers.[1-4] It is also associated with lower cognitive functioning and increased mortality.[5,6] Despite this, in many PD cases, depression is often not considered and is thus under-treated.[7,8] However, there is little evidence for drug-treatment in depression and apathy. Increasing our understanding of the underlying brain correlates of apathy and depression in PD therefore may provide rational targets for future novel drug therapies.

Epidemiology

Prevalence rates of depressive disorders in PD vary widely across different studies, ranging from 2.7% to more than 90%, depending on recruitment strategy and how depression is defined. In a systematic review we concluded that major depressive disorder was present in 17% of PD patients, minor depression in 22%, and dysthymia in 13%, whereas clinically significant depressive symptoms, irrespective of the presence of a DSM-defined depressive disorder, were present in 35%.[9]

Neither prevalence nor severity of depression is related to the course of PD. Interestingly, major depression may even predate the onset of the motor symptoms,[10] strongly arguing against depression being solely a reaction to the diagnosis and disability in PD. Little is known about the natural history of depression in PD. The existing longitudinal data suggest a chronic or variable course, with repeated remissions and relapses of depression.[11] Less severe depression is more likely to improve.[12]

Clinical Presentation

The neurotransmitter disturbances causing depression in PD may differ somewhat from those in 'common' depression regarding localization, distribution, and severity.[13] This may translate into a specific phenomenological symptom pattern with potential clinical implications. Early on, Friedrich Lewy described depressive patients with PD to be moody, irritable, and weepy from a clinical view.[14] Some authors have reported distinctive characteristics in PD-related depression with less classical 'endogenous' depressive symptoms such as feelings of guilt and suicidal ideation, but more somatic symptoms such as anxiety, sleep disturbances and concentration difficulties.[15-20] We found that patients with PD showed less anhedonia, energy loss, sadness, and feelings of guilt, but more severe concentration difficulties than depressed patients without PD.[21] This may shed light on underlying pathologies, since different symptoms of depression may have different biological underpinnings. According to one theory, behavioral functions like engagement, concentration, attention, motivation, and arousal may be linked to noradrenergic activity, whereas loss of energy and apathy may be linked to impaired dopaminergic activity, and finally affective reactivity, anxiety, suicidal ideation, and mood may be mediated by the serotonergic neurotransmitter system. Thus, applying the phenotype on this theory, we propose that noradrenergic depletion contributes to depression in PD by disrupting attentional processes and contributing to the dysexecutive syndrome observed in this patient group.

Diagnosis

Depression is difficult to assess in patients with PD due to the low specificity of the symptoms and cognitive impairment. Moreover, research has been hampered by the lack of diagnostic criteria for PD-related depression. As a consequence, cut-off values from different depression scales or DSM criteria have commonly been used to diagnose depression in PD. However, such criteria are difficult to use in PD and require attribution of specific symptoms to either the neurological disease or the depressive syndrome. Moreover, DSM criteria for major depression and dysthymia exclude up to 50% of PD patients with clinically significant depressive symptoms. Recently, provisional diagnostic criteria for depression in PD were provided,[22] recommending (1) a rather inclusive approach to symptom assessment to enhance reliability of ratings in PD and avoid the need to attribute symptoms to a particular cause; (2) the inclusion of subsyndromal depression in clinical research studies of depression of PD; (3) the specification of timing of assessments for PD patients with motor fluctuations; and (4) the use of informants for cognitively impaired patients. Key features such as "loss of pleasure" or "anhedonia" are more specific to depression, while "loss of interest" is considered a symptom of apathy often occurring in patients without depression.

Somatic symptoms are common in depression and included in depression rating scales, but may not necessarily represent depressive symptoms in patients with PD. Another diagnostic challenge is that the perception of depressive symptoms varies in *off* and *on* periods. Recently, an expert group recommended guidelines in using the most common depression scales in PD.[23] However, rating scales can only supplement but never substitute for the clinical diagnosis; thus, the diagnosis of depression should not be exclusively made by a score on a scale.

When using rating scales, patients should be instructed not to attribute their symptoms to either PD or depression, since an exclusive approach may lead to an underestimate of depression severity. There are no established instruments to identify minor or subsyndromal depression, recurrent brief depressive disorder, or dysthymia, which often occur in PD.[24] The impact of age, cognitive impairment, apathy, and cultural differences on the validity of depression scales has to be studied further.

Pathology and pathophysiology

Endogenous or reactive depression, or a combination?

Like de novo depression, depression in PD is a condition with heterogeneous etiology and can be explained on physiological, molecular, genetic, cellular, and behavioral levels. Modern research often focuses only on one level, and a comprehensive understanding and evaluation of the growing evidence from genetic, pathological, pathobiochemical and imaging studies is increasingly difficult to synthesize. Despite this, imaging studies and other methods have begun to elucidate the neurobiological abnormalities associated with major depression in people without neurological disease. Key mechanisms are neuroendocrine dysregulation and neurotrophic changes. Such changes interact with key brain structures in prefrontal cortex and limbic regions including the hippocampus, involving monoamine neurotransmitter systems such as serotonin and noradrenaline (Figure 8-1).

Several of these structures and systems are involved in PD, and thus it is believed that depression in PD and de novo depression have much in common. An additional component in PD is the psychological stress related to functional impairment, disability and poor prognosis. When treating a single individual, it is difficult to attribute the patient's depression to either 'biology' or 'psychology.'

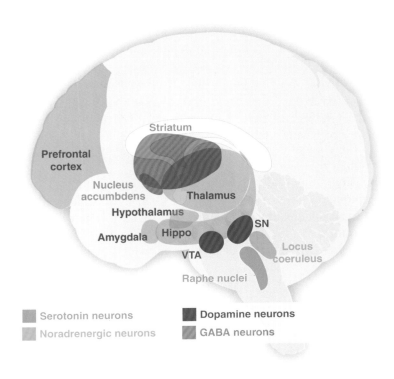

Figure 8-1. Brain structures and neurotransmitter systems involved in depression. Abbreviations: SN=substantia nigra; VTA=ventral tegmental area.

Several studies have aimed to disentangle psychological and biological factors contributing to depression in PD. However, a "mixed model," which takes both pathophysiological changes associated with PD and psychosocial aspects into account, seems more appropriate. Pathophysiological changes in PD lead to an increased vulnerability to negative emotional stimuli, and patients with more severe disease and a greater level of prefrontal cognitive dysfunction are more vulnerable to the distracting effects of external negative stimuli.[25] However, previous depression is associated with a higher risk for PD,[26] which can only be explained by biological mechanisms.

Reacting with depression is understandable when suffering from a chronic disabling disease, and even the patients themselves often attribute their sadness to disability. The high prevalence of depression especially in patients with early disease onset could be understood as the illness' negative effect on their job situation, economic security, and quality of life.[27] According to this hypothesis, depression should be more common and more severe in later stages of the disease. However, studies examining this relationship are conflicting. Robins found a group of PD patients much more depressed than chronically disabled control patients with an even more severe grade of physical handicap, and depression was unaffected by the severity of the disability in PD.[28] Similarly, Menza and Mark (1994) found that PD patients were more depressed than people with a similar level of disability, and functional disability explained only 9% of the variance in depression. Depression was correlated with "harm avoidance," a personality trait related to central serotonergic systems but not with novelty seeking, which is a trait related to dopaminergic pleasure and reward systems.[29] Nilsson et al showed in a large register study that PD patients had a higher risk of developing major depression compared to patients having other medical illnesses with a comparable degree of disability.[30] Cole et al found that depression was related to both illness severity and functional impairment in men, but not in women, and that depression was stronger in patients with early disease onset and those with right-sided PD, implicating a biological contribution.[31]

The best estimate of etiological factors can be drawn from longitudinal studies. Brown et al found that depression was more severe in patients with a rapid disease progression and functional impairment but rather independent of the absolute change in disability.[32] Schrag et al found similar results, i.e. higher depression scores associated with advancing disease severity, especially recent self-reported deterioration, akinesia, occurrence of falls, self-reported cognitive impairment, and the feeling of stigmatization.[33] Chronic pain may be another factor associated with depression in PD patients.[34] Psychological aspects in depression in PD were reviewed by Brown and Jahanshahi.[35]

Serotonin

Serotonergic pathways are involved in PD (Figure 8-2). Autopsy-studies have shown Lewy bodies and cell loss in the raphe nuclei (Figure 8-2), reduced 5HT concentrations and reuptake sites in the striatum and neocortex, and lower 5HT1a binding in the frontal cortex.[36] These and other key brainstem nuclei involved in monoaminergic neurotransmission are involved early in PD. Given the serotonergic model in depression,[37] it has been hypothesized that serotonergic disturbances may also cause depression in PD. Decreased concentrations of 5-hydroxyindolacetic acid (5-HIAA), a serotonin metabolite, in the cerebrospinal fluid of depressed PD patients was reported early, [38] and later replicated by the same group,[13] but not others.[39] However, several other neurochemical, neuropathological, and imaging studies support the serotonergic theory.

An over-representation of the short-allele form of a functional polymorphism in the serotonin transporter gene has been found in depressed PD patients.[40,41] More severe serotonergic neuronal cell loss in the dorsal raphe nucleus (DRN) was observed in PD patients with depression.[42] Reduced echogenicity using transcranial sonography (TCS) in the serotonergic mesencephalic raphe nuclei has been found.[43] Using postmortem immunohistochemical analysis, Halliday et al reported the first chemically-identified loss of serotonin neurons in the median raphe nucleus of the pons and of substance P-containing preganglionic neurons in the dorsal motor vagal nucleus.[44] Using PET, reduction in nucleus raphe 5-HT(1A) receptor binding in both depressed and non-depressed PD patients was found, but depressed patients had a greater reduction in cortical binding, reflecting post-synaptic 5-HT[1A] receptor dysfunction and supporting previous indirect evidence that serotonergic neurotransmission is decreased in PD.[45]

Noradrenaline

Greater degeneration within the locus coeruleus has been reported in depressed compared to non-depressed PD patients [46] (Figure 8-3). Increased $\alpha 1$ and $\beta 1$ receptors and decreased $\alpha 2$ receptors have been described in the prefrontal cortex of demented and depressed PD patients and seem to be related to the loss of the noradrenergic pathway from the locus coeruleus to the cortex,[47] although these findings were most pronounced in the caudal portion of the nucleus, which projects to the spinal cord. Remy et al employed PET to compare depressed with non-depressed PD patients.[48] The ligand[11]C-RTI-32 binds mainly to the dopamine transporter (DAT) in the striatum and decreased binding reflects loss of catecholaminergic innervation. In this study, the depressed group had lower binding in the locus coeruleus and in several regions of the limbic system including the anterior cingulate cortex, the thalamus, the amygdala, and the ventral

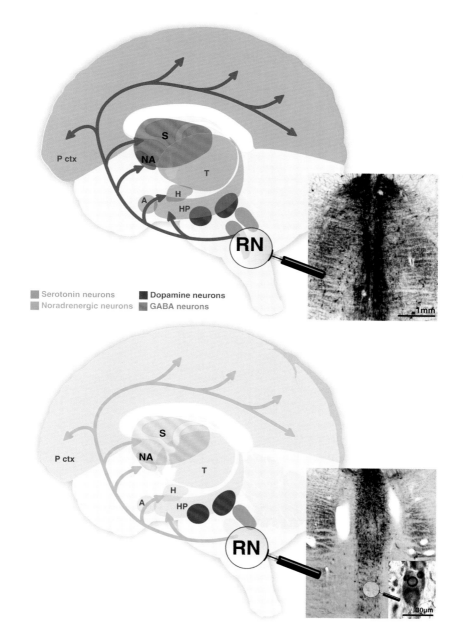

Figure 8-2. Diagram of the serotonergic pathways in non-depressed brain (top) versus Parkinson's disease (PD) and depression (bottom). Photomicrographs of serotoninergic neurons in both control and PD sections from human raphe nuclei (RN) showing marked cell loss in PD along with the presence of Lewy bodies (bottom figure). (Photomicrographs courtesy of Prof. G. Halliday). Abbreviations: A=amygdala; H=hypothalamus; HP=hippocampus; LC=locus coeruleus; P.Ctx=prefrontal cortex; S=striatum; SN=substantia nigra; T=thalamus; VTA=ventral tegmental area.

193

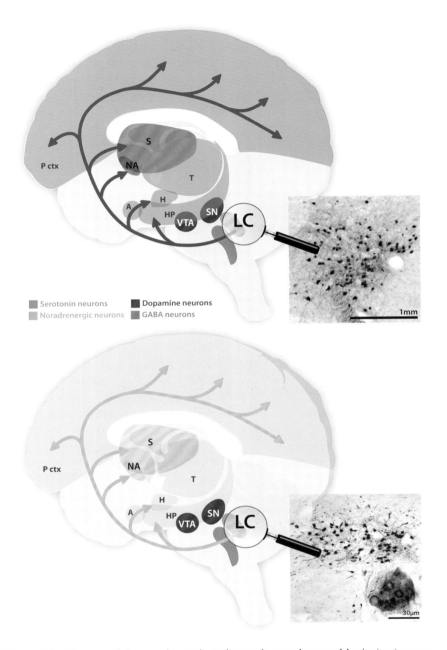

Figure 8-3. Diagram of the noradrenergic pathways in non-depressed brain (top) versus Parkinson's disease (PD) and depression (bottom). Photomicrographs of noradrenergic neurons in both control and PD sections from human locus coeruleus (LC) showing cell loss in PD along with the presence of Lewy bodies (bottom figure). (Photomicrographs courtesy of Prof. G. Halliday). Abbreviations: A=amygdala; H=hypothalamus; HP=hippocampus; P.Ctx=prefrontal cortex; RN=raphe nucleus; S=striatum; SN=substantia nigra; T=thalamus; VTA=ventral tegmental area.

striatum. The authors concluded that a specific loss of dopamine and nora-drenaline innervation in the limbic system may be crucial for the etiology of depression in PD (Figure 8-3).

Acetylcholine

Several studies[49-51] have found a relationship between depression and cognitive impairment in PD.[5,11,52-54] If depression is a risk factor for dementia, possible mechanisms are that (1) the comorbid mood disorder signals more widespread neurodegeneration, or (2) the treatment used for the depression itself affects the pathological process. Regarding the latter, tricyclic antidepressant with their anticholinergic-like properties may influence the accumulation of Alzheimer-like pathology. There is evidence that anticholinergic drugs are a risk factor for dementia in PD associated with cortical plaque and tangle densities.[55]

Using PET,[56] depression was found to be associated with cortical cho-linergic denervation in PD, even after controlling for cognitive impair-ment. The presence of dementia amplified this effect. Cholinergic dysfunction may play a role both for depression and cognitive impairment, which may explain why depression is a risk factor for dementia in PD.

A reduction in the activity of serotonergic and cholinergic systems can compensate for the dopaminergic lesions for some time, although these neurons begin to degenerate as well. These processes may be relevant for the development of depression and may also explain why depression often precedes the motor symptoms.

Dopamine

The "dopaminergic" hypothesis for depression was proposed by Fibiger. Not only nigrostriatal, but also mesocortical and mesolimbic dopaminer-gic projections degenerate in PD, although relatively spared compared with the nigrostriatal system.[57,58] These projections mediate self reward mechanisms. Damages here result in a reduced ability to experience plea-sure or reward (i.e. anhedonia), as recently shown in a PET study of people with idiopathic major depression.[59] However, nigral pathology may also contribute to depression in PD, a hypothesis supported recently in a study reporting nigral sonography changes in depressive disorders which were similar to those in PD.

The evidence for antidepressant efficacy of antiparkinsonian medica-tions is limited. This differs significantly from efficacy of medications in the more affected nigrostriatal system, suggesting limited deficits in the mesolimbic dopaminergic pathway.

The limbic system is a crucial anatomical substrate for emotions, and is supplied with dopaminergic innervation arising from the ventral tegmental area (field A10). In PD there is variable loss of dopaminergic neurons in the ventral tegmental area (VTA), which might affect the function of the limbic system and its prefrontal connections. Greater neuronal loss in the VTA has been associated with both mood disorder and dementia. Winter et al tested the influence of dopaminergic systems and their interrelationship with serotonergic systems in a rodent model. Lesions in the substantia nigra pars compacta (SNc) and VTA increased depressive-like behavior in rats. Both citalopram and l-dopa could reduce such behavior.[60] This suggests a direct involvement of dopaminergic lesions of either the SNc or the VTA but also serotonergic pathways in dopaminergic cell loss-induced depression.

Tyrosine hydroxylase is the enzyme responsible for catalyzing the conversion of the amino acid L-tyrosine to DOPA, a precursor for dopamine which in turn is a precursor for noradrenaline. The nigrostriatal loss of tyrosine hydroxylase, dopamine, and dopaminergic neurons in PD lead to changes which may directly or indirectly damage the forebrain catecholamine fibers and induce depression. Recent studies have found reduced striatal dopamine transporter activity, particularly in caudate, to correlate with depression in PD, supporting the involvement of nigro-striatal dopamine systems in the development of depression in PD.

Imaging (Structural and Functional)

Using diffusion tensor MRI (DTI), fractional anisotropy in the basal ganglia and frontal areas was found to differ between PD patients and healthy controls.[61] Furthermore, depressed PD subjects showed significant reductions in fractional anisotropy values in the bilateral anterior cingulate bundles compared to non-depressed subjects.[62]

A positron emission tomography study using 123I-beta-CIT failed to show a relationship between serotonergic median raphe HT1A binding and depression in PD.[63] In contrast, relative reductions in 5-HT1A binding were seen in depressed compared with euthymic PD patients in the anterior cingulate and superior/medial frontal gyrus. The finding of reduced frontal 5-HT1A binding in PD patients with depression supports former reports from Mayberg et al who found that regional cerebral glucose metabolism was reduced in depressed compared with nondepressed patients with PD.[64] The authors suggested that depression in PD is associated with dysfunction in the caudate and orbital-inferior area of the frontal lobe and that disruption of basal ganglia circuits involving the inferior region of the frontal lobe may affect the regulation of mood. They found that the temporal patterns of the midbrain and cerebellar activity were not significantly different from those in control subjects. In contrast, the specific striatal tracer volumes of distribution, V3, reflecting dopamine transporter (DAT) binding, were bilaterally reduced in all PD patients, being on average 32% lower than that of the control subjects. In PD patients, midbrain serotonin binding failed to correlate with striatal V3, motor, or Hamilton Depression Rating Scale scores. When the scans of 7 PD patients with depression were analyzed separately, midbrain 123I-beta-CIT uptake was found to be normal. These authors concluded that midbrain 5-HT transporter binding in early PD is unaffected and does not determine depressive symptoms.

Treatment Studies
In addition to alleviating depressive symptoms and improving quality of life for patients with PD and depression, the effect of different treatment modalities also offer insights into the underlying mechanisms of depression in PD, both with regard to neurochemical (drugs) as well as anatomical (brain stimulation) interventions.

Pharmacological Treatment
There is little empiric evidence to support the use of antidepressants in PD. In a review,[65] active treatment was found to be superior to placebo in depressed elderly patients without PD, but not in patients with PD. However, both active treatment and placebo had large effect sizes in PD. Older age and the diagnosis of major depression seem to improve the treatment response. Selective serotonin re-uptake inhibitors (SSRI) seem to be less effective in PD patients than in those without PD, which argues against an exclusively serotonergic hypothesis of depression in PD. On the other hand, a growing basic science literature suggests that SSRIs are not as selective as generally assumed.[66] They also activate directly biosynthesis of neurosteroids and modulate neurotransmitter- and voltage-gated neuronal ion channels. Conventional tricyclic antidepressants inhibit noradrenaline uptake and can be effective in depression in PD. Whether more selective noradrenergic drugs are effective in PD is not known.

The anxiolytic, antidepressive and antianhedonic effects, which dopamine agonists, especially pramipexole, have shown in experimental and clinical investigations,[67–70] are likely related to their specific action on D(2) and D(3) receptors in the mesolimbic system and prefrontal cortex.[71] Recently, pramipexol was even recommended as a first-line treatment in patients with PD and depression.[72] Treatment with dopaminergic drugs does not, however, consistently alleviate depression in PD.

Brain Stimulation

Electroconvulsive Therapy   There is some evidence supporting the hypothesis that ECT improves depression in PD, and even some motor improvement has been reported. As is the case in primary depression, the effect is transient and maintenance ECT or antidepressant drug therapy is needed for sustaining the benefit. At least part of the mechanism of action of ECT in PD may be enhanced dopamine function due to enhanced striatal D1 and D3 receptor upregulation.[73]

Transcranial Magnetic Stimulation   Transcranial magnetic stimulation (TMS) has been shown to improve depression in non-PD subjects, and there is evidence of antidepressive effects also in depressed PD patients, and even some motor improvement, during TMS, over the prefrontal cortex.[74] Although controlled studies exist,[74] comparisons with placebo have not yet been performed. TMS is primarily directed at surface cortical regions, and thus any effect on subcortical structures such as basal ganglia is probably indirect. Improvement on TMS has been shown to be associated with increased blood-flow in the prefrontal cortex and posterior and anterior cingulate gyrus.[75]

Deep Brain Stimulation   Deep brain stimulation (DBS) of brain structures including the subthalamic nucleus (STN) can successfully alleviate motor symptoms of PD. However, these procedures can acutely alter mood and behavior, and both acute depression[76,77] and mania[78] have been described, depending on the position of the electrodes. These reports provide evidence supporting the relevance for cortico-basal ganglionic system for mood regulation, and also the cortical segregation of motor and non-motor circuits. These findings, combined with functional imaging studies showing an association between depression and hyperactivity in the subcallosal cingulate gyrus have led to attempts to improve depression by directly modulating the output of the subcallosal cingulate gyrus by using DBS. Successful treatment of patients with treatment-resisting depression has been reported.[79] Whether DBS can be implemented to improve depression in patients with PD remains to be seen.

Psychosocial Therapies   Helping patients deal with the negative consequences of PD and manage their functional impairment, especially in late stages of the disease, is an important part of care. Negative consequences of the disease, like difficulty in dressing and turning, falls and autonomic disturbance (particularly urinary incontinence) are associated with depression and predict poor quality of life.[80] Adequate care can partly compensate for that. In addition, social support is important for sustaining humans' physical and mental health and dignity. Association between lack of social support and depression has been reported in elderly people.[81] Sufficient social support effectively buffers stress related to suffering.

Cheng et al investigated the correlation of social support, measured by a standardized scale, with depression in PD and corrected it for confounding clinical factors like disease severity and duration, and the results suggest that adequate social support may improve depression.[82] Thus, social support should be provided both by a professional and family caregivers.

Apathy

Definitions and Clinical Presentation

Challenges in Defining and Assessing Apathy

Apathy is derived from the Greek *pathos*, or passions, and is conventionally defined as absence or lack of feeling, emotion, interest, or concern.[83] In the early nineties, Marin proposed to define apathy as a primary lack of motivation that manifests itself as reduced goal-directed behavior (e.g. lack of initiative, productivity, and effort), reduced goal-directed cognition (e.g. lack of intellectual interest and curiosity), and reduced emotional concomitants of goal-directed behavior (e.g. flattened affect and lack of emotional response to positive or negative events).[84] He defined motivation as the direction, intensity, and persistence of goal-directed behavior. Marin also considered apathy to be a distinct neuropsychiatric syndrome if the primary lack of motivation was not attributable to diminished level of consciousness, cognitive impairment, or emotional distress. However, because apathy frequently occurs in patients with dementia or depression, Starkstein proposed to broaden Marin's criteria to include patients with apathy in the context of depression, dementia, or other neurodegenerative diseases.[85] Recently, inclusion of a time criterion was proposed to ascertain the persisting nature of apathy; it was recommended to require the symptoms to be present for at least 4 weeks during most of the day.[86]

Stuss et al argued that the definition and assessment of motivation is problematic, and suggested to define apathy as an absence of responsiveness to stimuli as demonstrated by a lack of self-initiated action.[87] They considered employing syndromal criteria for apathy to be potentially limiting, and suggested instead to divide apathy into separable types or states that differ in both functional disturbances underlying the clinical presentation and neural substrates of involvement. Recently, Levy and Dubois criticized lack of motivation to be an obscure psychological concept, and suggested to define apathy as an observable behavioral syndrome consisting in a quantitative reduction of voluntary (or goal-directed) behaviors.[88] They considered apathy to be related to disruption of emotional-affective, cognitive, and auto-activation processes in the prefrontal cortex-basal gan-glia circuits.

Several assessment scales have been developed to measure the severity of apathy in neurological and psychiatric disorders.[86,89] However, the study of apathy in neurology and psychiatry has been hampered by the lack of reliable and valid diagnostic criteria. In addition, the nosological relation of apathy to other neuropsychiatric syndromes such as abulia and akinetic syndromes remains uncertain.[86] At present, there is no consensus on diag-nostic criteria for an apathy syndrome. The only available are those formu-lated by Marin,[84] which have later been modified and organized into a standardized set of diagnostic criteria.[86]

Distinguishing Apathy from Depression

Apathy has traditionally been viewed as a feature of depression due to overlapping symptoms such as diminished interest, psychomotor retarda-tion, and poor concentration. In fact, DSM-IV allows the diagnosis of pri-mary major depression in the absence of depressed mood provided that markedly diminished interest or pleasure is accompanied by at least 4 other common depressive symptoms. Thus, there is a potential overlap between depression and apathy. For example, the category of minor depression has recently been shown to include a relatively large propor-tion of individuals with apathy rather than a "true" affective disorder in PD patients, suggesting that minor depression should be diagnosed using the DSM-IV criteria only when sad mood is present.[90] Thus, depressed mood is a key distinguishing feature between apathy and depression. Apathetic patients are emotionally indifferent, whereas dysphoric feelings (sadness, guilt, and pessimistic thoughts) are typical for depression. Despite the overlapping phenomenology between these two syndromes, several stud-ies have shown that apathy in PD can be distinguished from depression in the sense that some PD patients have apathy but not depression, and vice versa, some have depression but not apathy.[91–96] The potential neuroana-tomical differences underlying these two distinct syndromes in PD have yet to be determined. Interestingly, in a volumetric MRI-based study of the prefrontal cortex in 84 elderly subjects with or without major depres-sion, the depressed group had smaller orbitofrontal gray matter volumes compared to the age-matched normal comparison group, whereas apathy was associated with decreased gray matter volume in the right anterior cingulate gyrus.[97]

Relation to Cognition

Apathy is a key feature of subcortical dementia and dementia related to frontal lobe pathology,[98] and both subcortical and frontal lobe changes are common in PD.[99] Thus, not surprisingly, several studies have shown that apathy is associated with executive dysfunction in non-demented PD patients.[91,93,100] Three studies have reported a significant association between apathy and impaired global cognition in PD.[92,95,101] Whether cognitive deficits are necessary to produce apathy has not been specifically examined. As is the case with depression, some would argue that apathy should be included as part of a dysexecutive syndrome.

Epidemiology

Several studies of apathy in PD have been reported, with frequency rates ranging from 16.5% to 70%, depending upon the instruments used for assessment, different cut-off scores, and the selection of the samples examined (Table 8-1). In addition, frequency rates are affected by overlapping symptoms with mood disorders and variable degree of cognitive impairment in the study population. Most samples were not community-based, but rather were hospital-based samples recruited from outpatient neurological clinics, thus there is a considerable risk of selection bias. So far, the longitudinal course of apathy in PD has not been studied.

Pathology and Pathophysiology

Neurocircuitry of Apathy

The neurocircuitry of motivation and apathy is complex and current understanding is based on experimental neurocircuitry analysis in primates, human and animal lesion analyses, and neuropsychological and neuroanatomic studies in humans.

In a recent comprehensive review, the anterior cingulum (AC), nucleus accumbens (NA), ventral pallidum (VP), medial dorsal nucleus of the thalamus (MD), and the ventral tegmental area (VTA) were identified as important structures to establish and maintain the current motivational state (Figure 8-4). Disruption of the cortico-striatal-pallidal-thalamic circuit—which includes the AC, NA, VP and MD—produces akinetic mutism, abulia, or apathy depending on the severity of the dysfunction. Animal research has shown that initiation and maintenance of behavioral responses depends on the circuit composed of NA, VP and VTA.[108] The inclusion of AC in the motivational circuitry has been supported by experimental evidence showing that AC plays an important role in motivational aspects of decision making.[109,110] The amygdala and hippocampus, as well as the prefrontal cortex and the greater limbic lobe, are important structures that modulate information in the cortico-striatal-pallidal-thalamic circuit based on the current environment (reward processing).[111]

Table 8-1. Frequency of Apathy in Parkinson's Disease

Study (reference)	Sample	N	Instrument (cut-off)	% with apathy	% with depression#	% with dementia¶	Control group
Starkstein 1992[91]	Hospital-based	50	AS (≥14)	42	56	Unknown	No
Levy 1998[92]	Hospital-based	40	NPI (≥1)	32.5	55	Unknown	Other degenerative brain diseases
Aarsland 1999[102]	Selected community-based	139	NPI (≥1)	16.5	38	36–42	No
Ringman 2002[103]	Hospital-based	40	NPI (≥1)	40	Unknown	Unknown	Healthy
Isella 2002[93]	Hospital-based	30	AS (>14/16*)	70 (43.5*)	60	Unknown	Healthy
Pluck 2002[104]	Hospital-based	45	AES (≥38)	37.8	43	7	Osteoarthritis
Kirsch-Darrow 2006[94]	Hospital-based	80	AS (≥14)	51	26	Unknown	Dystonia
Aarsland 2007[105]	International multicentre	537	NPI (≥1/4**)	54.2 (37.8**)	22–58	100	No
Dujardin 2007[95]	Hospital-based	159	LARS (≥−16)	32.1	25	25	Healthy
Kulisevsky 2008[106]	Hospital-based	1351	NPI (≥1/4**)	48.3 (16.2**)	28–50	None (excluded)	No
Pedersen 2008[101]	Community-based	232	UPDRSI4 ≥ 2	37.9	30	26	No

MMSE = Mini-Mental State Examination; AS = Apathy Scale; AES = Apathy Evaluation Scale; NPI = Neuropsychiatric Inventory, apathy item; LARS = Lille Apathy Rating Scale; UPDRSI4 = Unified Parkinson's Disease Rating Scale, part I, item 4 (motivation/initiative).

#Depression diagnosed according to DSM criteria, depression rating scales, or both. See each study for more details.

¶Dementia diagnosed according to DSM criteria, except Pluck et al, who identified dementia based on the CAMCOG (the cognitive section of the Cambridge Examination for Mental Disorders in the Elderly [CAMDEX]) score.

*Adjusted cut-off score.

**An NPI apathy composite score of 4 or more is recommended to indicate clinical significant apathy in patients with PD. [107]

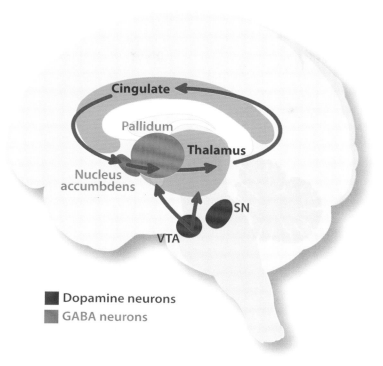

Figure 8-4. Brain circuitry important for motivational state highlighting the role of dopamine and non-dopamine pathways and of the cingulate loop. Abbreviations: NA=nucleus accumbdens; SN=substantia nigra; T=thalamus; VTA=ventral tegmented area.

Another approach to the underlying mechanisms of apathy is described by Bonelli and Cummings.[112] In their review of the neurocircuitry of behavior, apathy is hypothesized to be caused by loop dysfunction of the anterior cingulate circuit (Figure 8-4), which is one of the 5 major frontal-subcortical circuits.[113] Akinetic mutism, considered as the most severe disorder of diminished motivation,[111] has been closely related to lesions of the anterior cin~~~~~te [114] Neurons of the anterior cingulate serve as the origin of   'ate-subcortical circuit, and provide input to the ventral   ! limbic striatum). This area includes the ventromedia~   ~utamen, nucleus accumbens, and the olfactory tubercle. Proj~~~~~~~ ~~om the ventral striatum innervate the rostromedial globus pallidus interna (GPi), ventral pallidum, and the rostrodorsal substantia nigra.[115] The external pallidum then connects to the medial subthalamicus nucleus, which subsequently returns projections to the ventral pallidum.[116] There is some evidence that the ventral pallidum provides limited input to the magnocellular mediodorsal thalamus.[115] The anterior cingulate circuit is closed with projections from the dorsal portion of the magnocellular mediodorsal thalamus to the anterior cingulate.[117] Lesions to any one of the structures comprising the anterior cingulate circuit may thus potentially cause apathy.

Neurochemistry of Apathy in PD

The biological basis of apathy in PD has not been systematically examined, but several neurotransmitter systems of the brain may be considered as potential candidates. Dopamine, acetylcholine, and to a lesser degree noradrenaline and serotonin, appear to be the most important neurotransmitters involved in diminished motivation and apathy,[118] and are affected in PD.

Dopamine activity may influence the motivational state because of its role in reward, novelty seeking, and response to unexpected events.[111] In a recent study, apathy in PD was found to be inversely correlated with a marker of both dopamine and noradrenaline transporter in the ventral striatum.[48] Noradrenergic dysfunction may play an important role in the pathophysiology of apathy in PD because of an assumed relationship between bradyphrenia and neuronal loss in the locus coerulus. Another study demonstrated a significant difference in apathy scores between *off* and *on* states in fluctuating PD patients, suggesting that apathy in PD is at least partly a dopamine-dependent syndrome.[119] In addition, chronic administration of neuroleptics, which have strong dopamine receptor antagonist effects, has been associated with apathetic behavior.[120] In contrast, dose-dependent and reversible apathy has been reported in non-PD patients receiving selective serotonin reuptake inhibitors (SSRI) treatment.[121] Substantial improvement in apathy has been reported in some patients with PD dementia (PDD) using cholinesterase inhibitors,[122] which suggests that cholinergic deficits may at least partly be responsible for the development of apathetic behavior in PDD. Cholinergic and serotonergic pathways play a neuromodulatory role in the motivational circuitry, and several other neurotransmitters (including N-methyl-d-aspartate, AMPA, neurotensin, and substance P as well as nicotinic and opioid receptor agonists) are reported to modify the effect of dopamine on motivation.[120] A rare dominantly inherited syndrome of apathy, central hypoventilation, and parkinsonism is characterized by deficits of dopamine, serotonin, glutamate, and GABA with severe neuronal loss and gliosis of the substantia nigra.[123]

Treatment

Effects of DBS on Apathy

Several studies have reported changes in mood and apathy after DBS of the subthalamus (STN). In a comprehensive review of apathy following STN DBS surgery,[124] 4 studies reported increased apathy scores from pre-surgery to post-surgery, 2 reports did not find any change, and 1 study reported reduction in acute apathy when stimulators were switched from *off* to *on*. None of these reports found a significant reduction in mean apathy scores over time, leading to the conclusion that apathy is not improved by STN DBS surgery. Several hypotheses for apathy changes after STN DBS were proposed, including that motivational circuits may be affected by electrode placement or current spread. One study reported that apathetic patients had electrode placement more internally and ventrally in the STN than non-apathetic patients. Animal studies have shown that the limbic region of STN is located more ventrally and internally than the motor region, leading to the hypothesis that stimulation may have affected limbic circuits in the apathetic patients. Apathy change after STN DBS may also have been caused by reduction in levodopa medication after surgery, although none of the 3 studies examining this found a significant relationship between reductions in levodopa and apathy. Interestingly, one recent study of 8 PD patients who became apathetic after complete withdrawal of dopaminergic medication following STN stimulation [125] reported that treatment with small doses of a D2/D3 agonist markedly improved apathy in all but one of these patients. The authors suggested that apathy is associated with a dopaminergic deficit in associative-limbic areas of the brain.

General Strategies and Pharmacologic Treatment

Non-pharmacologic treatment includes educating caregivers about the symptoms of apathy to reduce misinterpretations of the patient's behavior as insensitive or laziness. Families may benefit from supportive therapy and help with problem solving. Patients will often benefit from structured environments, cueing, and simplification of tasks due to associated executive dysfunction.[126]

The pharmacologic treatment of apathy per se remains anecdotal and, to date, there are no formal studies on pharmacologic treatment of apathy in PD. The available treatments for apathy have only been tested in open trials or reported as case studies. At present, dopamine receptor agonists are regarded as the most effective treatment for apathy in neurological disorders.[127] Other dopaminergic agents (levodopa, selegeline, amantadine, and buproprion) have shown benefits in some cases.[119,128,129] In non-PD patients, older subjects with apathy may benefit from psychostimulants such as methylphenidate and dextroamphetamine.[129,130] To date, methylphenidate has only been described to be beneficial in a single case report of an older patient with PD.[131] Placebo-controlled studies with cholinesterase inhibitors have shown promising results on behavioral syndromes—including apathy—in dementia with Lewy bodies[132,133] and in PD.[122,134,135]

Summary

Depression and apathy are among the most common and characteristic neuropsychiatric symptoms in PD. Although depression and apathy frequently occur together, both syndromes can present independently as well. Both are probably linked to the key pathological features of PD, involving both dopaminergic and non-dopaminergic circuits, and can therefore be influenced by surgical manipulation of fronto-subcortical circuits. Although this has hitherto mainly been considered as a potential for adverse events, recent preliminary studies suggest that deep brain stimulation may represent a novel therapeutic potential. Several neurotransmitter-based pharmacological strategies exist, although systematic studies with serotonergic agents for depression have been negative, and systematic evidence of noradrenergic manipulation is lacking. Preliminary evidence of dopamine D3 agonists for depression is promising, whereas there is little evidence for the drug treatment of apathy. Although there is limited systematic evidence, preliminary studies and clinical practice suggest that counseling and psychoeducative approaches may be useful for patients with depression and apathy as well as their care givers.

References

1. Aarsland D, Larsen JP, Karlsen K, Lim NG, Tandberg E. Mental symptoms in Parkinson's disease are important contributors to caregiver distress. *Int J Geriatr Psychiatry*. 1999;14:866–74.
2. Karlsen KH, Larsen JP, Tandberg E, Maeland JG. Influence of clinical and demographic variables on quality of life in patients with Parkinson's disease. *J Neurol Neurosurg Psychiatry*. 1999;66:431–5.
3. Schrag A, Selai C, Jahanshahi M, Quinn NP. The EQ-5D–a generic quality of life measure-is a useful instrument to measure quality of life in patients with Parkinson's disease. *J Neurol Neurosurg Psychiatry*. 2000;69:67–73.

4. Weintraub D, Moberg PJ, Duda JE, Katz IR, Stern MB. Effect of psychiatric and other nonmotor symptoms on disability in Parkinson's disease. *J Am Geriatr Soc.* 2004;52:784–8.

5. Troster AI, Paolo AM, Lyons KE, Glatt SL, Hubble JP, Koller WC. The influence of depression on cognition in Parkinson's disease: a pattern of impairment distinguishable from Alzheimer's disease. *Neurology.* 1995;45:672–6.

6. Hughes TA, Ross HF, Mindham RH, Spokes EG. Mortality in Parkinson's disease and its association with dementia and depression. *Acta Neurol Scand.* 2004;110: 118–23.

7. Weintraub D, Moberg PJ, Duda JE, Katz IR, Stern MB. Recognition and treatment of depression in Parkinson's disease. *J Geriatr Psychiatry Neurol.* 2003;16:178–83.

8. Althaus A, Becker OA, Spottke A, et al. Frequency and treatment of depressive symptoms in a Parkinson's disease registry. *Parkinsonism Relat Disord.* 2008 Dec;14(8):626–32. Epub 2008 Apr 11

9. Reijnders JS, Ehrt U, Weber WE, Aarsland D, Leentjens AF. A systematic review of prevalence studies of depression in Parkinson's disease. *Mov Disord.* 2008;23:183–9; quiz 313.

10. Burn DJ. Depression in Parkinson's disease. *Eur J Neurol.* 2002;9 Suppl 3:44–54.

11. Starkstein SE, Mayberg HS, Leiguarda R, Preziosi TJ, Robinson RG. A prospective longitudinal study of depression, cognitive decline, and physical impairments in patients with Parkinson's disease. *J Neurol Neurosurg Psychiatry.* 1992;55:377–82.

12. Rojo A, Aguilar M, Garolera MT, Cubo E, Navas I, Quintana S. Depression in Parkinson's disease: clinical correlates and outcome. *Parkinsonism Relat Disord.* 2003;10:23–8.

13. Mayeux R, Stern Y, Sano M, Williams JB, Cote LJ. The relationship of serotonin to depression in Parkinson's disease. *Mov Disord.* 1988;3:237–44.

14. Lewy FH. *Die Lehre vom Tonus und der Bewegung.* Berlin: Julius Springer; 1923.

15. Gotham AM, Brown RG, Marsden CD. Depression in Parkinson's disease: a quantitative and qualitative analysis. *J Neurol Neurosurg Psychiatry.* 1986;49:381–9.

16. Schiffer RB, Kurlan R, Rubin A, Boer S. Evidence for atypical depression in Parkinson's disease. *Am J Psychiatry.* 1988;145:1020–2.

17. Starkstein SE, Preziosi TJ, Forrester AW, Robinson RG. Specificity of affective and autonomic symptoms of depression in Parkinson's disease. *J Neurol Neurosurg Psychiatry.* 1990;53:869–73.

18. Ehmann TS, Beninger RJ, Gawel MJ, Riopelle RJ. Depressive symptoms in Parkinson's disease: a comparison with disabled control subjects. *J Geriatr Psychiatry Neurol.* 1990;3:3–9.

19. Erdal KJ. Depressive symptom patterns in patients with Parkinson's disease and other older adults. *J Clin Psychol.* 2001;57:1559–69.

20. Merschdorf U, Berg D, Csoti I, et al. Psychopathological symptoms of depression in Parkinson's disease compared to major depression. *Psychopathology.* 2003;36: 221–5.

21. Ehrt U, Bronnick K, Leentjens AF, Larsen JP, Aarsland D. Depressive symptom profile in Parkinson's disease: a comparison with depression in elderly patients without Parkinson's disease. *Int J Geriatr Psychiatry.* 2006;21:252–8.

22. Marsh L, McDonald WM, Cummings J, Ravina B. Provisional diagnostic criteria for depression in Parkinson's disease: report of an NINDS/NIMH Work Group. *Mov Disord*. 2006;21:148–58.

23. Schrag A, Barone P, Brown RG, et al. Depression rating scales in Parkinson's disease: critique and recommendations. *Mov Disord*. 2007;22:1077–92.

24. Ehrt U, Bronnick K, De Deyn PP, et al. Subthreshold depression in patients with Parkinson's disease and dementia–clinical and demographic correlates. *Int J Geriatr Psychiatry*. 2007;22:980–5.

25. Serra-Mestres J, Ring HA. Vulnerability to emotionally negative stimuli in Parkinson's disease: an investigation using the Emotional Stroop task. *Neuropsychiatry Neuropsychol Behav Neurol*. 1999;12:52–7.

26. Leentjens AF, Van den Akker M, Metsemakers JF, Lousberg R, Verhey FR. Higher incidence of depression preceding the onset of Parkinson's disease: a register study. *Mov Disord*. 2003;18:414–8.

27. Taylor AE, Saint-Cyr JA. Depression in Parkinson's disease: reconciling physiological and psychological perspectives. *J Neuropsychiatry Clin Neurosci*. 1990;2:92–8.

28. Robins AH. Depression in patients with Parkinsonism. *Br J Psychiatry*. 1976;128: 141–5.

29. Menza MA, Mark MH. Parkinson's disease and depression: the relationship to disability and personality. *J Neuropsychiatry Clin Neurosci*. 1994;6:165–9.

30. Nilsson FM, Kessing LV, Sorensen TM, Andersen PK, Bolwig TG. Major depressive disorder in Parkinson's disease: a register-based study. *Acta Psychiatr Scand*. 2002;106:202–11.

31. Cole SA, Woodard JL, Juncos JL, Kogos JL, Youngstrom EA, Watts RL. Depression and disability in Parkinson's disease. *J Neuropsychiatry Clin Neurosci*. 1996;8:20–5.

32. Brown RG, MacCarthy B, Gotham AM, Der GJ, Marsden CD. Depression and disability in Parkinson's disease: a follow-up of 132 cases. *Psychol Med*. 1988;18:49–55.

33. Schrag A, Jahanshahi M, Quinn NP. What contributes to depression in Parkinson's disease? *Psychol Med*. 2001;31:65–73.

34. Starkstein SE, Preziosi TJ, Robinson RG. Sleep disorders, pain, and depression in Parkinson's disease. *Eur Neurol*. 1991;31:352–5.

35. Brown RG, Jahanshahi M, eds. Depression in Parkinson's disease. A psychological viewpoint. *Adv Neurol*. 1995;65:61–84.

36. Francis PT, Perry EK. Cholinergic and other neurotransmitter mechanisms in Parkinson's disease, Parkinson's disease dementia, and dementia with Lewy bodies. *Mov Disord*. 2007;22 Suppl 17:S351–7.

37. van Praag HM, de Haan S. Central serotonin metabolism and frequency of depression. *Psychiatry Res*. 1979;1:219–24.

38. Mayeux R, Stern Y, Cote L, Williams JB. Altered serotonin metabolism in depressed patients with parkinson's disease. *Neurology*. 1984;34:642–6.

39. Kuhn W, Muller T, Gerlach M, et al. Depression in Parkinson's disease: biogenic amines in CSF of "de novo" patients. *J Neural Transm*. 1996;103:1441–5.

40. Menza MA, Palermo B, DiPaola R, Sage JI, Ricketts MH. Depression and anxiety in Parkinson's disease: possible effect of genetic variation in the serotonin transporter. *J Geriatr Psychiatry Neurol*. 1999;12:49–52.

41. Mossner R, Henneberg A, Schmitt A, et al. Allelic variation of serotonin transporter expression is associated with depression in Parkinson's disease. *Mol Psychiatry.* 2001;6:350–2.

42. Paulus W, Jellinger K. The neuropathologic basis of different clinical subgroups of Parkinson's disease. *J Neuropathol Exp Neurol.* 1991;50:743–55.

43. Berg D, Supprian T, Hofmann E, et al. Depression in Parkinson's disease: brainstem midline alteration on transcranial sonography and magnetic resonance imaging. *J Neurol.* 1999;246:1186–93.

44. Halliday GM, Blumbergs PC, Cotton RG, Blessing WW, Geffen LB. Loss of brainstem serotonin- and substance P-containing neurons in Parkinson's disease. *Brain Res.* 1990;510:104–7.

45. Doder M, Rabiner EA, Turjanski N, Lees AJ, Brooks DJ. Tremor in Parkinson's disease and serotonergic dysfunction: an 11C-WAY 100635 PET study. *Neurology.* 2003;60:601–5.

46. Chan-Palay V. Depression and dementia in Parkinson's disease. Catecholamine changes in the locus ceruleus, a basis for therapy. *Adv Neurol.* 1993;60:438–46.

47. Cash R, Ruberg M, Raisman R, Agid Y. Adrenergic receptors in Parkinson's disease. *Brain Res.* 1984;322:269–75.

48. Remy P, Doder M, Lees A, Turjanski N, Brooks D. Depression in Parkinson's disease: loss of dopamine and noradrenaline innervation in the limbic system. *Brain.* 2005;128:1314–22.

49. Tandberg E, Larsen JP, Aarsland D, Cummings JL. The occurrence of depression in Parkinson's disease. A community-based study. *Arch Neurol.* 1996;53:175–9.

50. Sano M, Stern Y, Williams J, Cote L, Rosenstein R, Mayeux R. Coexisting dementia and depression in Parkinson's disease. *Arch Neurol.* 1989;46:1284–6.

51. Chia LG, Cheng LJ, Chuo LJ, Cheng FC, Cu JS. Studies of dementia, depression, electrophysiology and cerebrospinal fluid monoamine metabolites in patients with Parkinson's disease. *J Neurol Sci.* 1995;133:73–8.

52. Starkstein SE, Bolduc PL, Mayberg HS, Preziosi TJ, Robinson RG. Cognitive impairments and depression in Parkinson's disease: a follow up study. *J Neurol Neurosurg Psychiatry.* 1990;53:597–602.

53. Jacobs DM, Marder K, Cote LJ, Sano M, Stern Y, Mayeux R. Neuropsychological characteristics of preclinical dementia in Parkinson's disease. *Neurology.* 1995;45:1691–6.

54. Stern Y, Marder K, Tang MX, Mayeux R. Antecedent clinical features associated with dementia in Parkinson's disease. *Neurology.* 1993;43:1690–2.

55. Perry EK, Kilford L, Lees AJ, Burn DJ, Perry RH. Increased Alzheimer pathology in Parkinson's disease related to antimuscarinic drugs. *Ann Neurol.* 2003;54:235–8.

56. Bohnen NI, Kaufer DI, Hendrickson R, Constantine GM, Mathis CA, Moore RY. Cortical cholinergic denervation is associated with depressive symptoms in Parkinson's disease and parkinsonian dementia. *J Neurol Neurosurg Psychiatry.* 2007;78:641–3.

57. McRitchie DA, Cartwright HR, Halliday GM. Specific A10 dopaminergic nuclei in the midbrain degenerate in Parkinson's disease. *Exp Neurol.* 1997;144:202–13.

58. Damier P, Hirsch EC, Agid Y, Graybiel AM. The substantia nigra of the human brain. II. Patterns of loss of dopamine-containing neurons in Parkinson's disease. *Brain.* 1999;122 (Pt 8):1437–48.

59. Tremblay LK, Naranjo CA, Graham SJ, et al. Functional neuroanatomical substrates of altered reward processing in major depressive disorder revealed by a dopaminergic probe. *Arch Gen Psychiatry*. 2005;62:1228–36.
60. Winter C, von Rumohr A, Mundt A, et al. Lesions of dopaminergic neurons in the substantia nigra pars compacta and in the ventral tegmental area enhance depressive-like behavior in rats. *Behav Brain Res*. 2007;184:133–41.
61. Chan LL, Rumpel H, Yap K, et al. Case control study of diffusion tensor imaging in Parkinson's disease. *J Neurol Neurosurg Psychiatry*. 2007;78:1383–6.
62. Matsui H, Nishinaka K, Oda M, et al. Depression in Parkinson's disease. Diffusion tensor imaging study. *J Neurol*. 2007;254:1170–3.
63. Kim SE, Choi JY, Choe YS, Choi Y, Lee WY. Serotonin transporters in the midbrain of Parkinson's disease patients: a study with 123I-beta-CIT SPECT. *J Nucl Med*. 2003;44:870–6.
64. Mayberg HS, Starkstein SE, Sadzot B, et al. Selective hypometabolism in the inferior frontal lobe in depressed patients with Parkinson's disease. *Ann Neurol*. 1990;28:57–64.
65. Weintraub D, Morales KH, Moberg PJ, et al. Antidepressant studies in Parkinson's disease: a review and meta-analysis. *Mov Disord*. 2005;20:1161–9.
66. Bianchi MT. Non-serotonin anti-depressant actions: direct ion channel modulation by SSRIs and the concept of single agent poly-pharmacy. *Med Hypotheses*. 2008;70:951–6.
67. Reichmann H, Brecht HM, Kraus PH, Lemke MR. [Pramipexole in Parkinson disease. Results of a treatment observation]. *Nervenarzt*. 2002;73:745–50.
68. Barone P, Scarzella L, Marconi R, et al. Pramipexole versus sertraline in the treatment of depression in Parkinson's disease: a national multicenter parallel-group randomized study. *J Neurol*. 2006;253:601–7.
69. Lemke MR, Brecht HM, Koester J, Reichmann H. Effects of the dopamine agonist pramipexole on depression, anhedonia and motor functioning in Parkinson's disease. *J Neurol Sci*. 2006;248:266–70.
70. Aiken CB. Pramipexole in psychiatry: a systematic review of the literature. *J Clin Psychiatry*. 2007;68:1230–6.
71. Lemke MR. [Antidepressant effects of dopamine agonists : Experimental and clinical findings.]. *Nervenarzt*. 2007;78:31–8.
72. Lemke MR. Depressive symptoms in Parkinson's disease. *Eur J Neurol*. 2008;15 Suppl 1:21–5.
73. Strome EM, Zis AP, Doudet DJ. Electroconvulsive shock enhances striatal dopamine D1 and D3 receptor binding and improves motor performance in 6-OHDA-lesioned rats. *J Psychiatry Neurosci*. 2007;32:193–202.
74. Fregni F, Santos CM, Myczkowski ML, et al. Repetitive transcranial magnetic stimulation is as effective as fluoxetine in the treatment of depression in patients with Parkinson's disease. *J Neurol Neurosurg Psychiatry*. 2004;75:1171–4.
75. Fregni F, Ono CR, Santos CM, et al. Effects of antidepressant treatment with rTMS and fluoxetine on brain perfusion in PD. *Neurology*. 2006;66:1629–37.
76. Bejjani BP, Damier P, Arnulf I, et al. Transient acute depression induced by high-frequency deep-brain stimulation. *N Engl J Med*. 1999;340:1476–80.

77. Stefurak T, Mikulis D, Mayberg H, et al. Deep brain stimulation for Parkinson's disease dissociates mood and motor circuits: a functional MRI case study. *Mov Disord.* 2003;18:1508–16.

78. Kulisevsky J, Berthier ML, Gironell A, Pascual-Sedano B, Molet J, Pares P. Mania following deep brain stimulation for Parkinson's disease. *Neurology.* 2002;59: 1421–4.

79. Lozano AM, Mayberg HS, Giacobbe P, Hamani C, Craddock RC, Kennedy SH. Subcallosal cingulate gyrus deep brain stimulation for treatment-resistant depression. *Biol Psychiatry.* 2008;64:461–7.

80. Rahman S, Griffin HJ, Quinn NP, Jahanshahi M. Quality of life in Parkinson's disease: The relative importance of the symptoms. *Mov Disord.* 2008.

81. Koizumi Y, Awata S, Kuriyama S, et al. Association between social support and depression status in the elderly: results of a 1-year community-based prospective cohort study in Japan. *Psychiatry Clin Neurosci.* 2005;59:563–9.

82. Cheng Y, Liu C, Mao C, Qian J, Liu K, Ke G. Social support plays a role in depression in Parkinson's disease: a cross-section study in a Chinese cohort. *Parkinsonism Relat Disord.* 2008;14:43–5.

83. Marin RS. Differential diagnosis and classification of apathy. *Am J Psychiatry.* 1990;147:22–30.

84. Marin RS, Biedrzycki RC, Firinciogullari S. Reliability and validity of the Apathy Evaluation Scale. *Psychiatry Res.* 1991;38:143–62.

85. Starkstein SE, Manes F. Apathy and depression following stroke. *CNS Spectr.* 2000;5:43–50.

86. Starkstein SE, Leentjens AF. The nosological position of apathy in clinical practice. *J Neurol Neurosurg Psychiatry.* 2008;79:1088–92.

87. Stuss DT, Alexander MP. Executive functions and the frontal lobes: a conceptual view. *Psychol Res.* 2000;63:289–98.

88. Levy R, Dubois B. Apathy and the functional anatomy of the prefrontal cortex-basal ganglia circuits. *Cereb Cortex.* 2006;16:916–28.

89. Leentjens AF, Dujardin K, Marsh L, et al. Apathy and anhedonia rating scales in Parkinson's disease: critique and recommendations. *Mov Disord.* 2008;23:2004–14.

90. Starkstein SE, Merello M, Jorge R, et al. A validation study of depressive syndromes in Parkinson's disease. *Mov Disord.* 2008;23:538–46.

91. Starkstein SE, Mayberg HS, Preziosi TJ, Andrezejewski P, Leiguarda R, Robinson RG. Reliability, validity, and clinical correlates of apathy in Parkinson's disease. *J Neuropsychiatry Clin Neurosci.* 1992;4:134–9.

92. Levy ML, Cummings JL, Fairbanks LA, et al. Apathy is not depression. *J Neuropsychiatry Clin Neurosci.* 1998;10:314–9.

93. Isella V, Melzi P, Grimaldi M, et al. Clinical, neuropsychological, and morphometric correlates of apathy in Parkinson's disease. *Mov Disord.* 2002;17:366–71.

94. Kirsch-Darrow L, Fernandez HF, Marsiske M, Okun MS, Bowers D. Dissociating apathy and depression in Parkinson disease. *Neurology.* 2006;67:33–8.

95. Dujardin K, Sockeel P, Devos D, et al. Characteristics of apathy in Parkinson's disease. *Mov Disord.* 2007;22:778–84.

96. Pedersen KF, Larsen JP, Aarsland D. Validation of the Unified Parkinson's Disease Rating Scale (UPDRS) section I as a screening and diagnostic instrument for apathy in patients with Parkinson's disease. *Parkinsonism Relat Disord*. 2008;14: 183–6.

97. Lavretsky H, Ballmaier M, Pham D, Toga A, Kumar A. Neuroanatomical characteristics of geriatric apathy and depression: a magnetic resonance imaging study. *Am J Geriatr Psychiatry*. 2007;15:386–94.

98. Marin RS. Apathy: concept, syndrome, neural mechanisms, and treatment. *Semin Clin Neuropsychiatry*. 1996;1:304–14.

99. Braak H, Del Tredici K, Rub U, de Vos RA, Jansen Steur EN, Braak E. Staging of brain pathology related to sporadic Parkinson's disease. *Neurobiol Aging*. 2003;24:197–211.

100. Zgaljardic DJ, Borod JC, Foldi NS, et al. Relationship between self-reported apathy and executive dysfunction in nondemented patients with Parkinson disease. *Cogn Behav Neurol*. 2007;20:184–92.

101. Pedersen KF, Larsen JP, Alves G, Aarsland D. Prevalence and clinical correlates of apathy in Parkinson's disease: A community-based study. *Parkinsonism Relat Disord*. 2008.

102. Aarsland D, Larsen JP, Lim NG, et al. Range of neuropsychiatric disturbances in patients with Parkinson's disease. *J Neurol Neurosurg Psychiatry*. 1999;67:492–6.

103. Ringman JM, Diaz-Olavarrieta C, Rodriguez Y, Fairbanks L, Cummings JL. The prevalence and correlates of neuropsychiatric symptoms in a population with Parkinson's disease in Mexico. *Neuropsychiatry Neuropsychol Behav Neurol*. 2002;15:99–105.

104. Pluck GC, Brown RG. Apathy in Parkinson's disease. *J Neurol Neurosurg Psychiatry*. 2002;73:636–42.

105. Aarsland D, Bronnick K, Ehrt U, et al. Neuropsychiatric symptoms in patients with Parkinson's disease and dementia: frequency, profile and associated care giver stress. *J Neurol Neurosurg Psychiatry*. 2007;78:36–42.

106. Kulisevsky J, Pagonabarraga J, Pascual-Sedano B, Garcia-Sanchez C, Gironell A. Prevalence and correlates of neuropsychiatric symptoms in Parkinson's disease without dementia. *Mov Disord*. 2008.

107. Dubois B, Burn D, Goetz C, et al. Diagnostic procedures for Parkinson's disease dementia: recommendations from the movement disorder society task force. *Mov Disord*. 2007;22:2314–24.

108. Pierce RC, Kalivas PW. A circuitry model of the expression of behavioral sensitization to amphetamine-like psychostimulants. *Brain Res Rev*. 1997;25:192–216.

109. Bush G, Luu P, Posner MI. Cognitive and emotional influences in anterior cingulate cortex. *Trends Cogn Sci*. 2000;4:215–22.

110. Bush G, Vogt BA, Holmes J, et al. Dorsal anterior cingulate cortex: a role in reward-based decision making. *Proc Natl Acad Sci USA*. 2002;99:523–8.

111. Marin RS, Wilkosz PA. Disorders of diminished motivation. *J Head Trauma Rehabil*. 2005;20:377–88.

112. Bonelli RM, Cummings JL. Frontal-subcortical dementias. *Neurologist*. 2008;14: 100–7.

113. Alexander GE, DeLong MR, Strick PL. Parallel organization of functionally segregated circuits linking basal ganglia and cortex. *Annu Rev Neurosci.* 1986;9: 357–81.

114. Mega MS, Cohenour RC. Akinetic mutism: disconnection of frontal-subcortical circuits. *Neuropsychiatry Neuropsychol Behav Neurol.* 1997;10:254–9.

115. Critchley HD. Neural mechanisms of autonomic, affective, and cognitive integration. *J Comp Neurol.* 2005;493:154–66.

116. Smith Y, Bolam JP. The output neurones and the dopaminergic neurones of the substantia nigra receive a GABA-containing input from the globus pallidus in the rat. *J Comp Neurol.* 1990;296:47–64.

117. Goldman-Rakic PS, Porrino LJ. The primate mediodorsal (MD) nucleus and its projection to the frontal lobe. *J Comp Neurol.* 1985;242:535–60.

118. van Reekum R, Stuss DT, Ostrander L. Apathy: why care? *J Neuropsychiatry Clin Neurosci.* 2005;17:7–19.

119. Czernecki V, Pillon B, Houeto JL, Pochon JB, Levy R, Dubois B. Motivation, reward, and Parkinson's disease: influence of dopatherapy. *Neuropsychologia.* 2002;40:2257–67.

120. Shulman L. Apathy in patients with Parkinson's disease. *Intern Rev Psychiat.* 2000;12:298–306.

121. Barnhart WJ, Makela EH, Latocha MJ. SSRI-induced apathy syndrome: a clinical review. *J Psychiatr Pract.* 2004;10:196–9.

122. McKeith I. Dementia in Parkinson's disease: common and treatable. *Lancet Neurol.* 2004;3:456.

123. Perry TL, Wright JM, Berry K, Hansen S, Perry TL, Jr. Dominantly inherited apathy, central hypoventilation, and Parkinson's syndrome: clinical, biochemical, and neuropathologic studies of 2 new cases. *Neurology.* 1990;40:1882–7.

124. Kirsch-Darrow L, Mikos A, Bowers D. Does deep brain stimulation induce apathy in Parkinson's disease? *Front Biosci.* 2008;13:5316–22.

125. Czernecki V, Schupbach M, Yaici S, et al. Apathy following subthalamic stimulation in Parkinson disease: a dopamine responsive symptom. *Mov Disord.* 2008;23: 964–9.

126. Marsh L. Behavioral disturbances. In: Menza M, Marsh L, eds. *Psychiatric issues in Parkinson's disease - A practical guide.* London, New York: Taylor & Francis Group; 2006:193–218.

127. Campbell A, Villavicencio AT, Yeghiayan SK, Balikian R, Baldessarini RJ. Mapping of locomotor behavioral arousal induced by microinjections of dopamine within nucleus accumbens septi of rat forebrain. *Brain Res.* 1997;771:55–62.

128. Corcoran C, Wong ML, O'Keane V. Bupropion in the management of apathy. *J Psychopharmacol.* 2004;18:133–5.

129. Marin RS, Fogel BS, Hawkins J, Duffy J, Krupp B. Apathy: a treatable syndrome. *J Neuropsychiatry Clin Neurosci.* 1995;7:23–30.

130. Roccaforte WH, Burke WJ. Use of psychostimulants for the elderly. *Hosp Community Psychiatry.* 1990;41:1330–3.

131. Chatterjee A, Fahn S. Methylphenidate treats apathy in Parkinson's disease. *J Neuropsychiatry Clin Neurosci.* 2002;14:461–2.

132. McKeith I, Del Ser T, Spano P, et al. Efficacy of rivastigmine in dementia with Lewy bodies: a randomised, double-blind, placebo-controlled international study. *Lancet.* 2000;356:2031–6.

133. Edwards KR, Hershey L, Wray L, et al. Efficacy and safety of galantamine in patients with dementia with Lewy bodies: a 12-week interim analysis. *Dement Geriatr Cogn Disord.* 2004;17 Suppl 1:40–8.

134. Aarsland D, Hutchinson M, Larsen JP. Cognitive, psychiatric and motor response to galantamine in Parkinson's disease with dementia. *Int J Geriatr Psychiatry.* 2003;18:937–41.

135. Leroi I, Brandt J, Reich SG, et al. Randomized placebo-controlled trial of donepezil in cognitive impairment in Parkinson's disease. *Int J Geriatr Psychiatry.* 2004;19:1–8.

Chapter 9

Lesions Associated with Dyskinesias and the Dopamine Dysregulation Syndrome

Andrew H. Evans

Introduction

Parkinson's disease (PD) is a chronic progressive neurodegenerative disorder, the core neuropathological hallmark of which is the loss of the dopamine nigrostriatal pathway associated with the formation of α-synuclein-positive Lewy bodies. Dopamine depletion in the dorsal striatum results in the core motor features of PD, including bradykinesia and rigidity, once the degree of the main denervation has reached approximately 60%.[1] Attention on the nigrostriatal dopamine system in PD is justified by the success of the dopamine precursor levodopa and other dopamine agonists in alleviating motor symptoms. However, a broad range of non-motor symptoms also complicate PD and encompass neuropsychiatric, autonomic, sensory, and sleep disturbances.[2] Many of the non-motor symptoms reflect the evolution of non-dopamine lesions.

Conversely, the dopamine treatments used to ameliorate motor disability in PD can trigger, worsen, or be the primary cause of symptoms. Some of these medication-induced symptoms appear to be idiosyncratic, many are toxic or dose related, and others may arise only after long-term exposure to dopamine replacement drugs, thus reflecting drug-induced neuroplastic changes.

Motor-related complications of dopamine replacement treatments are the best understood medication-induced phenomena and include the progressive shortening of the duration of response to dopamine replacement drugs (i.e. the development of wearing-off phenomena) and the development of abnormal involuntary movements called dyskinesias. It has recently become apparent that medication-induced symptoms also include a set of complex disinhibitory behavioral pathologies that are linked by their repetitive, reward or incentive-based natures. These disinhibitory psychopathologies may evolve some time after the initiation of dopamine replacement therapies and encompass impulse control disorders (ICDs), punding, and the dopamine dysregulation syndrome (DDS). They often lead to negative consequences related to physical, psychological, social, legal or financial effects. In the clinic, early identification of these behaviors and understanding the specific individual vulnerabilities that may lead to the emergence of these behavioral phenomena would be expected to minimize the harm that results.

Dopamine agonists used to treat the motor symptoms of PD can engage a set of molecular mechanisms involving brain dopamine systems and related circuitry that are normally involved in learning and reward, lead to altered patterns of synaptic plasticity, and ultimately lead to persistent alterations in many neural systems, altering motor and many other psychological processes.[3] The expression of motor response complications and disinhibitory psychomotor behaviors is thought to arise from a complex interaction between individual disease processes and medication-induced neuroplastic changes. Pharmacotherapeutic approaches to the management of these psychomotor disorders are limited but successful management should aim to address neuroadaptive processes beyond the dopamine system that underlie these drug-induced psychomotor phenomena.

Dyskinesias

Phenomenology
Symptomatic treatment with levodopa is the most effective strategy in reducing the motor disability due to PD but levodopa has a short half-life, requiring it to be administered repeatedly in a chronic intermittent schedule. In some patients, abnormal involuntary movements (dyskinesias) can mar the long-term therapeutic response to chronic treatment with levodopa. Levodopa-induced dyskinesias typically present with an idiosyncratic mixture of chorea (abrupt movements that seem to flow from one body part to another) and dystonia (slow twisting movements). It is the pulsatile treatment pattern that underpins the evolution of the dyskinesias, which

are usually most severe during the 2 hours that follow a drug dose when the plasma and brain levels of exogenous levodopa reach their peak. Dyskinesias are highly responsive to stress.[4]

Prevalence and risk factors

Disease factors

Approximately 30% of PD patients experience dyskinesias after 4 to 6 years of levodopa treatment and close to 90% show dyskinesias after 9 years.[5] Clinical and epidemiological studies have identified young age at PD onset, disease severity and duration, higher initial levodopa dose, and duration of levodopa treatment as prominent risk factors for dyskinesias.[6–9] The association of dyskinesias with the severity and duration of PD relates to the extent of striatal dopamine depletion.[10] In disorders not associated with dopamine denervation, such as dopa-responsive dystonia, dyskinesias do not usually develop with levodopa treatment.[11] In asymmetrically affected parkinsonian patients, dyskinesias usually appear first and are more severe on the most affected side.[12] In patients with severe untreated PD or massive relatively acute degeneration of dopamine nigrostriatal neurons due to MPTP-induced parkinsonism, dyskinesias develop within months of levodopa treatment.[13,14] Differences in individual responses to "dopamine replacement" is also relevant; a greater amplitude of motor effect from levodopa in dopa-naïve patients predicts a greater augmentation in levodopa's motor effects, and the earlier development of dyskinesias.[15]

Examination of the *in vivo* effects of dopamine denervation and levodopa treatment in PD patients is limited by the nature of the pathological process and variations in individual treatment regimens. By contrast, animal models allow for detecting the impact of the specific elements under strictly controlled conditions. Incomplete lesions of the rat nigrostriatal dopamine system mobilizes a variety of neuroplastic responses in surviving dopamine neurons, including increased dopamine synthesis and release, a reduced rate of dopamine inactivation, and a vigorous axonal sprouting in the terminal arbours[16] which would normally be inhibited by a tonic stimulation of D2 autoreceptors.[17] The homeostatic capacity of the nigrostriatal dopamine system decompensates when >70% of nigral dopamine neurons are lost.[16] Consistent with clinical observations, the severity of the nigrostriatal dopamine lesion in animals strongly influences the threshold at which an acute dose of levodopa can induce dyskinesia.[18]

Medication Factors

In human studies of levodopa-induced dyskinesias, risk factors include levodopa dose and treatment duration. In animal models of dyskinesia, cumulative dose of levodopa has been suggested to be more important for the induction of dyskinesias than the amount of levodopa given with each dose.[19]

Presynaptic Plasticity

Levodopa-induced plasticity invokes changes in presynaptic mechanisms of levodopa or dopamine uptake, conversion, and metabolism. Using the 6-OHDA lesion model of PD, the surge in extracellular dopamine levels in the striatum elicited by a peripheral dose of levodopa can be augmented or sensitized by a prior course of levodopa treatment.[20] In PD patients, levodopa induced surges in extracellular dopamine in the dorsal striatum have also been correlated to dyskinesia severity and provide evidence for medication-induced sensitization of dorsal striatal systems.[21]

Brain serotonin projections may contribute to unregulated striatal levodopa-induced dopamine release observed in advanced PD.[3] Severe dopamine denervation alters the routes of levodopa uptake and metabolism in the brain; for instance, serotonin neurons and other neuronal elements can become capable of decarboxylating levodopa to dopamine. Serotonin neurons can store dopamine in synaptic vesicles and release it together with serotonin but lack both dopamine autoreceptors and the dopamine transporter. This can provide a source of unregulated dopamine efflux into the extracellular space following administration of exogenous levodopa.[3] Serotonin lesions or combined treatment with agonists at 5HT1A and 5HT1B autoreceptors (which reduce transmitter release from serotonin axons) block the expression of dyskinesia in rat models.[22]

Post-synaptic Plasticity

In rodents with near complete nigrostriatal denervation, dyskinesias are much more tightly correlated with long-lasting changes in gene expression in striatal neurons (i.e. prodynorphin [preproenkephalin-B] mRNA and FosB-related transcription factors) than markers of presynaptic dopamine denervation.[23] The signaling pathway through which levodopa induces these changes primarily involves upregulation of D1-dependent dopamine receptor signaling pathways rather than D2 receptor pathways.

In the normal brain, the D3 receptor is predominantly expressed in the nucleus accumbens and limbic regions and is largely absent from the rat motor striatum. 6-OHDA induced nigrostriatal lesions do not affect D3 receptor expression. However, D3 receptor expression is increased in the nucleus accumbens and induced in the caudate and putamen by levodopa treatment, and parallels the development of behavioral sensitization to levodopa.[24] Behavioral sensitization to levodopa can be blocked by D3 receptor antagonists and D3 receptor agonists can potentiate behavioral sensitization induced by D1 receptor agonists.[25] The striatal D3 receptor induction is ablated by deprivation of brain-derived neurotrophic factor normally synthesized by dopamine neurons.[26]

Plasticity in the induction of levodopa-induced dyskinesias also involves structural changes within the basal ganglia. Hypertrophy within the internal globus pallidus (GPi) and substantia nigra pars reticulata (SNR),[27] which together represent the output nuclei of the basal ganglia, along with profound changes in neuronal firing patterns and alterations in the microvasculature,[28] all contribute to levodopa-induced dyskinesias.

This ultimately leads to alterations in the neuronal firing patterns in the basal ganglia and cortex. Consistent with models of basal ganglia functioning, the onset of levodopa-induced dyskinesias correlates with both an over-reduction of the firing frequency of the GPi and abnormal firing patterns that lead, through reduced inhibition of motor thalamic nuclei, to the subsequent overactivation of cortical motor areas.[29]

GABAergic and Glutamatergic Mechanisms

Exuberant post-synaptic responses to dopamine are also important in dyskinesias. Dopamine receptors are expressed on striatal medium spiny neurons that constitute the efferent GABAergic pathways from the striatum to GPi/SNR (direct pathway) and to the external segment of the globus pallidus (GPe) (indirect pathway). Dopamine exerts opposing effects on these 2 neuronal populations based on their preferential expression of 2 subclasses of dopamine receptor. The D1 dopamine receptor predominates in the direct pathway, where it mediates facilitatory responses to fast neurotransmitters, whereas the D2 subtype is the main subtype in the indirect pathway, where it is proposed to decrease neuronal excitability. In addition to nigrostriatal dopamine projections, these GABAergic neurons also receive glutamatergic projections from most cortical areas as well as terminals from other extrinsic (such as serotonin) and intrinsic (such as cholinergic) pathways.[30] Pulsatile stimulation of striatal dopamine receptors can induce downstream changes in striatal proteins and genes, and abnormalities in non-dopamine transmitter systems.

Long-term potentiation (LTP), a model of hippocampal memory/learning, has been demonstrated in cortical and subcortical areas involved in motor behavior and learning. The activity-dependent increase in synaptic efficacy that is characteristic of LTP appears to depend largely on enhanced sensitivity of glutamate receptors, including the N-methyl-D-aspartate (NMDA) subtype.[31] Type 5 metabotropic glutamate receptors (mGluR5) have been shown to modulate D1 receptor-dependent signaling and are implicated in the intracellular processes responsible for upregulation of FosB. The tight functional interaction between glutamate and dopamine inputs on GABAergic striatal neurons is thought to allow the plasticity of corticospinal transmission to be modulated and is pivotal to the learning and storage of both adaptive and maladaptive behaviors.[3]

Non-dopamine Modulators

Adenosine A2A receptors also play a modulatory role in dopamine innervated brain regions where they can form complexes with both D2 receptors and mGluR5. Dyskinetic PD patients have been shown to have increased adenosine A2A receptors in the GPe[32]; however, the mechanism of receptor over-expression remains unclear. A2A antagonists and targeted A2A receptor depletion attenuate the development of sensitized responses to levodopa in mouse PD models of levodopa-induced dyskinesias.[33] A2A antagonists represent a promising treatment for levodopa-induced dyskinesias in humans.[34]

Disinhibitory Psychopathologies

Impulse Control Disorders (ICDs)

Phenomenology

ICDs typically involve pleasurable or hedonic behaviors that are performed repetitively, excessively, and/or compulsively, and to an extent that interferes in normal life function. ICDs have been conceptualized as "behavioral" addictions.[35] ICDs identified in PD encompass a range of compulsive appetitive behaviors and include hypersexuality, compulsive shopping, binge or compulsive eating,[36] kleptomania, reckless driving,[37] and compulsive generosity.

Pathological gambling is the most extensively studied ICD in PD and non-PD populations and is defined as persistent and recurrent maladaptive gambling behavior. Hypersexuality was the earliest recognized PD-related ICD and may cause serious sexual assault.[38] It is characterised by a preoccupation with sexual thoughts, demands for sex, desire for frequent genital stimulation, promiscuity, habitual use of telephone sex lines, and Internet pornography or contact with sex workers. Paraphilias may accompany hypersexuality or occur in isolation in the form of transvestic fetishism,[39] pedophilia,[40] sadomasochism,[41] and zoophilia.[42] Compulsive buying is defined by the presence of repetitive impulsive and excessive buying of goods that are not needed and may lead to financial stress.[43] Binge eating refers to discrete episodes of increased eating and compulsive eating is characterized by uncontrollable consumption of a larger amount of food than normal and in excess of that which is necessary to alleviate hunger and may occur without binge eating.[44]

Prevalence and Risk Factors

The greatest risk factor for ICDs in PD is dopamine agonist drugs. Studies particularly highlight the link not only with total dopamine agonist dose but also total levodopa dose (especially when given in combination). ICDs are often under-recognized in routine clinical practice.[45] Systematic prevalence estimates for common ICDs in treated PD patients are around 14.0% and increase to 17.1% in patients treated with dopamine agonists.[45–48] Univariate analysis in different studies has also found younger age, history of ICD symptoms prior to development of PD, amantadine use, unmarried status, and family history of gambling problems to be associated with the presence of an ICD.[47–49] There is also a general association between the presence of an ICD and higher measures of impulsivity and depression.[50,51] One-third or more of patients with an ICD have more than one ICD.[47,48,50]

Punding

Phenomenology

Punding was first described in psychostimulant addicts.[52] There is a continuum of punding behavior ranging from excessive "hobbyism" to prolonged, disabling, highly stereotyped ritualistic behavior. Activities may include collecting or hoarding items, cleaning, repairing things, gardening, writing and categorizing information, artistic drawing or craft-making, singing or playing a musical instrument, playing cards, fishing, and excessive computer and Internet use.[53] Punders may neglect their physiological needs, such as sleep, hunger, and thirst, as well as their social responsibilities. They may or may not retain insight regarding the inappropriateness of their behavior. Some patients report the activity as soothing and may become irritated when interrupted; others report no joy or satisfaction in their activities or even become agitated while carrying out the activity.

Prevalence and Risk Factors

There are conflicting data about prevalence estimates of punding. Using a semistructured interview, one study found the rate to be surprisingly high: punding occurred in nearly 14% of consecutive PD outpatients, and in about 30 % of patients receiving a medication dose of greater than 800 levodopa equivalence units daily.[53] A subsequent self-administered questionnaire survey found the prevalence of punding to be one-tenth of that estimate (1.4% of PD patients). A figure of 8% in another prospective survey may be more congruent with the experience of most PD clinics.[48] Higher impulsivity, poorer disease-related quality of life, younger age of disease onset, and concomitant daily medication dosage from dopamine receptor agonists have been found to independently predict punding-like behaviors in PD patients.[54]

Dopamine Dysregulation Syndrome (DDS)

Phenomenology
DDS refers to the compulsive use of dopamine agonist medications well beyond the dose needed to optimally control motor disability and in the face of a mounting number of harmful physical, psychiatric, and social sequelae.[55–57] Many individuals with DDS report the avoidance of aversive off-period non-motor symptoms as the reason for the compulsive use of medications and fulfill ICD-10 criteria for "addiction."[58] Disability due to DDS may improve with medication reductions but there is an enduring tendency for the individual to relapse.[57] Impulsive aggression is often encountered in individuals with DDS in the context of aggressive demands for medications or sexual intercourse.[55] Self-injury ideation/behavior and hypomanic behavior may feature during medication binges.

Prevalence and Risk Factors
Addiction to dopamine replacement drugs is uncommon, but has been reported to occur in up to 4% of PD patients in tertiary referral centers. DDS patients have been found to have a significantly younger age of disease onset, longer disease duration, higher dopamine drug intake, greater past experimental drug use, more depressive symptoms, score higher on impulsivity ratings, and tend to have higher alcohol intake than PD controls. Compared to healthy controls, DDS patients have higher impulsivity, more depressive symptoms, and are more likely to have used illicit drugs in the past.[59]

Overlaps Between Medication-induced Psychopathologies
Behavioral data implicate common neurobiological systems in mediating the emergence of disinhibitory psychopathologies. ICDs, DDS, and punding have not been described in untreated PD patients and frequently coexist in treated PD patients—indicating that dopamine drugs can potentially "sensitize" a range of appetitive or repetitive behaviors.[57] ICDs are a common source of morbidity in patients with DDS but far fewer patients with ICDs will use their dopamine drugs compulsively.[46,60,61] Increased or new substance addictions (tobacco, alcohol or other recreational drugs)

have also occasionally been reported [61–63] in PD patients displaying ICDs. ICD patients without DDS often exhibit multiple ICDs.[61,62,64–68] Moreover, there is significant overlap in risk factors for ICDs, punding, and DDS except the duration of treatment may be longer for DDS or punding compared to pathological gambling (PG) (Table 9-1).[60] Patients with DDS

Table 9-1. Medication, Disease and Individual Factors Reported to be Relevant to the Emergence of DDS, ICDs and Punding

Dopamine dysregulation syndrome (DDS)	Impulse control disorders (ICDs)	Punding	Pathological or problem gambling	Hypersexuality
Medication Factors				
Dopamine agonist use	No	Yes	Yes	Yes
Longer agonist therapy		Probable		
Agonist dose		Probable	Probable	Probable
Total medication dose	Yes	Probable	Probable	Yes
Disease Factors				
Early PD onset	Yes	Yes	Yes	Yes
Disease duration	9.5 years (59)	7.8 years (60)	9.6 years	?longer
Cognitive dysfunction	Possible			
Individual Factors				
Impulsivity	Yes	Yes	Yes	Yes
Male gender	No	Yes	Yes	Modifies phenomenology
Marital status		Yes	Yes	
Prior substance use	Yes	Yes	No	
Depression	Yes	Possible	Yes	Assoc. with poorer disease-related QoL
Medication-induced mania		Yes	No	
Family History		Yes		

QoL = quality of life

frequently report idiosyncratic and highly ritualized medication dosing routines and punding is frequently reported in the setting of DDS.[53,59,69–71]

Neuroplastic Events Underlying the Disinhibitory Psychopathologies

Giving dopamine-receptor agonists to rats or monkeys with normal nigrostriatal systems also produces excess movements, but these are not dyskinesias. The development of such abnormally repetitive motor actions (and perhaps of relatively invariable thought patterns) coincides with a breakdown in the ability to initiate normal adaptive responses. Specific behaviors sensitized in rodents depend upon drug dose, with stimulant-induced locomotion enhanced following sensitization with low doses of stimulant drug. At higher drug doses, sensitization of stereotyped behaviors emerges.

The emergence of drug-induced stereotypies is mediated by drug effects on the ventral tegmental area (VTA) and its targets. The VTA is the origin of dopamine cell bodies and comprises the mesocorticolimbic dopamine system, and is widely implicated in the drug and natural reward circuitry of the brain, cognition, motivation, drug addiction, and several psychiatric disorders (Figure 9-1). The VTA contains neurons that project to numerous areas of the brain, including the ventral striatum (nucleus accumbens), the prefrontal cortex (PFC), and caudal brainstem.

The nucleus accumbens plays an important role in reward, laughter, pleasure, addiction, fear, and the placebo effect. The GABAergic output neurons of the nucleus accumbens send axon projections to the GPi which projects to the mediodorsal nucleus of the thalamus with a projection on to the prefrontal cortex. Other efferents from the nucleus accumbens include connections with the substantia nigra and pontine reticular formation. Major inputs to the nucleus accumbens include prefrontal association cortices and basolateral amygdala, as well as the previously mentioned dopamine neurons located in the VTA, which connect via the mesolimbic pathway (Figure 9-1).

Dopamine Drug "Reward"

Repeated administration of directly acting dopamine-receptor agonists (such as apomorphine) and the indirectly acting dopamine-receptor agonists such as amphetamine and cocaine, lead to a variety of behavioral phenomena in animals with intact dopamine systems. There are few data on the activation of accumbens-related reward pathways by dopamine therapies used to treat PD. Conditioned place-preference (CPP) in animals is used as one index of reward. Rewards such as food, sexual stimuli, and psychostimulant drugs cause conditioned place preferences to occur.[72]

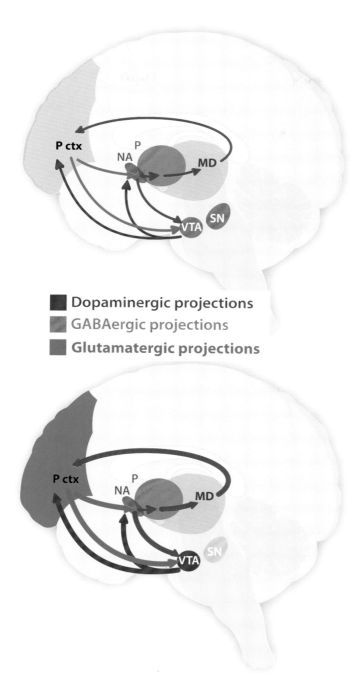

Figure 9-1. Simplified schematic diagram of the main reward pathways in the brain (top) and their relative dysregulation in PD (bottom). MD=mediodorsal nucleus of the thalamus; NA=nucleus accumbens; P=putamen; P cortex=prefrontal cortex; SN=substantia nigra; VTA=ventral tegmental area

When psychostimulant drugs (unconditioned stimulus; UCS) are administered reliably and repeatedly in one distinct environment, the associated cues (conditioned stimuli; CS) take on attributes of the UCS. CPP assesses the strength of CS–UCS associations and, thus, can reflect the rewarding effects of certain drugs. Neuroplastic changes within regions of the mesolimbic dopamine system, including the hippocampus and basolateral amygdala, play important roles in associations between conditioned stimuli and drug reward.[73] In rats, levodopa combined with the catechol-*O*-methyltransferase inhibitor entacapone induces a CPP similar to that induced by psychostimulants such as amphetamine.[74] This effect is also produced by the dopamine agonists apomorphine[75,76] and bromocriptine,[77] suggesting they are "rewarding." Such CPP is accompanied by increased dopamine stimulation in the accumbens, and lesions to the accumbens disrupt apomorphine preference[76] and self-administration.[78] Pramipexole increases activity in accumbens-related circuitry.[79] Therefore, dopamine replacement therapies used in PD are able to act as unconditioned stimuli and share at least some of the properties of potentially addictive drugs.

DDS: Reward Related Learning?

DDS in PD may be conceptualized as a manifestation of a form of aberrant learning. The premise of habit models of addiction is that, despite beginning as a goal-directed action, there is an eventual progression to a form of automatic behavior in which voluntary control over drug use is lost. In addition, stimuli consistently present in the environment gain motivational power through their predictive association with drugs. This view is supported by the finding that dopamine neurons signal errors in reward prediction that are critical for associative learning.[80] Drugs of addiction and drugs that act on dopamine systems can usurp molecular and cellular mechanisms that underlie long-term associative memories in several forebrain circuits (involving the ventral and dorsal striatum and prefrontal cortex) that receive input from midbrain dopamine neurons.[81] Repeated exposure to psychostimulants can give rise to both long term depression (LTD) and LTP in the VTA, and also in the nucleus accumbens and other targets of VTA dopamine neurons.[82] Striatal dopamine is also clearly involved in the development and reinforcement of automatic stimulus-response habits.[83]

Dopamine replacement drugs also influence various forms of learning in humans with intact brain dopamine systems.[84,85] Excessive doses of levodopa have the propensity to increase the reinforcing effect of wins in an instrumental learning task, but not losses as measured by ventral striatum blood-oxygen level-dependent activity.[86] In PD patients under dopamine agonist treatment, increased impulsivity and abnormal harm avoidance behavior has been found.[87,88] PD patients off medication display impaired learning from positive feedback, but enhanced learning to avoid choices that lead to negative outcomes. After an acute challenge with dopamine agonist medication, this bias is reversed, making patients more sensitive to positive than negative outcomes and leading to an impaired ability to avoid negative outcomes.[89] Moreover, pramipexole, a commonly used dopamine D2/D3 receptor agonist in PD, has been found to produce significant dose-dependent decreases in rCBR in the orbitofrontal, cingulate, and insular cortices as measured by H2[15]O PET in monkeys.[79] Recent data also highlight the role of the subthalamic nucleus in decision-making processes.[90–93] Subthalamic lesions increase premature anticipatory responding to cues signaling reward, and contribute to impulsivity.[94–100]

These observations provide a good explanation for the stereotypical behaviors seen in punding—a common feature of compulsive dopamine drug use in PD. In DDS patients, stereotyped behaviors develop from prepotent, habitual routines (e.g., grooming[53]), which are homologous to the complex stereotyped responses seen in rats during hyperdopaminergic states.[101] Strong stimulus-response habits form the basis of such routine activities. Stereotypy can be considered to represent the culmination of a continuous process of psychomotor stimulation and behavioral competition.[102] Smaller doses of psychostimulant drugs potentiate the approach responses to rewards, which is mediated by accumbens dopamine.[103] With increased doses, prepotent stimulus-response habits—mediated by the dorsal striatal structures—are potentiated and gain control over behavior.[104] Punding or excessive hobbyism often develops from prepotent habits, which are idiosyncratic, depending on individual life histories (e.g., office workers stereotypically shuffle papers, a seamstress will stereotypically collect and arrange buttons[53]). Individuals become unable to control automatic stimulus response selection mechanisms (i.e., stereotypies are often purposeless, and there is a dissociation between knowledge and behavior).

Disabling punding has been linked to higher daily requirements of dopamine agonists[53] and punding-like behavior has been linked to concomitant daily medication dosage from dopamine receptor agonists.[105] Case series also highlight improvement in punding behavior after reduction or cessation of dopamine agonist therapy.[66,106] In PD, dyskinesias overlap with punding behaviors and have been linked to punding behaviors independently of medication dose.[107] Punding can also develop in individuals with intact dopamine systems.[108]

However, automatic stimulus response processes cannot in themselves confer compulsive qualities to drug seeking and intake, and cannot easily explain the apparently flexible goal-directed actions that patients with PD use to obtain dopamine medications (e.g., faking akinetic states[55–57]).

The habit model does not explain why most patients with PD are not addicted to their medications. Moreover, the ability to modulate stimulus-response and conditioned responses can be impaired in some patients with PD, and such deficits can be exacerbated by levodopa.[88,109]

Compulsive Drug-taking: Sensitized Incentive Salience

Repeated administration of drugs of abuse producing sensitization (i.e. an increase in drug effect) typically involve measures of the psychomotor activating effects of drugs, such as their ability to enhance locomotor activity, rotational behavior, or stereotyped motor patterns. Behavioral sensitization is the progressive and enduring augmentation of these behaviors following repetitive drug use. In animal models of addiction, behavioral sensitization is hypothesised to index the neuroadaptive changes that occur in the nucleus accumbens in response to compulsive drug self-administration.[110] The development of psychomotor sensitization by psychostimulants in animal models of PD is favored by the same schedule of drug dosing as that necessary to induce dyskinesias in animal models of PD. This is associated with persistent[111] neurochemical changes in the nucleus accumbens including increased D1 receptor electrophysiological responsiveness[112,113] and upregulation of cyclic adenosine monophosphate (cAMP) signal transduction.[114] NMDA and α-amino-3-hydroxy-5-methyl-4-isoxazole propionate (AMPA) metabotropic glutamate receptors all participate in the development of sensitization, while maintenance of the sensitized state involves alterations in serotonin, noradrenaline and GABA function as well as in the expression and changes in intracellular signaling pathways of these AMPA and NMDA receptors.[115] The neuronal protein, alpha-synuclein, interacts with the dopamine transporter, and regulates dopamine content, neurotransmission, and the synaptic strength of dopamine neurons. Alpha-synuclein levels are elevated in the serum and dopamine neurons of chronic cocaine abusers, and the expression of alpha-synuclein expression is related to measures of addiction severity.[116,117] This suggests a role for alpha-synuclein in psychostimulant-induced behavioral effects.

Another consistently demonstrated change in the nucleus accumbens is that of augmentation of the increase in extracellular dopamine elicited by stimulants which requires a period of drug withdrawal.[118] D3 overexpression in the nucleus accumbens is another neuroadaptation involved in compulsive drug use.[26] There are even persistent changes in the physical structure of GABAergic medium spiny neurons of the nucleus accumbens and dorsolateral caudate-putamen. The neurochemical changes of sensitization may therefore contribute to some of the persistent behavioral and psychological consequences of repeated exposure to psychostimulant drugs by broadly reorganizing synapses at the site of dopamine-glutamate interaction in the striatum, and altering dopamine-glutamate signaling.[119]

In the incentive sensitization theory (IST) of addiction, the critical neuroadaptations for addiction render brain reward systems hypersensitive ("sensitized") to drugs and drug associated stimuli. The brain systems that are sensitized do not mediate the pleasurable or euphoric effects of drugs (drug "liking"), but instead they are proposed to mediate a subcomponent of reward termed incentive salience or drug "wanting." It is the psychological process of incentive salience specifically that is responsible for instrumental drug-seeking and drug-taking behavior (drug "wanting").[118]

There is in vivo evidence for a central role of sensitization of brain reward systems in compulsive dopamine drug use in PD. PD patients with DDS have been shown to exhibit enhanced levodopa-induced ventral striatal dopamine release compared with levodopa treated patients with PD not compulsively taking dopamine drugs. The sensitized ventral striatal dopamine neurotransmission produced by levodopa in these individuals has been positively correlated with self-reported compulsive drug "wanting" but not "liking" and related to heightened psychomotor activation (punding).[120]

ICDs and Sensitization
A global sensitization or "cross-sensitization" of appetitive behaviors may account for symptoms of hypersexuality and compulsive eating in PD. Both money[121,122] and consumer goods[123] activate the accumbens circuitry, indicating that symptoms of compulsive shopping and gambling could also be explained by IST. These findings are also relevant to the debate as to whether or not behavioral and chemical addictions share the same substrates.[35]

In PD, chronic dopamine replacement therapy has been shown to sensitize certain psychomotor effects of different dopamine drugs.[124] In treated PD patients, there is also a strong and dose-dependent association between dopamine agonist therapy and ICDs[61,63,125–127]; and between daily levodopa equivalent dose and DDS. ICDs, DDS, and punding all typically arise after many years of dopamine drug treatment implicating underlying neuroplastic mechanisms in their genesis (Figure 9-1). However, ICDs appear to differ from DDS in that dopamine agonist use is almost invariably associated, whereas DDS may be associated with high doses of levodopa and higher total daily levodopa equivalent doses.[60] It is unclear whether it is the uncontrolled effects of dopaminergic agonism that leads to ICDs (i.e. by bypassing the normal mechanisms of cellular release) or whether oral agonists cause ICDs via more D3 receptor mechanisms.

Loss of Inhibitory Control of Behavior

Behavioral decision-making tasks consistently demonstrate impairments in decision making in patients with addictions compared with controls. Orbitofrontal cortex activity has been implicated in cue reactivity and craving. Studies during acute withdrawal reveal hyperactivation of the orbitofrontal cortex, whereas studies during abstinence demonstrate hypo-activation of this region and structural abnormalities in individuals with substance use disorders.[128] In PD, cognitive functions associated with the frontal cortex modulated by dopamine systems may be further disrupted by disease processes, and frontal cortical pathology could cause additional loss of regulation of habitual or sensitized behaviors.[129]

The Iowa Gambling task emphasizes the learning of reward and punishment associations in order to guide ongoing decision-making. The task is sensitive to dysfunction of the ventromedial prefrontal cortex in which individuals do not acquire a preference for the safe decks but instead prefer the risky decks for the duration of the task.[130] PD patients without pathological gambling and pathological gamblers without PD have been found to be impaired on the Iowa Gambling Task compared to healthy controls.[131,132]

Individual Risk Factors

Individuals with PD receiving drugs that act on brain dopamine systems show variable susceptibility to the development of impulsive and compulsive behaviors. Relevant factors can be categorized as pharmacological, sex-related, age-related, temperamental, activity-level dependent, personality, experiential, and social factors.

Dopamine neurons fire in response to novelty. In epidemiological studies there is a high degree of correlation between addiction disorders and novelty-seeking personality traits. These traits describe an individual's tendency toward excitement in response to novel stimuli or cues for potential rewards, leading to frequent exploratory activity in pursuit of such experiences, often with rapid reactions to internal or external stimuli and diminished regard to the negative consequences of these reactions (i.e., impulsivity). Novelty-seeking scores decline with increasing age in adult non-PD subjects.[133] Higher novelty seeking traits have been associated with ICDs in non-PD populations,[134] and with ICDs[51] and DDS[59] in PD patients, and may explain some of the increased susceptibility to drug-induced disinhibitory psychopathologies seen in younger PD patients.

Experiential risk factors include cross-sensitization between stress and psychostimulants, and cross-sensitization between different drugs.[135] For instance, stress, corticosterone, and midbrain dopamine neurons seem to be organized in a pathophysiological chain determining a vulnerability to addiction. The mesolimbic dopamine system has been shown to have a stimulatory action upon the hypothalamic-pituitary-adrenal axis and visa versa.[136] Thus, corticosterone itself is readily self-administered by animals and stimulates dopamine release.[137] Moreover, these effects are mediated by individual differences in responses to novelty.[138] Genetic influences, including dopamine transporter[139] and D2 receptor[140] polymorphisms, and individual differences in D3 receptor alternative splicing and expression, appear to be relevant in mediating stimulant-induced behavioral sensitization.[141]

Concluding Remarks

Dopamine therapies used to treat PD can engage synaptic plasticity mechanisms in key brain circuits. The brain adaptations that underlie neuroplasticity associated with dyskinesias in PD and drug addictions in non PD populations are complex and involve drug-induced changes in gene transcription, membrane excitability, and neuronal morphology. The neuroplastic changes are likely strongly modified by differences in individual disease processes and individual variations in susceptibilities to the psychomotor activating effects of dopamine agonists. The data discussed in this chapter suggest that the neural mechanisms involved in the plastic effects underlying motor response complications, stereotypical behaviors, and addictions are similar and that the substrate that mediates the psychomotor-activating effects of dopamine drugs at least overlaps with the neural substrate for reward effects of drugs (Figure 9-1). However, there may be important differences—the most obvious being that dyskinesias are induced by levodopa whereas dopamine agonists are particularly linked to reward-related behaviors.

The neuroadaptations that cause dyskinesias and punding are similar to those seen after psychomotor sensitization by, for example, amphetamine.[81,135,142] They occur, however, in the dorsolateral striatum, rather than the accumbens-related circuitry.[142] Although there is evidence of a role for "motor" structures such as the dorsolateral striatum in reward processing[143–145] and that whilst both motor and incentive phenomena share key characteristics, there are clear dissociations between them. Locomotor sensitization that follows chronic amphetamine administration in rats does not necessarily predict incentive sensitization.[146] Furthermore, even though compulsive dopamine drug use in PD is associated with dyskinesias, few dyskinetic patients are compulsive dopamine drug users. Changes at the neuronal level induced by chronic levodopa may be region specific and involve primarily the dorsolateral striatum.[147]

There are significant gaps in understanding of the relevance of animal models to the observations made in patients with a progressive neurodegenerative process such as PD as well as significant challenges remaining to understand and potentially modify the neuroplastic changes that give rise to harmful psychomotor phenomena such as dyskinesias and addiction. Greater understanding of the non-dopamine processes engaged by dopamine drugs has the potential to substantially improve management of PD.

References

1. Hornykiewicz O, Kish SJ. Biochemical pathophysiology of Parkinson's disease. In: Yahr MD, Bergmann KJ, eds. *Advances in Neurology*. New York: Raven Press, 1986.
2. Chaudhuri KR, Martinez-Martin P, Schapira AH, et al. International multicenter pilot study of the first comprehensive self-completed nonmotor symptoms questionnaire for Parkinson's disease: the NMSQuest study. *Mov Disord*. 2006 Jul;21:916–923.
3. Cenci MA, Lindgren HS. Advances in understanding L-DOPA-induced dyskinesia. *Curr Opin Neurobiol*. 2007 Dec;17:665–671.
4. Durif F, Vidailhet M, Debilly B, Agid Y. Worsening of levodopa-induced dyskinesias by motor and mental tasks. *Mov Disord*. 1999 Mar;14:242–245.
5. Ahlskog JE, Muenter MD. Frequency of levodopa-related dyskinesias and motor fluctuations as estimated from the cumulative literature. *Mov Disord*. 2001 May;16: 448–458.
6. Blanchet PJ, Allard P, Gregoire L, Tardif F, Bedard PJ. Risk factors for peak dose dyskinesia in 100 levodopa-treated parkinsonian patients. *Can J Neurol Sci*. 1996 Aug;23:189–193.
7. Grandas F, Galiano ML, Tabernero C. Risk factors for levodopa-induced dyskinesias in Parkinson's disease. *J Neurol*. 1999 Dec;246:1127–1133.
8. Peppe A, Dambrosia JM, Chase TN. Risk factors for motor response complications in L-dopa-treated parkinsonian patients. *Adv Neurol*. 1993;60:698–702.
9. Schrag A, Quinn N. Dyskinesias and motor fluctuations in Parkinson's disease. A community-based study. *Brain*. 2000 Nov;123 (Pt 11):2297–2305.
10. Seibyl JP, Marek KL, Quinlan D, et al. Decreased single-photon emission computed tomographic [123I]beta-CIT striatal uptake correlates with symptom severity in Parkinson's disease. *Ann Neurol*. 1995 Oct;38:589–598.
11. Blau N, Bonafe L, Thony B. Tetrahydrobiopterin deficiencies without hyperphenylalaninemia: diagnosis and genetics of dopa-responsive dystonia and sepiapterin reductase deficiency. *Mol Genet Metab*. 2001 Sep;74:172–185.
12. .Horstink MW, Zijlmans JC, Pasman JW, Berger HJ, van't Hof MA. Severity of Parkinson's disease is a risk factor for peak-dose dyskinesia. *J Neurol Neurosurg Psychiatry*. 1990 Mar;53:224–226.
13. Ballard PA, Tetrud JW, Langston JW. Permanent human parkinsonism due to 1-methyl-4-phenyl-1,2,3,6-tetrahydropyridine (MPTP): seven cases. *Neurology*. 1985 Jul;35:949–956.

14. Barbeau A. Importance and pathogenesis of abnormal movements during L-dopa therapy of Parkinson's disease. *Neurology.* 1970 Apr;20:377.

15. McColl CD, Reardon KA, Shiff M, Kempster PA. Motor response to levodopa and the evolution of motor fluctuations in the first decade of treatment of Parkinson's disease. *Mov Disord.* 2002 Dec;17:1227–1234.

16. Finkelstein DI, Stanic D, Parish CL, Tomas D, Dickson K, Horne MK. Axonal sprouting following lesions of the rat substantia nigra. *Neuroscience.* 2000;97:99–112.

17. Parish CL, Stanic D, Drago J, Borrelli E, Finkelstein DI, Horne MK. Effects of long-term treatment with dopamine receptor agonists and antagonists on terminal arbor size. *Eur J Neurosci.* 2002 Sep;16:787–794.

18. Jenner P. Factors influencing the onset and persistence of dyskinesia in MPTP-treated primates. *Ann Neurol.* 2000 Apr;47:S90–S99.

19. Tsironis C, Marselos M, Evangelou A, Konitsiotis S. The course of dyskinesia induction by different treatment schedules of levodopa in Parkinsonian rats: is continuous dopaminergic stimulation necessary? *Mov Disord.* 2008 May 15;23:950–957.

20. Meissner W, Ravenscroft P, Reese R, et al. Increased slow oscillatory activity in substantia nigra pars reticulata triggers abnormal involuntary movements in the 6-OHDA-lesioned rat in the presence of excessive extracellular striatal dopamine. *Neurobiol Dis.* 2006 Jun;22:586–598.

21. Pavese N, Evans AH, Tai YF, et al. Clinical correlates of levodopa-induced dopamine release in Parkinson disease: a PET study. *Neurology.* 2006 Nov 14;67:1612–1617.

22. Carta M, Lindgren HS, Lundblad M, Stancampiano R, Fadda F, Cenci MA. Role of striatal L-DOPA in the production of dyskinesia in 6-hydroxydopamine lesioned rats. *J Neurochem.* 2006 Mar;96:1718–1727.

23. Andersson M, Hilbertson A, Cenci MA. Striatal fosB expression is causally linked with l-DOPA-induced abnormal involuntary movements and the associated upregulation of striatal prodynorphin mRNA in a rat model of Parkinson's disease. *Neurobiol Dis.* 1999 Dec;6:461–474.

24. Bordet R, Ridray S, Schwartz JC, Sokoloff P. Involvement of the direct striatonigral pathway in levodopa-induced sensitization in 6-hydroxydopamine-lesioned rats. *Eur J Neurosci.* 2000 Jun;12:2117–2123.

25. Bordet R, Ridray S, Carboni S, Diaz J, Sokoloff P, Schwartz JC. Induction of dopamine D3 receptor expression as a mechanism of behavioural sensitization to levodopa. *Proc Natl Acad Sci U S A.* 1997 Apr 1;94:3363–3367.

26. Gullin O, Diaz J, Carroll P, Griffon N, Schwarz J-C, Sokoloff P. BDNF controls dopamine D3 receptor expression and triggers behavioural sensitization. *Nature.* 2001;411:86–89.

27. Tomiyama M, Mori F, Kimura T, et al. Hypertrophy of medial globus pallidus and substantia nigra reticulata in 6-hydroxydopamine-lesioned rats treated with L-DOPA: implication for L-DOPA-induced dyskinesia in Parkinson's disease. *Neuropathology.* 2004 Dec;24:290–295.

28. Westin JE, Lindgren HS, Gardi J, et al. Endothelial proliferation and increased blood-brain barrier permeability in the basal ganglia in a rat model of 3,4-dihydroxyphenyl-L-alanine-induced dyskinesia. *J Neurosci.* 2006 Sep 13;26:9448–9461.

29. Boraud T, Bezard E, Bioulac B, Gross CE. Dopamine agonist-induced dyskinesias are correlated to both firing pattern and frequency alterations of pallidal neurones in the MPTP-treated monkey. *Brain*. 2001 Mar;124:546–557.

30. Metman LV, Konitsiotis S, Chase TN. Pathophysiology of motor response complications in Parkinson's disease: hypotheses on the why, where, and what. *Mov Disord*. 2000 Jan;15:3–8.

31. Nicoll RA, Malenka RC. Contrasting properties of two forms of long-term potentiation in the hippocampus. *Nature*. 1995 Sep 14;377:115–118.

32. Calon F, Dridi M, Hornykiewicz O, Bedard PJ, Rajput AH, Di PT. Increased adenosine A2A receptors in the brain of Parkinson's disease patients with dyskinesias. *Brain*. 2004 May;127:1075–1084.

33. Xiao D, Bastia E, Xu YH, et al. Forebrain adenosine A2A receptors contribute to L-3,4-dihydroxyphenylalanine-induced dyskinesia in hemiparkinsonian mice. *J Neurosci*. 2006 Dec 27;26:13548–13555.

34. Stacy M, Silver D, Mendis T, et al. A 12-week, placebo-controlled study (6002-US-006) of istradefylline in Parkinson disease. *Neurology*. 2008 Jun 3;70:2233–2240.

35. Holden C. 'Behavioural' addictions: do they exist? *Science*. 2001 Nov 2;294: 980–982.

36. Voon V, Potenza MN, Thomsen T. Medication-related impulse control and repetitive behaviours in Parkinson's disease. *Curr Opin Neurol*. 2007 Aug;20:484–492.

37. Avanzi M, Baratti M, Cabrini S, Uber E, Brighetti G, Bonfa F. The thrill of reckless driving in patients with Parkinson's disease: an additional behavioural phenomenon in dopamine dysregulation syndrome? *Parkinsonism Relat Disord*. 2008;14:257–258.

38. Cannas A, Solla P, Floris GL, Serra G, Tacconi P, Marrosu MG. Aberrant sexual behaviours in Parkinson's disease during dopaminergic treatment. *J Neurol*. 2007 Jan;254:110–112.

39. Quinn NP, Toone B, Lang AE, Marsden CD, Parkes JD. Dopa dose-dependent sexual deviation. *Br J Psychiatry*. 1983;142:296–298.

40. Berger C, Mehrhoff FW, Beier KM, Meinck HM. [Sexual delinquency and Parkinson's disease]. *Nervenarzt*. 2003 Apr;74:370–375.

41. Miller BL, Cummings JL, McIntyre H, Ebers G, Grode M. Hypersexuality or altered sexual preference following brain injury. *J Neurol Neurosurg Psychiatry*. 1986 Aug;49:867–873.

42. Jimenez-Jimenez FJ, Sayed Y, Garcia-Soldevilla MA, Barcenilla B. Possible zoophilia associated with dopaminergic therapy in Parkinson disease. *Ann Pharmacother*. 2002 Jul;36:1178–1179.

43. McElroy SL, Keck PE, Jr., Pope HG, Jr., Smith JM, Strakowski SM. Compulsive buying: a report of 20 cases. *J Clin Psychiatry*. 1994 Jun;55:242–248.

44. American Psychiatric Association. *Diagnostic and Statistical Manual of Mental Disorders, Fourth Edition, Text Revision* ed. Washington, DC: American Psychiatric Press, 2000.

45. Weintraub D, Siderowf AD, Potenza MN, et al. Association of dopamine agonist use with impulse control disorders in Parkinson disease. *Arch Neurol*. 2006 Jul;63: 969–973.

46. Voon V, Hassan K, Zurowski M, et al. Prevalence of repetitive and reward-seeking behaviours in Parkinson disease. *Neurology*. 2006 Oct 10;67:1254–1257.

47. Weintraub D, Koester J, Potenza MN, et al. Dopaminergic Therapy and Impulse Control Disorders in Parkinson's Disease: Top Line Results of a Cross-Sectional Study of Over 3,000 patients. *Mov Disord*. 2008;23:LB4.

48. Weiss HD, Hirsch E, Swerigen L, et al. Impulse control disorders in Parkinson's disease patients followed in a community-based neurology practice. *Mov Disord*. 2008;23:S281.

49. Ondo WG, Lai D. Predictors of impulsivity and reward seeking behaviour with dopamine agonists. *Parkinsonism Relat Disord*. 2008;14:28–32.

50. Isaias IU, Siri C, Cilia R, De GD, Pezzoli G, Antonini A. The relationship between impulsivity and impulse control disorders in Parkinson's disease. *Mov Disord*. 2008 Feb 15;23:411–415.

51. Voon V, Thomsen T, Miyasaki JM, et al. Factors associated with dopaminergic drug-related pathological gambling in Parkinson disease. *Arch Neurol*. 2007 Feb;64: 212–216.

52. Rylander G. Psychoses and the punding and choreiform syndromes in addiction to central stimulant drugs. *Psychiatr Neurol Neurochir*. 1972;75:203–12.

53. Evans AH, Katzenschlager R, Paviour D, et al. Punding in Parkinson's disease: its relation to the dopamine dysregulation syndrome. *Mov Disord*. 2004 Apr;19:397–405.

54. Lawrence AJ, Blackwell AD, Barker RA, et al. Predictors of punding in Parkinson's disease: results from a questionnaire survey. *Mov Disord*. 2007 Dec;22:2339–2345.

55. Giovannoni G, O'Sullivan JD, Turner K, Manson AJ, Lees AJ. Hedonistic homeostatic dysregulation in patients with Parkinson's disease on dopamine replacement therapies. *J Neurol Neurosurg Psychiatry*. 2000;68:423–8.

56. Evans AH, Lees AJ. Dopamine dysregulation syndrome in Parkinson's disease. *Curr Opin Neurol*. 2004 Aug;17:393–398.

57. Lawrence AD, Evans AH, Lees AJ. Compulsive use of dopamine replacement therapy in Parkinson's disease: reward systems gone awry? *Lancet Neurol*. 2003 Oct;2: 595–604.

58. Bearn J, Evans A, Kelleher M, Turner K, Lees A. Recognition of a dopamine replacement therapy dependence syndrome in Parkinson's disease: a pilot study. *Drug Alcohol Depend*. 2004 Dec 7;76:305–310.

59. Evans AH, Lawrence AD, Potts J, Appel S, Lees AJ. Factors influencing susceptibility to compulsive dopaminergic drug use in Parkinson disease. *Neurology*. 2005 Nov 22;65:1570–1574.

60. Gallagher DA, O'Sullivan SS, Evans AH, Lees AJ, Schrag A. Pathological gambling in Parkinson's disease: risk factors and differences from dopamine dysregulation. An analysis of published case series. *Mov Disord*. 2007 Sep 15;22:1757–1763.

61. Nirenberg MJ, Waters C. Compulsive eating and weight gain related to dopamine agonist use. *Mov Disord*. 2006 Apr;21:524–529.

62. Dodd ML, Klos KJ, Bower JH, Geda YE, Josephs KA, Ahlskog JE. Pathological gambling caused by drugs used to treat Parkinson disease. *Arch Neurol*. 2005 Sep;62:1377–1381.

63. Klos KJ, Bower JH, Josephs KA, Matsumoto JY, Ahlskog JE. Pathological hyper-sexuality predominantly linked to adjuvant dopamine agonist therapy in Parkinson's disease and multiple system atrophy. *Parkinsonism Relat Disord*. 2005 Sep;11: 381–386.

64. McKeon A, Josephs KA, Klos KJ, et al. Unusual compulsive behaviours primarily related to dopamine agonist therapy in Parkinson's disease and multiple system atrophy. *Parkinsonism Relat Disord*. 2007 Dec;13:516–519.

65. Kimber TE, Thompson PD, Kiley MA. Resolution of dopamine dysregulation syndrome following cessation of dopamine agonist therapy in Parkinson's disease. *J Clin Neurosci*. 2008 Feb;15:205–208.

66. Miyasaki JM, Al HK, Lang AE, Voon V. Punding prevalence in Parkinson's disease. *Mov Disord*. 2007 Jun 15;22:1179–1181.

67. Shapiro MA, Chang YL, Munson SK, Okun MS, Fernandez HH. Hypersexuality and paraphilia induced by selegiline in Parkinson's disease: report of 2 cases. *Parkinsonism Relat Disord*. 2006 Sep;12:392–395.

68. Wong SH, Cowen Z, Allen EA, Newman PK. Internet gambling and other pathological gambling in Parkinson's disease: a case series. *Mov Disord*. 2007 Mar 15;22: 591–593.

69. Kumar S. Punding in Parkinson's disease related to high-dose levodopa therapy. *Neurol India*. 2005 Sep;53:362.

70. Bonvin C, Horvath J, Christe B, Landis T, Burkhard PR. Compulsive singing: another aspect of punding in Parkinson's disease. *Ann Neurol*. 2007 Nov;62:525–528.

71. Serrano-Duenas M. Chronic Dopamimetic Drug Addiction and Pathologic Gambling in Patients with Parkinson's Disease - Presentation of Four Cases. *German J Psychiatry*. 2002 May 15;5:62–66.

72. Bardo MT, Bevins RA. Conditioned place preference: what does it add to our preclinical understanding of drug reward? *Psychopharmacology. (Berl)* 2000 Dec;153: 31–43.

73. Rademacher DJ, Kovacs B, Shen F, Napier TC, Meredith GE. The neural substrates of amphetamine conditioned place preference: implications for the formation of conditioned stimulus-reward associations. *Eur J Neurosci*. 2006 Oct;24:2089–2097.

74. Katajamaki J, Honkanen A, Piepponen TP, Linden IB, Zharkovsky A, Ahtee L. Conditioned place preference induced by a combination of L-dopa and a COMT inhibitor, entacapone, in rats. *Pharmacol Biochem Behav*. 1998 May;60:23–26.

75. Papp M. Different effects of short- and long-term treatment with imipramine on the apomorphine- and food-induced place preference conditioning in rats. *Pharmacol Biochem Behav*. 1988 Aug;30:889–893.

76. van der Kooy D, Swerdlow NR, Koob GF. Paradoxical reinforcing properties of apomorphine: effects of nucleus accumbens and area postrema lesions. *Brain Res*. 1983;259:111–118.

77. Hoffman DC, Dickson PR, Beninger RJ. The dopamine D2 receptor agonists, quinpirole and bromocriptine produce conditioned place preferences. *Prog Neuropsychopharmacol Biol Psychiatry*. 1988;12:315–322.

78. Zito KA, Vickers G, Roberts DC. Disruption of cocaine and heroin self-administration following kainic acid lesions of the nucleus accumbens. *Pharmacol Biochem Behav*. 1985 Dec;23:1029–1036.

79. Black KJ, Hershey T, Koller JM, et al. A possible substrate for dopamine-related changes in mood and behaviour: prefrontal and limbic effects of a D3-preferring dopamine agonist. *Proc Natl Acad Sci U S A*. 2002 Dec 24;99:17113–17118.
80. Waelti P, Dickinson A, Schultz W. Dopamine responses comply with basic assumptions of formal learning theory. *Nature*. 2001 Jul 5;412:43–48.
81. Berke JD, Hyman SE. Addiction, dopamine, and the molecular mechanisms of memory. *Neuron*. 2000;25:515–532.
82. Hyman SE, Malenka RC, Nestler EJ. Neural mechanisms of addiction: the role of reward-related learning and memory. *Annu Rev Neurosci*. 2006;29:565–598.
83. Everitt BJ, Dickinson A, Robbins TW. The neuropsychological basis of addictive behaviour. *Brain Res Brain Res Rev*. 2001;36:129–138.
84. Knecht S, Breitenstein C, Bushuven S, et al. Levodopa: faster and better word learning in normal humans. *Ann Neurol*. 2004 Jul;56:20–26.
85. Mehta MA, Swainson R, Ogilvie AD, Sahakian J, Robbins TW. Improved short-term spatial memory but impaired reversal learning following the dopamine D(2) agonist bromocriptine in human volunteers. *Psychopharmacology (Berl)*. 2001 Dec;159: 10–20.
86. Pessiglione M, Seymour B, Flandin G, Dolan RJ, Frith CD. Dopamine-dependent prediction errors underpin reward-seeking behaviour in humans. *Nature*. 2006 Aug 31;442:1042–1045.
87. Thiel A, Hilker R, Kessler J, Habedank B, Herholz K, Heiss WD. Activation of basal ganglia loops in idiopathic Parkinson's disease: a PET study. *J Neural Transm*. 2003 Nov;110:1289–1301.
88. Cools R, Barker RA, Sahakian BJ, Robbins TW. L-Dopa medication remediates cognitive inflexibility, but increases impulsivity in patients with Parkinson's disease. *Neuropsychologia*. 2003;41:1431–1441.
89. Frank MJ, Seeberger LC, O'reilly RC. By carrot or by stick: cognitive reinforcement learning in parkinsonism. *Science*. 2004 Dec 10;306:1940–1943.
90. Anderson KE, Mullins J. Behavioural changes associated with deep brain stimulation surgery for Parkinson's disease. *Curr Neurol Neurosci Rep*. 2003 Jul;3:306–313.
91. Houeto JL, Mesnage V, Mallet L, et al. Behavioural disorders, Parkinson's disease and subthalamic stimulation. *J Neurol Neurosurg Psychiatry*. 2002 Jun;72:701–707.
92. Hershey T, Revilla FJ, Wernle A, Gibson PS, Dowling JL, Perlmutter JS. Stimulation of STN impairs aspects of cognitive control in PD. *Neurology*. 2004 Apr 13;62:1110-1114.
93. Frank MJ, Samanta J, Moustafa AA, Sherman SJ. Hold your horses: impulsivity, deep brain stimulation, and medication in parkinsonism. *Science*. 2007 Nov 23;318:1309–1312.
94. Baunez C, Nieoullon A, Amalric M. In a rat model of parkinsonism, lesions of the subthalamic nucleus reverse increases of reaction time but induce a dramatic premature responding deficit. *J Neurosci*. 1995 Oct;15:6531–6541.
95. Baunez C, Robbins TW. Bilateral lesions of the subthalamic nucleus induce multiple deficits in an attentional task in rats. *Eur J Neurosci*. 1997 Oct;9:2086–2099.
96. Baunez C, Humby T, Eagle DM, Ryan LJ, Dunnett SB, Robbins TW. Effects of STN lesions on simple vs choice reaction time tasks in the rat: preserved motor readiness, but impaired response selection. *Eur J Neurosci*. 2001 Apr;13:1609–1616.

97. Florio T, Capozzo A, Cellini R, Pizzuti G, Staderini EM, Scarnati E. Unilateral lesions of the pedunculopontine nucleus do not alleviate subthalamic nucleus-mediated anticipatory responding in a delayed sensorimotor task in the rat. *Behav Brain Res.* 2001 Nov 29;126:93–103.

98. Phillips JM, Brown VJ. Reaction time performance following unilateral striatal dopamine depletion and lesions of the subthalamic nucleus in the rat. *Eur J Neurosci.* 1999 Mar;11:1003–1010.

99. Uslaner JM, Robinson TE. Subthalamic nucleus lesions increase impulsive action and decrease impulsive choice - mediation by enhanced incentive motivation? *Eur J Neurosci.* 2006 Oct;24:2345–2354.

100. Winstanley CA, Baunez C, Theobald DE, Robbins TW. Lesions to the subthalamic nucleus decrease impulsive choice but impair autoshaping in rats: the importance of the basal ganglia in Pavlovian conditioning and impulse control. *Eur J Neurosci.* 2005 Jun;21:3107–3116.

101. Berridge KC, Aldridge JW. Super-stereotypy I: enhancement of a complex movement sequence by systemic dopamine D1 agonists. *Synapse.* 2000 Sep 1;37:194–204.

102. Toates F. The interaction of cognitive and stimulus-response processes in the control of behaviour. *Neurosci Biobehav Rev.* 1998;22:59–83.

103. Ikemoto S, Panksepp J. The role of nucleus accumbens dopamine in motivated behaviour: a unifying interpretation with special reference to reward-seeking. *Brain Res Brain Res Rev.* 1999 Dec;31:6–41.

104. Whishaw IQ, Fiourino D, Mittleman G, Castaneda E. Do forebrain structures compete for behavioural expression? Evidence from amphetamine-induced behaviour, microdialysis, and caudate-accumbens lesions in medial frontal cortex damaged rats. *Brain Res.* 1992 Mar 27;576:1–11.

105. Lawrence AJ, Blackwell AD, Barker RA, et al. Predictors of punding in Parkinson's disease: results from a questionnaire survey. *Mov Disord.* 2007 Dec;22:2339–2345.

106. Kimber TE, Thompson PD, Kiley MA. Resolution of dopamine dysregulation syndrome following cessation of dopamine agonist therapy in Parkinson's disease. *J Clin Neurosci.* 2008 Feb;15:205–208.

107. Silveira-Moriyama L, Evans AH, Katzenschlager R, Lees AJ. Punding and dyskinesias. *Mov Disord.* 2006 Dec;21:2214–2217.

108. Evans AH, Stegeman JR. Punding in patients on dopamine agonists for restless leg syndrome. *Mov Disord.* 2008 Oct 14.

109. Cools R, Barker RA, Sahakian BJ, Robbins TW. Enhanced or Impaired Cognitive Function in Parkinson's Disease as a Function of Dopaminergic Medication and Task Demands. *Cereb Cortex.* 2001;11:1136–1143.

110. Samaha AN, Mallet N, Ferguson SM, Gonon F, Robinson TE. The rate of cocaine administration alters gene regulation and behavioural plasticity: implications for addiction. *J Neurosci.* 2004 Jul 14;24:6362–6370.

111. Wolf ME. The role of excitatory amino acids in behavioural sensitization to psychomotor stimulants. *Prog Neurobiol.* 1998 Apr;54:679–720.

112. Henry DJ, White FJ. Repeated cocaine administration causes persistent enhancement of D1 dopamine receptor sensitivity within the rat nucleus accumbens. *J Pharmacol Exp Ther.* 1991 Sep;258:882–890.

113. Higashi H, Inanaga K, Nishi S, Uchimura N. Enhancement of dopamine actions on rat nucleus accumbens neurones in vitro after methamphetamine pre-treatment. *J Physiol.* 1989 Jan;408:587–603.
114. Nestler EJ, Terwilliger RZ, Walker JR, Sevarino KA, Duman RS. Chronic cocaine treatment decreases levels of the G protein subunits Gi alpha and Go alpha in discrete regions of rat brain. *J Neurochem.* 1990 Sep;55:1079–1082.
115. Wolf ME. The role of excitatory amino acids in behavioural sensitization to psychomotor stimulants. *Prog Neurobiol.* 1998 Apr;54:679–720.
116. Mash DC, Ouyang Q, Pablo J, et al. Cocaine abusers have an overexpression of alpha-synuclein in dopamine neurons. *J Neurosci.* 2003 Apr 1;23:2564–2571.
117. Mash DC, Adi N, Duque L, Pablo J, Kumar M, Ervin FR. Alpha synuclein protein levels are increased in serum from recently abstinent cocaine abusers. *Drug Alcohol Depend.* 2008 Apr 1;94:246–250.
118. Robinson TE, Berridge KC. The neural basis of drug craving: an incentive-sensitization theory of addiction. *Brain Res Brain Res Rev.* 1993;18:247–91.
119. Li Y, Kolb B, Robinson TE. The location of persistent amphetamine-induced changes in the density of dendritic spines on medium spiny neurons in the nucleus accumbens and caudate-putamen. *Neuropsychopharmacology.* 2003 Jun;28:1082–1085.
120. Evans AH, Pavese N, Lawrence AD, et al. Compulsive drug use linked to sensitized ventral striatal dopamine transmission. *Ann Neurol.* 2006 May;59:852–858.
121. Knutson B, Adams CM, Fong GW, Hommer D. Anticipation of increasing monetary reward selectively recruits nucleus accumbens. *J Neurosci.* 2001 Aug 15;21:RC159.
122. Koepp MJ, Gunn RN, Lawrence AD, et al. Evidence for striatal dopamine release during a video game. *Nature.* 1998 May 21;393:266–268.
123. Erk S, Spitzer M, Wunderlich AP, Galley L, Walter H. Cultural objects modulate reward circuitry. *Neuroreport.* 2002 Dec 20;13:2499–2503.
124. Evans AH, Lawrence AD, Lees AJ. Changes in psychomotor effects of L-dopa and methylphenidate after sustained dopaminergic therapy in Parkinson disease. *J Neurol Neurosurg Psychiatry.* 2008 Oct 31.
125. Courty E, Durif F, Zenut M, Courty P, Lavarenne J. Psychiatric and sexual disorders induced by apomorphine in Parkinson's disease. *Clin Neuropharmacol.* 1997;20:140–7.
126. Uitti RJ, Tanner CM, Rajput AH, Goetz CG, Klawans HL, Thiessen B. Hypersexuality with antiparkinsonian therapy. *Clin Neuropharmacol.* 1989;12:375-83.
127. Voon V, Hassan K, Zurowski M, et al. Prospective prevalence of pathologic gambling and medication association in Parkinson disease. *Neurology.* 2006 Jun 13;66:1750–1752.
128. Dom G, Sabbe B, Hulstijn W, van den BW. Substance use disorders and the orbitofrontal cortex: systematic review of behavioural decision-making and neuroimaging studies. *Br J Psychiatry.* 2005 Sep;187:209–220.
129. Jentsch JD, Taylor JR. Impulsivity resulting from frontostriatal dysfunction in drug abuse: implications for the control of behaviour by reward-related stimuli. *Psychopharmacology (Berl).* 1999;146:373–390.

130. Bechara A, Damasio AR, Damasio H, Anderson SW. Insensitivity to future consequences following damage to human prefrontal cortex. *Cognition*. 1994;50:7–15.
131. Cavedini P, Riboldi G, Keller R, D'Annucci A, Bellodi L. Frontal lobe dysfunction
in pathological gambling patients. *Biol Psychiatry*. 2002 Feb 15;51:334–341.
132. Pagonabarraga J, Garcia-Sanchez C, Llebaria G, Pascual-Sedano B, Gironell A,
Kulisevsky J. Controlled study of decision-making and cognitive impairment in
Parkinson's disease. *Mov Disord*. 2007 Jul 30;22:1430–1435.
133. Heiman N, Stallings MC, Hofer SM, Hewitt JK. Investigating age differences in the
genetic and environmental structure of the tridimensional personality questionnaire
in later adulthood. *Behav Genet*. 2003 Mar;33:171–180.
134. Potenza MN, Voon V, Weintraub D. Drug Insight: impulse control disorders and
dopamine therapies in Parkinson's disease. *Nat Clin Pract Neurol*. 2007 Dec;3:
664–672.
135. Robinson TE, Berridge KC. The psychology and neurobiology of addiction: an
incentive-sensitization view. *Addiction*. 2000;95 Suppl 2:91–117.
136. Piazza PV, Le Moal ML. Pathophysiological basis of vulnerability to drug abuse:
role of an interaction between stress, glucocorticoids, and dopaminergic neurons.
Annu Rev Pharmacol Toxicol. 1996;36:359–378.
137. Piazza PV, Deroche V, Deminiere JM, Maccari S, Le Moal M, Simon H. Corticosterone
in the range of stress-induced levels possesses reinforcing properties: implications
for sensation-seeking behaviours. *Proc Natl Acad Sci U S A*. 1993;90:11738–42.
138. Dellu F, Piazza PV, Mayo W, Le Moal M, Simon H. Novelty-seeking in rats–biobe-
havioural characteristics and possible relationship with the sensation-seeking trait in
man. *Neuropsychobiology*. 1996;34:136–45.
139. Lott DC, Kim SJ, Cook EH, Jr., de WH. Dopamine transporter gene associated with
diminished subjective response to amphetamine. *Neuropsychopharmacology*. 2005
Mar;30:602–609.
140. Blum K, Braverman ER, Holder JM, et al. Reward deficiency syndrome: a bioge-
netic model for the diagnosis and treatment of impulsive, addictive, and compulsive
behaviours. *J Psychoactive Drugs*. 2000 Nov;32 Suppl:i–112.
141. Pritchard LM, Logue AD, Taylor BC, et al. Relative expression of D3 dopamine
receptor and alternative splice variant D3nf mRNA in high and low responders to
novelty. *Brain Res Bull*. 2006 Oct 16;70:296–303.
142. Graybiel AM, Canales JJ, Capper-Loup C. Levodopa-induced dyskinesias and
dopamine-dependent stereotypies: a new hypothesis. *Trends Neurosci*. 2000
Oct;23:S71–S77.
143. Ito R, Robbins TW, Everitt BJ. Differential control over cocaine-seeking behaviour
by nucleus accumbens core and shell. *Nat Neurosci*. 2004 Apr;7:389–397.
144. Salamone JD, Correa M, Mingote S, Weber SM. Nucleus accumbens dopamine and
the regulation of effort in food-seeking behaviour: implications for studies of natural
motivation, psychiatry, and drug abuse. *J Pharmacol Exp Ther*. 2003 Apr;305:1–8.
145. Volkow ND, Wang GJ, Fowler JS, et al. "Nonhedonic" food motivation in humans
involves dopamine in the dorsal striatum and methylphenidate amplifies this effect.
Synapse. 2002 Jun 1;44:175–180.

146. Nocjar C, Panksepp J. Chronic intermittent amphetamine pretreatment enhances future appetitive behaviour for drug- and natural-reward: interaction with environmental variables. *Behav Brain Res.* 2002 Jan 22;128:189–203.

147. Mura A, Mintz M, Feldon J. Behavioural and anatomical effects of long-term L-dihydroxyphenylalanine (L-DOPA) administration in rats with unilateral lesions of the nigrostriatal system. *Exp Neurol.* 2002 Sep;177:252–264.

Chapter 10

Lesions Associated with Visual Hallucinations and Psychoses

David R. Williams and Werner Poewe

Definitions

Psychosis in Parkinson's disease (PD) is defined by the presence of at least one of a number of characteristic symptoms including paranoid delusions, illusions, false sense of presence, and hallucinations.[1] Illusions are misperceptions of real stimuli which in PD are usually visual in nature. By contrast, hallucinations refer to abnormal perceptions that, as defined in DSM-IV,[2] have a compelling sense of reality of a true perception but that occur without external stimulation of the relevant sensory system. Hallucinations may involve any sensory modality, but in PD they again mainly consist of visual perceptions. Minor forms of these include passage hallucinations where subjects experience vague and fleeting images in their peripheral vision, or a sense of presence where patients experience the presence of someone when nobody is there. Delusions are false beliefs that are maintained despite compelling evidence or proof to the contrary.

Clinical Phenomenology

Visual hallucinations (VH) are the by far the most common type of hallucinations that occur in patients with PD.[3–5] They are typically well-formed

242

and rich in detail and color and mostly consist of familiar or unfamiliar persons, animals, or, less commonly, objects.[6,7] Insight into the hallucinatory nature of these perceptions may be retained, particularly in patients with a clear sensorium and without marked degrees of cognitive decline. They can occur any time during the day but sometimes may be particularly prominent in the evening or in dim lighting conditions. VH in PD can appear and vanish suddenly multiple times during a day and hallucinatory images are seen against the normal visual background (see Figure 10-1). The hallucinatory

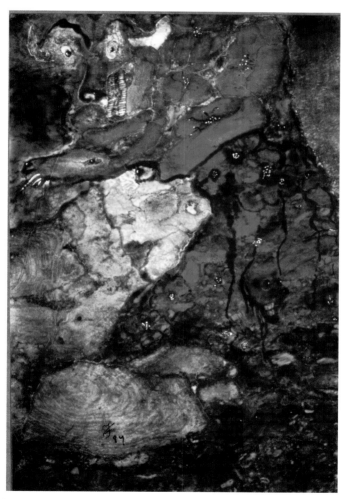

Figure 10-1. Recurring visual hallucination as experienced and painted by a PD patient who called this "the marble woman!" (Courtesy of Dr. Georg Ebersbach, Beelitz-Heilstätten, Germany)

content tends to be stereotyped and recurring in a given patient. VH in PD are often non-frightening and do not seem to cause major concern or distress. Hallucinations of single persons or groups of people are observed from the position of a spectator rather then an actor, but patients may sometimes speak to these people enquiring about their whereabouts or asking them to leave. In such instances it is common for the hallucinated persons to remain silent. Patients with more marked degrees of cognitive dysfunction or dementia often lose insight and may feel threatened or annoyed by their hallucinations or go on to develop florid paranoid psychosis. This may result in verbal or physical aggression or the police getting called in. Occasionally the content of VH themselves may be frightening, for example in the form of distorted and unreal figures or animals. One of the authors' patients who had recurring evening appearances of huge bird-like animals with human faces sitting in the trees of his garden would regularly fire at those images with his shotgun—much to the concern of his family and neighbors.

Minor visual misperceptions and hallucinatory phenomena in PD include visual illusions, passage hallucinations, and sense of presence. Visual illusions in PD most often consist of seeing inanimate objects as living beings—for example a vase as a human head or breadcrumbs on a plate as insects. Passage hallucinations are brief visual perceptions in the periphery of the visual field creating the impression of a person or an animal passing by the patient, who is usually specific about the perception, identifying it as a familiar or unfamiliar person or specific type of animal.[3,8] Sense of presence refers to a vivid experience of somebody being present nearby, when there is actually nobody there. These persons are usually precisely localized as behind or by the side of the subject and can again be unfamiliar or familiar, like living or deceased relatives or friends.

Selective diplopia is an as yet poorly defined type of visual perceptual dysfunction in PD, which is akin to VH but unique in that only isolated parts of a visual scene appear duplicated. This peculiar type of double vision comes on and ceases abruptly, is usually recurrent, short-lasting, and not explained by oculomotor or refractory abnormalities. It thus shares many similarities with VH and also occurs in temporal relation to PD medication change.[9]

Patients with PD dementia (PDD) and VH may also independently display different types of misidentification syndromes, including beliefs that familiar persons have been replaced by an identical looking impostor (Capgras syndrome) or that familiar persons (often relatives) have disguised themselves into unfamiliar people (Fregoli illusion). Different forms of reduplicative paramnesia may also occur, including the belief that one has been placed into an identical appearing duplicate place from home or that an identical double of another person exists.[10]

These phenomena are distinct from VH but—like VH—are strongly associated with cognitive dysfunction and dementia (see below) in PD and are also core clinical features of dementia with Lewy bodies (DLB). The distinction between PDD and DLB has, however, remained controversial, since it currently rests only on differences of temporal onset of dementia in relation to clinical parkinsonism.[11] The underlying brain pathology is indistinguishable between the two disorders as is the clinical profile of dementia itself. This includes the phenomenology of VH[12] as well as the relative frequencies of visual versus non-visual hallucinations,[13] which are also similar in PDD and DLB. Furthermore, patterns of visuo-perceptual dysfunction in non-hallucinating inpatients were identical between PDD and DLB but different from those in Alzheimer's disease.[12,14]

Hallucinations in non-visual sensory domains are uncommon in PD—unlike those in schizophrenia which usually involve auditory or sensory-tactile perceptions. Auditory hallucinations have been reported to occur in up to 22% of PD patients,[3,4,15,16] but in the majority occur together with VH, where acoustic phenomena are part of the hallucinated scene—like the voices of unreal people. Isolated acoustic hallucinations have been reported to occur in less than 10% of patients in most hospital-based series,[15] but were noted in 16% in another.[17] Rarely such auditory phenomena may occur as schizophrenia-like paranoid perceptions of voices making negative comments or threatening remarks about the patient.[18] Similar to their auditory counterparts, tactile hallucinations in PD usually occur as part of VH, when they include sensations of being touched by hallucinated animals or people. A typical history obtained from one of the authors' patients was as follows:

A 64-year-old retired civil servant with a 5 year history of PD and combined treatment with levodopa and a dopamine agonist reported about the regular appearance of four black cats which would suddenly show up when he was about to go bed and then stay until he had fallen asleep. They would always follow him into his bed and cuddle by his legs where he could feel their warm and soft fur. They would never scratch and he carefully observed the details of their paws, which, instead of claws had small soft buds. He also could see that they had no teeth and when they nagged at his legs he could feel their gums. In contrast to his wife, he was not alarmed by these phenomena, but rather enjoyed what he found were pleasant companions.

Prevalence

There are few systematic and prospective studies of the prevalence or incidence of psychosis and specifically VH in PD. Most of the available

Table 10-1. Prevalence of VH in PD*

Authors	N	% with VH	Type of study
Sanchez-Ramos et al, 1996[83]	214	25.7	hospital-based
Graham et al, 1997[4]	129	24.8	hospital-based
Inzelberg et al, 1998[14]	121	29	hospital-based
Fènelon et al, 2000[3]	216	40	hospital-based
Holroyd et al, 2001[85]	102	26.5	hospital-based
Pacchetti et al, 2005[86]	289	30	hospital-based
Paleacu et al, 2005[87]	276	32	hospital-based
Williams et al, 2008[16]	115	75	hospital-based
Aarsland et al, 1999[18]	235	15.8	community-based
Schrag et al, 2002[19]	124	23	community-based
Williams + Lees, 2005[15]	445	50	retrospective autopsy-based

*(series including >100 patients)

information comes from hospital-based series in PD centers and may not accurately reflect the true prevalence of these phenomena in the community. Nevertheless, reported figures from different series are remarkably consistent and suggest a cross-sectional prevalence of VH in clinic-based samples of between 20% and 30% (see Table 10-1). The largest population based set of data comes from a study of 254 patients with PD ascertained by standard diagnostic criteria in a defined geographical area in Norway.[19] Of these patients, 235 had assessments of the thought disorder item on the UPDRS part I. Based on this criterion, 10% were identified as having VH with retained insight and an additional 6% had more severe degrees of hallucinations and delusions according to item 2 of the UPDRS part I. A similar figure of 23% for all types of hallucinations was reported in a smaller population-based sample of 124 PD patients from the London area in the UK.[20]

When minor forms, like visual illusions, sense of passage, or presence hallucinations are included, the cross-sectional prevalence rises to close to 40%.[3] In addition, the observed prevalence of VH in PD is dependent on assessment periods: Inzelberg and colleagues found that 37% of their patients had experienced complex VH over the previous 2 years.[15] Hely and colleagues, when longitudinally and prospectively following a cohort of 149 patients with PD, reported a prevalence of VH of 50% in those surviving after 15 years of follow-up and of 74% among 30 survivors after 20 years of disease duration.[21,22] In a large series of 788 cases with different types of parkinsonism archived at the Queen Square Brain Bank for Neurological Diseases, 50% of 445 patients with pathologically confirmed

PD had experienced VH as assessed by retrospective chart review—including minor forms like sense of presence, passage, or visual illusions.[16] These figures suggest that VH become increasingly common with prolonged disease duration and follow-up. Cognitive dysfunction is one of the cardinal risk factors for the development of VH and—not surprisingly—prevalence of VH has been found greatest in series of patients with PDD, where VH were found in about 70% of cases.[3,16,17]

Natural History of VH and Psychosis

Few studies have prospectively assessed outcomes in PD patients with VH or other features of psychosis.[23–26]. As a rule, VH and psychosis in PD tend to follow a chronic and progressive course and are associated with the development of dementia and the need for nursing home care.[27,28] A one year follow-up study of 127 outpatients originally included in a cross-sectional outpatient survey of hallucinations in PD has confirmed the chronic course of VH.[23] Less than 10% of subjects with any type of hallucinations at first visit were no longer hallucinating after one year of follow-up. Overall prevalence rates for all types of hallucinations increased over one year in this clinic-based sample with the greatest increase being related to the new onset of visual illusions or sense of presence or passage. The study showed that 26% of patients who had been free of hallucinations at baseline developed those after one year. In a longer follow-up study of 89 PD patients over 4 years, 50% of those not experiencing hallucinations at baseline had developed them after 4 years of follow-up and the overall prevalence of hallucinations rose from 33% at baseline to 44% at 18 months and 63% at 48 months.[25]

There is also some suggestion that VH with retained insight—sometimes termed benign hallucinations—once established in PD patients, tend to progress to more troublesome psychotic behavior. A recent study of 48 PD outpatients scoring for "benign hallucinations with retained insight" on the thought disorder item of the UPDRS part I at study entry has provided data on the evolution of hallucinosis over a 3 year period. More than 80% of these patients progressed to scores of 3 or 4, signifying persistent hallucinations, delusions, or florid psychosis.[26] There was a higher percentage of new onset dementia in those patients declining on their hallucinosis scores as compared to the small group of patients remaining stable at 3 years. Time intervals to progression to more maligned degrees of psychosis were short with a mean of 16 months.

The ominous prognostic significance of VH and psychosis for the natural history of PD is also highlighted by follow up data from the PSYCLOPS study, a short-term trial on the antipsychotic efficacy of clozapine in 60 PD patients. Two year follow-up data of 59 of these patients revealed that 25% had died, 42%—as compared to 12% at baseline—had been admitted to nursing homes, and dementia was diagnosed in 68% as compared to 56% at baseline. Despite continued antipsychotic treatment 69% of this cohort had persistent psychosis.[24]

Finally the adverse prognostic significance of VH is illustrated by post-mortem series which have noted short survival times of less than 4 years after the onset of VH.[16,29] These studies have also suggested that the timing of onset of VH can predict the time of death—irrespective of disease duration.

Clinical Correlations

Persistent VH, particularly in the absence of delirium, are exceedingly rare in movement disorders other than Lewy body parkinsonism (incorporating PD and DLB).[16] There are only a few reports of VH in clinically and pathologically-diagnosed progressive supranuclear palsy, multiple system atrophy, and corticobasal degeneration, and in many of these cases the disorders of visual perception were related directly to medications or delirium.[30-33] These cases contrast with PD where VH often develop independent of medication changes, remain persistent despite medication alterations and progress to more malignant forms.[16,23,34] The presence of persistent VH has been suggested as a clinical indicator of underlying Lewy body pathology and may be helpful in differentiating these conditions from other bradykinetic rigid syndromes.[16,17]

Many centrally-acting medications are recognized to cause alterations in perception and in particular hallucinations, but the association between VH and medications in PD is complex.[5,34] VH are not an inevitable consequence of dopaminergic medications, and there does not appear to be a direct link between these drugs and hallucinations in PD, but rather a complex interaction between medications, the stage of disease and the extent of underlying Lewy body neurodegeneration.[16] Dopaminergic medications used in other conditions without neurodegeneration, including restless legs syndrome, dopa responsive dystonia, and pituitary tumors do not provoke VH. In non-Lewy body neurodegeneration, for example in progressive supranuclear palsy and multiple system atrophy, these medications are much less likely to provoke VH than in PD, suggesting a unique physiological interaction with Lewy body pathologies.[16,17]

The distribution of this pathology appears to be important and clinical correlations provide further clues to the underlying pathophysiology. Visual hallucinations have consistently been associated with older age, older age at disease onset, and the presence of cognitive dysfunction.[16,17,23] Alzheimer's type pathology is not usually implicated and several studies have found no difference between the MMSE of hallucinators and non-hallucinators.[16,17,23] Multivariate analyses have identified an association between VH and clinical indicators of more widespread Lewy body pathology, including autonomic dysfunction, symmetrical disease, and axial rigidity.[16,17,23] In these studies, VH occur less frequently in patients with unilateral signs at disease onset, normal cognition, and normal autonomic function.

Visual hallucinations rarely present in the earliest stages of PD and their emergence usually indicates progression into the second half of the overall disease duration.[16] They often herald a phase of accelerated disability and loss of independence and together this probably indicates a progression of the neurodegeneration.[29] Proposed models of pathological spread in PD predict that cortical regions are affected by Lewy body pathology only after more caudal structures in the basal ganglia and brainstem.[35] While it is tempting to implicate pathological spread to cortical regions as the primary cause of VH, understanding of the pathophysiology is far from complete. It remains unclear whether their emergence is related to physiological changes specific to Lewy body pathology or whether the distribution of that pathology is the more important factor.

Disease Characteristics Contributing to Hallucinations

Accurate visual perception and interpretation requires intact neurological systems in the retina, optic nerve, optic radiation, occipital lobe, and the dorsal and ventral cortical visual pathways. Lewy body neurodegeneration can disrupt the visual input system at all of these different levels (Figure 10-2). Defective visual input promotes visual misinterpretation and the most florid example of this is the Charles Bonnett syndrome, described in elderly people with cataracts but without dementia.[36] These people experience hallucinatory experiences very similar to PD, consisting of well-formed, stereotyped, persistent, and repetitive VH. It is thought that a relative sensory deprivation caused by ocular pathology permits re-emergence or release of previously recorded visual percepts.

Blurring of vision or diplopia is not uncommon and can be a relatively early feature of PD.[9,23,37] These alterations are thought to relate to bradykinesia of eye movements and can manifest as reduced convergence or divergence. Deficits in color vision, and in particular discrimination along the red-green axis, are progressive in PD, and have been found to change with levodopa therapy.[38] Levodopa-related motor fluctuations also affect

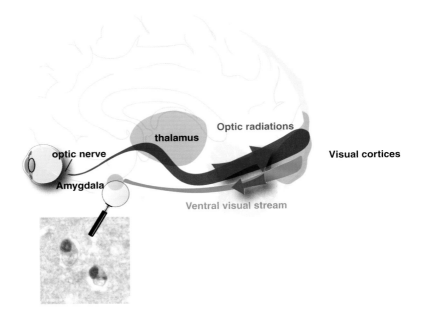

Figure 10-2. Diagram of the major visual pathways implicated pathologically in VH in PD.

contrast sensitivity, and a significant reduction in contrast sensitivity has been demonstrated in PD hallucinators.[38,39] Reduced dopaminergic innervation around the fovea and thinning of the retinal nerve fiber layer is reported in PD, and would alter the visual processing at the level of the ganglion cells.[40]

Higher level disturbances of visual perception have also been identified in PD, using a number of different testing paradigms. Most compelling is the finding of altered processing of visual memory and imagery in PD hallucinators, implicating dysfunction of the ventral or occipitotemporal visual pathway.[41]

Disorders of sleep are common in PD, in particular REM behavior disorder (RBD), excessive daytime somnolence, and vivid dreaming.[37] These non-motor phenomena appear to be related to VH, but their relationship is not simple.[42] For example, vivid dreaming has been associated with a greater severity of VH, but the two do not necessarily occur together in the same patient and vivid dreaming does not appear to predict the onset of VH.[43] A single study using 24-hour polysomnographic recordings reported non-REM sleep EEG changes during the day at the same time that VH were occurring.[44] A longitudinal study has linked the severity and frequency of RBD with VH and others have suggested that hallucinations represent exported fragments of REM sleep during wakefulness.[45,46] This hypothesis doesn't explain the phenomenological differences between dreams, which are often incongruous and difficult to recall, and VH that are repetitive and stereotyped.

Fluctuations in consciousness are a hallmark of DLB and PDD. They are thought to be caused by changes in the reticular activating system, leading to reduced maintenance of alertness through the reticulo-thalamo-cortical pathways.[47,48] It is likely that these alterations gradually evolve, and even before fluctuations in cognition are apparent, smaller amplitude or more focal fluctuations in cortical activity may allow the intrusion of hallucinatory objects into scene perception.

Deiderich argues that to produce the spectrum of VH experienced in PD, reduced activation has to occur in combination with dysfunctional sensory gating of internal and external stimuli, as well as altered attentional vigilance.[49] This "three dimensional model" is attractive because it integrates data on visual deficiencies, sleep abnormalities, and the triggering effects of medications in PD. In addition to the ventral visual pathway, it also implicates the pedunculopontine nucleus and the frontal forebrain as regions of disordered activity related to VH.

Pathological Correlations

The predicted anatomical substrates for VH have, to some extent, been confirmed using functional imaging techniques. Although conflicting results make firm conclusions difficult, changes are consistently seen in the temporal, frontal, and occipital lobes. One of the most consistent findings in PD hallucinators have been of decreased blood flow in the ventral visual processing pathways.[50,51] Interestingly, in the Charles Bonnett syndrome an increase of activation is reported in this region when patients hallucinate about landscapes and figures.[52] The amygdala is the final processing center in this ventral stream of the cortical visual system that subserves conscious visual identification and discrimination and the extrageniculostriate (colliculo-thalamo-amygdala) visual system, which appears to subserve automatic, non-conscious emotional visual processing.[53]

Volumetric analyses suggest a reduction in the grey matter volume of the lingual and fusiform gyri in PD hallucinators, implying structural changes in the ventral visual system.[54] These patients also had a loss of volume in the superior parietal lobe, the end point of the dorsal visual pathway.

Cerebral metabolic activity, measured using [^{18}F] fluorodeoxyglucose PET, was shown to be decreased in the ventral visual system in one study of PD hallucinators,[55] but in other studies of hallucinations in DLB cerebral metabolic activity was preserved or increased in the ventral temporal lobe regions.[56–58] A paradoxical increase in metabolism in the superior frontal region has also been reported and is thought to indicate a disinhibition of frontal cortical processing.[55]

Functional MRI studies have the advantage of assessing brain function in the active state, in contrast to the "resting state" analyzed in PET studies. Although no fMRI studies have been published that tested patients during their hallucinations, a study in PD patients performing basic visual tests found that hallucinators had reduced function in the ventral and dorsal visual pathways compared to non-hallucinators.[59]

The seemingly contradictory results from different functional imaging studies are probably related to differences in study protocols, patient characteristics and imaging ligands. It may be that these contrasting results reflect the dynamic nature of hallucinatory experiences. Testing paradigms that do not assess function or blood flow during a VH will only partially reflect the pathophysiology of these spontaneous visual experiences. Nevertheless, results from these studies consistently indicate an alteration in the ventral visual pathway along with disordered cortical inhibition.

Few histopathological studies have examined the pathological basis for VH in PD. In one study, using retrospective case notes analysis without a standardized clinical assessment protocol, additional pathological diagnoses were compared between hallucinators and non-hallucinators.[60] There were no differences in the frequency of age-related changes, Alzheimer's disease pathology, vascular disease, or other pathological diagnoses amongst the two groups. Interestingly, the extent of Lewy body pathology in PD patients with and without dementia was similar. The close relationship between PDD and VH suggest that more detailed regional studies are needed to identify the pathological substrate.[61]

The ventral temporal lobe has been identified as a region likely to provide pathological clues related to VH because of its proposed functional role in visual recognition,[62–64] the regional abnormalities identified by functional imaging, and the importance of parahippocampal Lewy bodies in differentiating PD from DLB.[65] The degree of neuronal loss and Lewy body pathology in amygdale subnuclei has been examined using stereological methods in 18 prospectively studied, non-demented patients with

PD and 16 age- and sex-matched controls. They found that patients who had experienced VH had nearly double the density of Lewy bodies and proportion of neurons containing Lewy bodies in the basolateral nucleus, compared to non-hallucinators.[65] They did not find, however, any difference in the degree of neuronal loss between these groups. While the functional implication of the presence of Lewy bodies is uncertain, the absence of neuronal loss in this study would suggest neuronal dysfunction rather than loss of function. The finding of increased densities of Lewy bodies implies a disruption of the amygdala's ability to integrate coordinated behavioral responses between the 2 visual systems (see Figure 10-2).

Management of VH and Psychosis

Minor forms of visual misperception in PD, like recurring brief sense of passage or presence, brief complex VH with fully retained insight, or visual illusions and selective diplopia do not necessarily require treatment in all cases. Patients and caregivers, after proper counseling, may be unconcerned and able to cope with these more benign features of PD psychosis. In cases of troublesome VH, in particular with loss of insight or additional features of psychosis, identification and removal of aggravating or triggering factors becomes paramount. This includes control of medical conditions like infections, dehydration, and electrolyte disturbances or reductions of polypharmacy with antiparkinsonian and other centrally-active drugs like antimuscarinic antidepressants, anxiolytics, and sedatives.[66] In cases of new onset confusion and delirium not readily explained by any of these triggers or medication changes, brain imaging should be used liberally to exclude new structural brain pathology like subdural hematomas or stroke. When reducing and simplifying antiparkinsonian combination therapy, drugs with high-risk benefit ratios regarding cognitive side effects versus antiparkinsonian efficacy should be tapered first, i.e. anticholinergics and amantadine, but also MAO-B inhibitors, before reducing dopamine agonists and levodopa. Similarly, dopamine agonists by virtue of their greater potential to induce psychosis should be tapered before levodopa.[7] Dose reductions of anti-parkinsonian drugs to a level that will lead to a resolution of hallucinosis and other psychotic symptoms, while maintaining sufficient symptomatic motor control, is not always feasible and start of antipsychotic therapy becomes necessary.

In recent years a number of atypical antipsychotic drugs with low potential of causing extrapyramidal adverse reactions have been tested in the setting of psychosis in patients with PD in order to control psychiatric symptoms without reducing motor function. Clozapine remains the only atypical antipsychotic agent with consistent evidence for efficacy from open-label and randomized controlled studies.[43] Two randomized placebo-controlled trials have documented antipsychotic efficacy without worsening of UPDRS motor scores after 4 weeks of double-blind treatment.[67,68] Open label extensions of these studies provided evidence for maintained efficacy of clozapine over an additional 12 weeks.[69] Consistently reported side effects even with low-dose clozapine in these studies include sedation, dizziness, increased drooling, orthostatic hypotension, and weight gain. In addition, clozapine is associated with the rare (0.38% according to Honigfeld et al[70]) but serious and potentially life-threatening occurrence of agranulocytosis. By contrast, olanzapine has consistently failed to show antipsychotic efficacy in several randomized controlled trials,[70–72] but was associated with significant motor worsening in all. Four randomized controlled trials have assessed the efficacy of quetiapine to treat psychosis in PD.[74–77] Two of these failed to show superiority of quetiapine over placebo on the primary outcome measures,[76,77] while the other two trials[74,75] found similar efficacy of quetiapine and clozapine. On the other hand, quetiapine was generally associated with improvement in some 70% to 80% of patients in open-label studies and some motor worsening was reported at one point during prolonged treatment in up to one-third of patients by Fernandez et al.[78] One study compared efficacy and safety of quetiapine between parkinsonian patients with and without dementia and found demented patients to have a higher propensity for worsening of motor symptoms. More recently, several open label studies have reported antipsychotic efficacy of rivastigmine,[78,80] donepezil,[81,82] or galantamine[83] in demented and non-demented PD patients. In addition, post-hoc analysis of a large placebo-controlled study of rivastigmine in PD dementia showed improvement of VH on rivastigmine.[84,85]

In routine clinical practice and when there is a clear need for antipsychotic therapy for VH and other psychotic manifestations, quetiapine, although not formally established as efficacious in randomized controlled trials, should be a pragmatic first choice due to its improved safety profile as compared to clozapine. Treatment should start with 25–50mg at bedtime, increasing to 200mg/d if needed. Clozapine is the only antipsychotic agent with proven efficacy based on randomized controlled trials and should be used in all cases failing treatment with quetiapine, but can also be considered as first-line option, despite onerous weekly blood count monitoring. It should be started with 6.25 mg/d at bedtime and increased by the same amount every other day until psychosis remits or adverse events occur. Rivastigmine and donepezil may be another treatment option for psychotic behavior specifically in patients with PD and dementia.

Unknown Aspects of Hallucinations

There are many aspects of the clinicopathological relationship between Lewy body pathology and VH that remain unanswered. The overwhelming preponderance of hallucinations in the visual system suggests very specific regional susceptibility to Lewy body sensory disturbance (Figure 10-2). The pathophysiological basis of this regional susceptibility is unclear, and currently our functional measures of these regions are imperfect and have given somewhat contradictory results. The presymptomatic stage of VH is currently untested, although interest in the ocular dysfunction and subtle cognitive changes that precede VH may provide some clues. At present the tools for assessing VH are blunt. Several structured questionnaires have been developed to assess the presence of minor and major VH[17] or neuropsychiatric accompaniments of VH.[86] While these questionnaires can be helpful in the routine clinical setting, for research purposes a validated measure of the severity of VH and disorders of visual processing is needed to better track the natural history of this phenomenon. Finally, the best treatment of VH in PD is not clear. The relative benign nature of early hallucinations does not, in many cases, warrant specific therapy.

References

1. Ravina B, Marder K, Fernandez HH et al. Diagnostic criteria for psychosis in Parkinson's disease: report of an NINDS, NIMH work group. *Mov Disord.* 2007;22: 1061–1068.
2. American Psychiatric A. *Diagnostic and Statistical Manual of Mental Disorders.* Vol. 4th edition. Washington DC, 1994.
3. Fenelon G, Mahieux F, Huon R, Ziegler M. Hallucinations in Parkinson's disease: prevalence, phenomenology and risk factors. *Brain.* 2000;123 (Pt 4):733–745.
4. Graham JM, Grunewald RA, Sagar HJ. Hallucinosis in idiopathic Parkinson's disease. *J Neurol Neurosurg Psychiatry.* 1997;63:434–440.
5. Papapetropoulos S, Argyriou AA, Ellul J. Factors associated with drug-induced visual hallucinations in Parkinson's disease. *J Neurol.* 2005;252:1223–1228.
6. Barnes J, David AS. Visual hallucinations in Parkinson's disease: a review and phenomenological survey. *J Neurol Neurosurg Psychiatry.* 2001;70:727–733.
7. Poewe W. Psychosis in Parkinson's disease. *Mov Disord.* 2003;18 Suppl 6:S80–S87.
8. Fenelon G. Psychosis in Parkinson's disease: phenomenology, frequency, risk factors, and current understanding of pathophysiologic mechanisms. *CNS Spectr.* 2008;13: 18–25.
9. Nebe A, Ebersbach G. Selective diplopia in Parkinson's disease: a special subtype of visual hallucination? *Mov Disord.* 2007;22:1175–1178.

10. Pagonabarraga J et al. A prospective study of delusional misidentification syndromes in Parkinson's disease with dementia. *Mov Disord.* 2008;23:443–448.

11. McKeith I, Mintzer J, Aarsland D et al. Dementia with Lewy bodies. *Lancet Neurol.* 2004;3:19–28.

12. Mosimann UP, Rowan EN, Partington CE et al. Characteristics of visual hallucinations in Parkinson disease dementia and dementia with Lewy bodies. *Am J Geriatr Psychiatry.* 2006;14:153–160.

13. Aarsland D, Litvan I, Salmon D et al. Performance on the dementia rating scale in Parkinson's disease with dementia and dementia with Lewy bodies: comparison with progressive supranuclear palsy and Alzheimer's disease. *J Neurol Neurosurg Psychiatry.* 2003;74:1215–1220.

14. Mosimann UP, Mather G, Wesnes KA et al. Visual perception in Parkinson disease dementia and dementia with Lewy bodies. *Neurology.* 2004;63:2091–2096.

15. Inzelberg R, Kipervasser S, Korczyn AD. Auditory hallucinations in Parkinson's disease. *J Neurol Neurosurg Psychiatry.* 1998;64:533–535.

16. Williams DR, Lees AJ. Visual hallucinations in the diagnosis of idiopathic Parkinson's disease: a retrospective autopsy study. *Lancet Neurol.* 2005;4:605–610.

17. Williams DR, Warren JD, Lees AJ. Using the presence of visual hallucinations to differentiate Parkinson's disease from atypical parkinsonism. *J Neurol Neurosurg Psychiatry.* 2008;79:652–655.

18. Todes CJ. At the receiving end of the lisuride pump. *Lancet.* 1986;2:36–37.

19. Aarsland D, Larsen JP, Cummins JL, Laake K. Prevalence and clinical correlates of psychotic symptoms in Parkinson disease: a community-based study. *Arch Neurol.* 1999;56:595–601.

20. Schrag A, Ben-Shlomo Y, Quinn N. How common are complications of Parkinson's disease? *J Neurol.* 2002;249:419–423.

21. Hely MA, Morris JG, Reid WG, Trafficante R. Sydney Multicenter Study of Parkinson's disease: non-L-dopa-responsive problems dominate at 15 years. *Mov Disord.* 2005;20:190–199.

22. Hely MA, Reid WG, Adena MA et al. The Sydney multicenter study of Parkinson's disease: the inevitability of dementia at 20 years. *Mov Disord.* 2008;23: 837–844.

23. de Maindreville AD, Fenelon G, Mahieux F. Hallucinations in Parkinson's disease: a follow-up study. *Mov Disord.* 2005;20:212–217.

24. Factor SA, Feustel PJ, Friedman JH et al. Longitudinal outcome of Parkinson's disease patients with psychosis. *Neurology.* 2003;60:1756–1761.

25. Goetz CG, Leurgans S, Pappert EJ et al. Prospective longitudinal assessment of hallucinations in Parkinson's disease. *Neurology.* 2001;57:2078–2082.

26. Goetz CG, Fan W, Leurgans S et al. The malignant course of "benign hallucinations" in Parkinson disease. *Arch Neurol.* 2006;63:713–716.

27. Aarsland D, Larsen JP, Tandberg E, Laake K. Predictors of nursing home placement in Parkinson's disease: a population-based, prospective study. *J Am Geriatr Soc.* 2000;48:938–942.

28. Goetz CG, Stebbins GT. Risk factors for nursing home placement in advanced Parkinson's disease. *Neurology.* 1993;43:2227–2229.

29. Kempster PA, Williams DR, Selikhova M et al. Patterns of levodopa response in Parkinson's disease: a clinico-pathological study. *Brain.* 2007;130:2123–2128.

30. Aarsland D, Litvan I, Larsen JP. Neuropsychiatric symptoms of patients with progressive supranuclear palsy and Parkinson's disease. *J Neuropsych Clinical Neurosciences.* 2001;13:42–49.

31. Lees AJ, Bannister R. The use of lisuride in the treatment of multiple system atrophy with autonomic failure (Shy-Drager syndrome). *J Neurol Neurosurg Psychiatry.* 1981;44:347–351.

32. Nagaoka K, Ookawa S, Maeda K. [A case of corticobasal degeneration presenting with visual hallucination]. Rinsho shinkeigaku = *Clinical Neurology.* 2004;44:193–197.

33. Shimo Y, Takanashi M, Ohta S et al. [A-56-year-old woman with parkinsonism, whose mother had Parkinson's disease]. No to shinkei = *Brain and Nerve.* 2001;53:495–505.

34. Cummings JL. Behavioral complications of drug treatment of Parkinson's disease. *J Am Geriatr Soc.* 1991;39:708–716.

35. Braak H, Rub U, Jansen Steur EN et al. Cognitive status correlates with neuropathologic stage in Parkinson disease. *Neurology.* 2005;64:1404–1410.

36. Teunisse RJ, Cruysberg JR, Hoefnagels WH et al. Visual hallucinations in psychologically normal people: Charles Bonnet's syndrome. *Lancet.* 1996;347:794–797.

37. Chaudhuri KR, Martinez-Martin P, Schapira AH et al. International multicenter pilot study of the first comprehensive self-completed nonmotor symptoms questionnaire for Parkinson's disease: the NMSQuest study. *Mov Disord.* 2006;21:916–923.

38. Biousse V, Skibell BC, Watts RL et al. Ophthalmologic features of Parkinson's disease. *Neurology.* 2004;62:177–180.

39. Pieri V, Diederich NJ, Raman R, Goetz CG. Decreased color discrimination and contrast sensitivity in Parkinson's disease. *J Neurol Sci.* 2000;172:7–11.

40. Nguyen-Legros J. Functional neuroarchitecture of the retina: hypothesis on the dysfunction of retinal dopaminergic circuitry in Parkinson's disease. *Surg Radiol Anat.* 1988;10:137–144.

41. Barnes J, Boubert L, Harris J et al. Reality monitoring and visual hallucinations in Parkinson's disease. *Neuropsychologia.* 2003;41:565–574.

42. Pappert EJ, Goetz CG, Niederman FG et al. Hallucinations, sleep fragmentation, and altered dream phenomena in Parkinson's disease. *Mov Disord.* 1999;14:117–121.

43. Goetz CG, Poewe W, Rascol O, Sampaio C. Evidence-based medical review update: pharmacological and surgical treatments of Parkinson's disease: 2001 to 2004. *Mov Disord.* 2005;20:523–539.

44. Comella CL, Tanner CM, Ristanovic RK. Polysomnographic sleep measures in Parkinson's disease patients with treatment-induced hallucinations. *Ann Neurol.* 1993;34:710–714.

45. Sinforiani E, Zangaglia R, Manni R et al. REM sleep behavior disorder, hallucinations, and cognitive impairment in Parkinson's disease. *Mov Disord.* 2006;21:462–466.

46. Sinforiani E, Pacchetti C, Zangaglia R et al. REM behavior disorder, hallucinations and cognitive impairment in Parkinson's disease: a two-year follow up. *Mov Disord.* 2008;23:1441–1445.

47. Stuss DT, Murphy KJ, Binns MA, Alexander MP. Staying on the job: the frontal lobes control individual performance variability. *Brain.* 2003;126:2363–2380.

48. Walker MP, Ayre GA, Perry EK et al. Quantification and characterization of fluctuating cognition in dementia with Lewy bodies and Alzheimer's disease. *Dement Geriatr Cogn Dis*. 2000;11:327–335.

49. Diederich NJ, Goetz CG, Stebbins GT. Repeated visual hallucinations in Parkinson's disease as disturbed external/internal perceptions: focused review and a new integrative model. *Mov Disord*. 2005;20:130–140.

50. Matsui H, Nishinaka K, Oda M et al. Hypoperfusion of the auditory and prefrontal cortices in Parkinsonian patients with verbal hallucinations. *Mov Disord*. 2006;21: 2165–2169.

51. Okada K, Suyama N, Oguro H et al. Medication-induced hallucination and cerebral blood flow in Parkinson's disease. *J Neurol*. 1999;246:365–368.

52. Ffytche DH, Howard RJ. The perceptual consequences of visual loss: 'positive' pathologies of vision. *Brain*. 1999;122 (Pt 7):1247–1260.

53. Morris JS, DeGelder B, Weiskrantz L, Dolan RJ. Differential extrageniculostriate and amygdala responses to presentation of emotional faces in a cortically blind field. *Brain*. 2001;124:1241–1252.

54. Ramirez-Ruiz B, Marti MJ, Tolosa E et al. Cerebral atrophy in Parkinson's disease patients with visual hallucinations. *Eur J Neurol*. 2007;14:750–756.

55. Boecker H, Ceballos-Baumann AO, Volk D et al. Metabolic alterations in patients with Parkinson disease and visual hallucinations. *Arch Neurol*. 2007;64:984–988.

56. Higuchi M, Tashiro M, Arai H et al. Glucose hypometabolism and neuropathological correlates in brains of dementia with Lewy bodies. *Exp Neurol*. 2000;162: 247–256.

57. Imamura T, Ishii K, Hirono N et al. Visual hallucinations and regional cerebral metabolism in dementia with Lewy bodies (DLB). *Neuroreport*. 1999;10:1903–1907.

58. Lobotesis K, Fenwick JD, Phipps A et al. Occipital hypoperfusion on SPECT in dementia with Lewy bodies but not AD. *Neurology*. 2001;56:643–649.

59. Stebbins GT, Goetz CG, Carrillo MC et al. Altered cortical visual processing in PD with hallucinations: an fMRI study. *Neurology*. 2004;63:1409–1416.

60. Colosimo C, Hughes AJ, Kilford L, Lees AJ. Lewy body cortical involvement may not always predict dementia in Parkinson's disease. *J Neurol Neurosurg Psychiatry*. 2003;74:852–856.

61. Kovari E, Gold G, Herrmann FR et al. Lewy body densities in the entorhinal and anterior cingulate cortex predict cognitive deficits in Parkinson's disease. *Acta Neuropathologica*. 2003;106:83–88.

62. Halgren E, Dale AM, Sereno MI et al. Location of human face-selective cortex with respect to retinotopic areas. *Hum Brain Mapp*. 1999;7:29–37.

63. Santhouse AM, Howard RJ, ffytche DH. Visual hallucinatory syndromes and the anatomy of the visual brain. *Brain*. 2000;123 (Pt 10):2055–2064.

64. Tanaka K. Inferotemporal cortex and object vision. *Ann Rev Neurosci*. 1996;19: 109–139

65. Harding AJ, Broe GA, Halliday GM. Visual hallucinations in Lewy body disease relate to Lewy bodies in the temporal lobe. *Brain*. 2002;125:391–403.

66. Poewe W, Seppi K. Treatment options for depression and psychosis in Parkinson's disease. *J Neurol*. 2001;248 Suppl 3:III12-III21.

67. Low-dose clozapine for the treatment of drug-induced psychosis in Parkinson's disease. The Parkinson Study Group. *N Engl JMed.* 1999;340:757–763.
68. Pollak P, Tison F, Rascol O et al. Clozapine in drug induced psychosis in Parkinson's disease: a randomised, placebo controlled study with open follow up. *J Neurol Neurosurg Psychiatry.* 2004;75:689–695.
69. Factor SA, Friedman JH, Lannon MC et al. Clozapine for the treatment of drug-induced psychosis in Parkinson's disease: results of the 12 week open label extension in the PSYCLOPS trial. *Mov Disord.* 2001;16:135–139.
70. Honigfeld G, Arellano F, Sethi J, Bianchini A, Schein J. Reducing clozapine-related morbidity and mortality: 5 years of experience with the Clozaril National Registry. *J Clin Psychiatry.* 1998;59 Suppl 3:3–7.
71. Breier A, Sutton VK, Feldman PD et al. Olanzapine in the treatment of dopamimetic-induced psychosis in patients with Parkinson's disease. *Biol Psychiatry.* 2002;52: 438–445.
72. Goetz CG, Blasucci LM, Leurgans S, Pappert EJ. Olanzapine and clozapine: comparative effects on motor function in hallucinating PD patients. *Neurology.* 2000;55: 789–794.
73. Ondo WG, Levy JK, Vuong KD et al. Olanzapine treatment for dopaminergic-induced hallucinations. *Mov Disord.* 2002;17:1031–1035.
74. Merims D, Balas M, Peretz C et al. Rater-blinded, prospective comparison: quetiapine versus clozapine for Parkinson's disease psychosis. *Clin Neuropharmacol.* 2006;29:331–337.
75. Morgante L, Epifanio A, Spina E et al. Quetiapine and clozapine in parkinsonian patients with dopaminergic psychosis. *Clin Neuropharmacol.* 2004;27:153–156.
76. Ondo WG, Tintner R, Voung KD et al. Double-blind, placebo-controlled, unforced titration parallel trial of quetiapine for dopaminergic-induced hallucinations in Parkinson's disease. *Mov Disord.* 2005;20:958–963.
77. Rabey JM, Prokhorov T, Miniovitz A et al. Effect of quetiapine in psychotic Parkinson's disease patients: a double-blind labeled study of 3 months' duration. *Mov Disord.* 2007;22:313–318.
78. Fernandez HH, Friedman JH, Jacques C, Rosenfeld M. Quetiapine for the treatment of drug-induced psychosis in Parkinson's disease. *Mov Disord.* 1999;14:484–487.
79. Bullock R, Cameron A. Rivastigmine for the treatment of dementia and visual hallucinations associated with Parkinson's disease: a case series. *Curr Med Res Opin.* 2002;18:258–264.
80. Reading PJ, Luce AK, McKeith IG. Rivastigmine in the treatment of parkinsonian psychosis and cognitive impairment: preliminary findings from an open trial. *Mov Disord.* 2001;16:1171–1174.
81. Bergman J, Lerner V. Successful use of donepezil for the treatment of psychotic symptoms in patients with Parkinson's disease. *Clin Neuropharmacol.* 2002;25:107–110.
82. Fabbrini G, Barbanti P, Aurilia C et al. Donepezil in the treatment of hallucinations and delusions in Parkinson's disease. *Neurol Sci.* 2002;23:41–43.
83. Aarsland D, Hutchinson M, Larsen JP. Cognitive, psychiatric and motor response to galantamine in Parkinson's disease with dementia. *Int J Geriatr Psychiatry.* 2003;18:937–941.

84. Emre M, Aarsland D, Albanese A et al. Rivastigmine for dementia associated with Parkinson's disease. *N Engl J Med.* 2004;351:2509–2518.

85. Sanchez-Ramos JR, Ortoll R, Paulson GW. Visual hallucinations associated with Parkinson disease. *Arch Neurol.* 1996;53:1265–1268.

86. Brandstaedter D, Spieker S, Ulm G et al. Development and evaluation of the Parkinson Psychosis Questionnaire A screening-instrument for the early diagnosis of drug-induced psychosis in Parkinson's disease. *J Neurol.* 2005;252:1060–1066.

87. Holroyd S, Currie L, Wooten GF. Prospective study of hallucinations and delusions in Parkinson's disease. *J Neurol Neurosurg Psychiatry.* 2001;70:734–738.

88. Pacchetti C, Manni R, Zangaglia R et al. Relationship between hallucinations, delusions, and rapid eye movement sleep behavior disorder in Parkinson's disease. *Mov Disord.* 2005;20:1439–1448.

89. Paleacu D, Schechtman E, Inzelberg R. Association between family history of dementia and hallucinations in Parkinson disease. *Neurology.* 2005;64:1712–1715.

Chapter 11

Lesions Associated with Cognitive Impairment and Dementia

Jonathan Evans, Tamas Revesz, and Roger A. Barker

Introduction

Whilst Parkinson's disease (PD) continues to be defined clinically in terms of its motor features, recognition of the spectrum of non-motor deficits seen in the syndrome is improving. Cognitive impairment, progressing in some cases to overt dementia, is a common non-motor symptom and one which has a major impact both upon the individual, being a major determinant of quality of life, and health care economies, given it is the strongest predictor of the need for nursing home placement.[1]

The pathophysiology of impaired cognition in PD is incompletely understood. It is now generally recognized that the neurodegenerative process in PD is not one confined to the nigrostriatal system, nor one which has an exclusive effect upon dopaminergic neurons. The histopathological hallmark of PD, the Lewy body, is found in widespread cortical and subcortical loci at post-mortem.[2] Indeed, according to the recently proposed classification system for the staging of PD pathology by Braak et al,[3] the pathological process begins in the caudal brainstem, progressing cranially to involve the substantia nigra only at a later stage. As cognitive dysfunction in PD is not, in general, ameliorated by dopamine replacement therapy, degeneration in such extra-nigral, non-dopaminergic loci presents a plausible pathogenic mechanism for PD dementia (PDD). But this hypothesis itself generates a number of further questions: Which neuroanatomical systems are affected? Which neurotransmitters are involved? What molecular processes are at work? And, most pertinently, how can we use the answers to these questions to suggest and develop novel therapies for this most disabling of PD complications?

Our aim in this chapter is to review the evidence by which degeneration of non-dopaminergic systems has been implicated in the cognitive dysfunction of PD. This evidence is drawn from histopathological, molecular biological and neuropsychological studies and the challenge will be to synthesize this information into a plausible model of PDD as encountered in clinical practice.

Epidemiology of PDD

There are wide variations in both the reported incidence and prevalence of cognitive impairment in PD. These discrepancies can be ascribed, at least in part, to variations in the study population (hospital versus community-based, age structure of cohort) and study methodology (diagnostic criteria used for PD, definition of dementia). Thus incidence rates of 95.3,[4] 107.1,[5] and 112.5[6] per 1000 patient years have been reported from community-based studies, implying that approximately 10% of a given PD population will develop dementia per year. However, dementia risk is correlated with disease duration[7] and thus it is difficult to generalize these results without reference to the age stratification of study populations and length of follow up. This problem can be circumvented by following patients longitudinally from diagnosis.[8] One such study showed that 3 to 5 years after diagnosis the incidence of dementia was 30 /1000 patient years, indicating a relative risk of dementia of 5 times that seen in an age-matched control population.[9]

Relationship of PDD to Dementia with Lewy Bodies

The current consensus view is that PDD and dementia with Lewy bodies (DLB) should be regarded, along with non-demented PD, as related entities along a clinicopathological spectrum of Lewy body disorders.[10] Whilst the temporal course and symptom profile of these disorders differs, both are characterized neuropathologically by the Lewy body and as such these differences could be regarded as quantitative not qualitative.[11] It follows that experimental observations resulting from studies of one of these clinical conditions might reasonably be extrapolated to the other.

Neuropsychological Profile of PDD

Appreciating the nature and pattern of neuropsychological deficits in PD and PDD provides an insight into which cortical-subcortical networks are likely to be involved pathophysiologically. The cognitive dysfunction which develops in patients with Mendelian forms of PD (especially those affected by PARK1 and PARK 8 mutations in the α-synuclein and LRRK2 genes respectively) has the same profile as that seen in patients with sporadic disease, providing evidence that we are dealing with a distinct clinicopathological entity.[12,13] This profile is, however, heterogeneous, and in an elderly at-risk population the interference of other age-related or age-dependent neurodegenerative processes may further complicate interpretation.

A task force commissioned by The Movement Disorder Society has recently endeavored to synthesize clinical and neuropsychological data into a set of diagnostic criteria for PDD.[14] Although a useful synthesis of this area, there are still a number of unresolved issues, not least the significance of deficits in executive function.

Much has been written about executive impairment—incorporating the ability to plan, to order complex behaviors, and to understand abstract concepts—in PD. Certainly there is compelling evidence that, early in the disease course, patients with PD do demonstrate executive impairment, with this impairment being more pronounced than that seen in cases of Alzheimer's disease (AD) matched for disease duration.[15] In a cohort of newly diagnosed, non-demented patients with PD, selective impairment of executive function was seen in 14 out of 106 patients studied.[8] However, the testing of executive function is problematic in that standard paradigms require that other neuropsychological faculties, such as memory, attention, and language abilities are broadly intact. This is most easily understood through analogy with the "neuropsychological pyramid" (Figure 11-1). Many neuropsychological tests probe a number of different domains simultaneously, and poor performance may be attributable to deficits in one or more different areas (generally those positioned towards the base of the pyramid). As executive abilities sit atop the pyramid, their assessment is highly susceptible to confounding from deficits elsewhere. This is evident in the literature, where the terms "executive function" and "attention" are often used interchangeably when in reality they describe quite distinct faculties.

Dysfunction in other, non-executive, neuropsychological domains has been repeatedly described in PD and PDD. Impairment in attention is well recognized, just as it is one of the defining characteristics of dementia with Lewy bodies (DLB).[16–18] Fluctuations in levels of attention, which has been objectively demonstrated in tasks measuring serial reaction times,[19] are recognized in clinical practice as features of the PDD syndrome, and

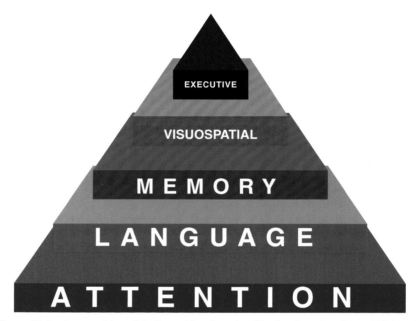

Figure 11-1. A pyramid model of cognitive domains. Testing domains situated high up in the pyramid in isolation requires that the domains below it are intact. For example, the results of a memory test are only valid if the subject can attend to the task and understand the instructions given to him (language).

are incorporated into the diagnostic criteria referred to above. One study has compared PDD and DLB with AD directly, finding subjects with the former conditions performed significantly worse on attention tests, and correspondingly better on tests of memory.[20]

Notwithstanding this, memory impairment is the presenting feature in over half of patients diagnosed with PDD[20] (memory difficulties are perhaps more overt both to patients and caregivers). Some investigators have described memory deficits which improve with retrieval cues, implying preservation of encoding and storage faculties. It has been suggested, therefore, that memory deficits in PD relate predominantly to difficulties with memory retrieval, a task generally regarded as requiring the use of an appropriate search strategy and thus being more executive in nature.[21] Whilst this may be the case in the early stages of the disease, in patients meeting criteria for dementia there is growing evidence that recognition memory per se is also deficient,[22] although this deficit may not be as prominent as that observed in the comparable stages of AD.[20] Semantic memory is relatively preserved, and in general language function in PD and PDD remains intact; clinically evident aphasia is rare.[23]

Whilst tests of construction ability and praxis are subject to confounding in PD due to motor symptoms, the available evidence suggests that on tasks such as the clock-drawing test patients with PDD show impairments greater than those seen in AD.[24] Performance on such tasks also draws upon both executive abilities and visuospatial function, and there is additional independent evidence to support specific impairment of visuoperceptual abilities in PDD.[25]

In summary, the cognitive profile of PDD may typically incorporate impairment in the domains of attention, visuo-spatial function, memory, and executive function. Given this heterogeneous pattern of deficits it is incorrect to refer to PDD purely, or even primarily, as a dysexecutive syndrome. Whilst isolated executive deficits may be seen in non-demented PD patients, with time involvement of other modalities is invariably seen, and these later changes may then evolve so as to dominate the clinical picture. Janvin et al have sought to classify the dementia syndrome using a different algorithm, defining it as a "subcortical" dementia based on the pre-eminence of attentional and visuo-perceptual deficits over faculties that localize to the cerebral cortex, such as language and delayed memory,[26] given that aphasia, apraxia, and agnosia are uncommon in PDD.[27] PDD, as we might expect, shows a similar profile to DLB and both can be distinguished from AD with reasonable accuracy using such an approach, although a considerable amount of overlap still exists. It follows that the involvement of subcortico-cortical networks is likely to be important in the pathophysiology of PDD, an observation which will inform our later discussion.

The Clinical Phenotype of PDD: Biomarkers of Dementia Risk

Whilst the clinical syndrome of "parkinsonism" predictably results from nigrostriatal degeneration, it has not hitherto been possible to definitively map particular symptoms on to dysfunction of particular neuroanatomical loci.[28] There is a great deal of symptomatic heterogeneity in patients with PD, particularly early in the disease course,[8,29] and it is well recognized that some symptoms respond better to dopamine replacement therapy than others. A number of studies have sought to investigate the relationship between motor and non-motor symptoms, particularly cognitive impairment, in PD. This is helpful for two reasons. First, symptoms which co-exist might reasonably share a neuro-anatomical or neuro-chemical substrate, and this can inform our understanding of the functional basis of the disorder. Secondly, as motor parameters can be measured quickly and easily, especially compared with cognitive parameters, motor biomarkers indicative or predictive of cognitive dysfunction might be of clinical utility both in defining prognosis and guiding therapy.

Features of PD which respond poorly to dopamine, such as the axial symptoms of gait dysfunction, postural impairment, and deficits in balance, have repeatedly been shown to correlate with the risk of prevalent dementia.[30,31] In longitudinal studies the risk of developing dementia has been associated with speech and axial symptoms, and in several studies with the so-called postural instability/gait disorder ("PIGD") phenotype as defined by Zetusky et al.[9,32,33] Postural symptoms have been postulated to originate from dysfunction in the brainstem cholinergic system,[34] but a precise locus has yet to be identified. Dementia risk, by contrast, is reduced in those patients exhibiting a tremor-dominant phenotype.

The Neuropathological Substrate of PDD

The morphological substrate of dementia associated with Lewy body disorders has been a matter of considerable controversy. Unlike the situation in AD, where cognitive impairment correlates strongly with the extent of macroscopic cortical atrophy and, histologically, with the extent of neurofibrillary tangles,[35,36] no consistent pattern has yet emerged in PDD. Some of this may be due to the inherent heterogeneity of the condition, but methodological problems (e.g. the underestimation of Lewy bodies prior to the availability of α-synuclein immunohistochemistry) may also have contributed. The variability of these results has driven the development of numerous theories of the neuropathological etiology of dementia in PD.

Both DLB and PDD patients may show brain atrophy which, in comparison with other dementias, is usually of limited extent.[37] Subcortical atrophy is not especially prominent in neuropathologically confirmed cases, but mild frontal and medial temporal lobe atrophy are regular findings.[38,39]

As previously stated, the heterogeneous neuropsychological profile of PDD is best modeled as arising from dysfunction in subcortico-cortical networks. Such a clinical picture can best be represented by the co-occurrence of both subcortical and cortical pathologies, which are well recognized components of the neuropathological spectrum in PD.[40] Theories as to the morphological changes underlying dementia in PD can be largely classified into 3 main types (Figure 11-2). According to one proposition, cognitive impairment is primarily due to involvement of subcortical and brainstem structures, while an extension of Lewy body pathology into limbic or higher cortical association areas is accepted by others as a plausible substrate for the dementia in Lewy body disorders. The third proposition is that concurrent AD-type pathology underlies the cognitive decline in PDD.

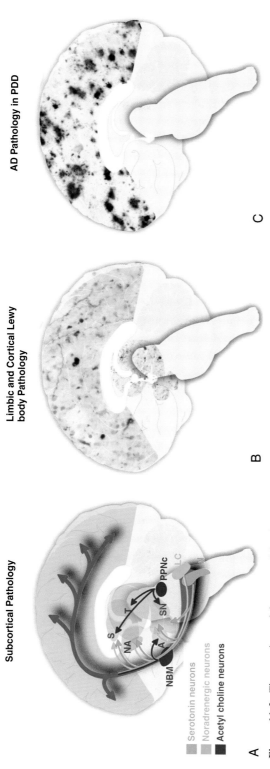

Figure 11-2. Three main models proposed for the pathogenesis of PD dementia. A) Dementia results from the degeneration of cortically-projecting (red line) acetyl choline, serotonin, and noradrenaline-producing neurons located in subcortical and brainstem loci. B) Dementia results from the spread of Lewy body pathology to limbic and neocortical areas. C) Dementia results from concurrent Alzheimer's disease (AD)-type changes in the neocortex. These 3 different models are not mutually exclusive. Pathophysiological interactions between these mechanisms may be occurring in PDD. A=amygdala, H=hippocampus, LC=locus coeruleus, NA=nucleus accumbens, NBM=nucleus basalis, PPNc=pedunculopontine tegmental nucleus pars compacta, RN=raphe nuclei, S=striatum, SN=substantia nigra, T=thalamus.

Subcortical Pathology

A stereotypic progression of Lewy body pathology in 6 consecutive stages, taking place along axonal pathways interconnecting vulnerable brain regions, has been proposed by Braak et al.[3] According to this scheme α-synuclein pathology first appears in lower brainstem nuclei and olfactory pathways and further progresses, initially to higher brainstem structures and thence to the basal forebrain and cerebral cortex. In pathological series the majority of PD cases appear to follow this pattern of disease spread,[41–43] although it has been proposed that DLB and a subset of PDD cases may not.[44,45] Despite the overlapping pathologies of DLB and PDD, it has been proposed that there is a difference in the selective vulnerability of affected neuronal populations in the early stages of the disease process.[46] It has been suggested that limbic and basal forebrain structures may be involved differentially in DLB, with brainstem nuclei affected earlier and more extensively in PDD. The few quantitative morphological studies comparing PDD and DLB have, however, failed to differentiate these syndromes on the grounds of Lewy body load by neuroanatomical region.[46–48]

Distinct pathological involvement of several brainstem nuclear groups is well recognized in PD, in line with the theory of Braak et al. Nuclei contributing to noradrenergic, serotonergic, and cholinergic neurotransmitter systems are all clearly involved in PD, and we shall review the evidence for their contribution to the syndrome of PDD in due course.

Limbic and Cortical Lewy Body Pathology

The notion that dementia in PD is associated with the extension of Lewy body pathology into cortical areas has gained widespread support in recent years.[49,50] This concept is underpinned by observations made by a number of clinicopathological studies which have demonstrated that the most common and consistent pathological finding in PDD is Lewy body pathology in limbic and, in a significant proportion of cases, also in neocortical regions. Cortical and, in particular, limbic Lewy body load has been shown to correlate with cognitive impairment in both PDD and DLB.[44,50–52] Community-based clinicopathological studies of well-characterized elderly individuals with PD have also indicated that cortical Lewy body disease with or without associated AD-type changes is likely to affect cognition.[53,54] It is of note, however, that both well-documented PD cases and elderly individuals without clinical evidence of either parkinsonism or cognitive decline in life may also show cortical Lewy body pathology,[43,55] the severity of which may be comparable to that seen in PDD.[10,48,56]

Conversely, although the risk of dementia generally increases with the progression of α-synuclein pathology signified by higher Braak stages, it has been recognized that some individuals with cognitive impairment may show only mild cortical Lewy body pathology.[43]

AD Pathology in PDD

The presence of increased amyloid-β plaque burden is a common finding in both DLB and PDD, although co-existing neurofibrillary tangle (NFT) pathology is rarely severe enough to meet the diagnostic criteria of AD.[11,41,46,57,58] Community-based pathological studies have documented that patients with dementia usually have multiple pathologies, and that patients with combined AD and Lewy body pathologies have more severe cognitive impairment than those with pure Lewy body pathology.[59] Morphological studies have shown a correlation between cortical Lewy body load and neuritic plaque load in DLB and PD,[47,60,61] and, as we might therefore anticipate, the degree of AD pathology in both the diseases is more marked than in non-demented PD.[46] Although the precise mechanism by which co-existing amyloid-β pathology may influence the pathogenesis of DLB and PDD is not known, there are *in vivo* and *in vitro* data to suggest a synergistic interaction between the amyloid- β peptide and α-synuclein,[62] which are also supported by neuropathological studies.[47,63] More recent studies have shown a significant negative correlation between the duration of the parkinsonian state prior to dementia and the quantitative plaque burden, with cases of parkinsonism pre-dating dementia by more than 9.5 years showing proportionally less plaque pathology.[11] In another study, an increased striatal amyloid-β burden, independent of the degree of cortical AD pathology, has been reported to be a good marker of dementia in PD.[64,65] Although a putative mechanism by which co-existing amyloid plaques could influence the pathogenesis of PDD has not been established, there is evidence, provided by in vivo transgenic and in vitro studies, to suggest a synergistic interaction between β-amyloid and α-synuclein.[62]

An Emerging Role for Tau in the Pathophysiology of PDD

Few large scale studies of genetic risk factors for dementia in PD have been conducted. As yet, no polymorphisms in genes involved in either dopaminergic or non-dopaminergic systems influencing PDD risk have been identified. Goris et al, studying an incident cohort of PD cases followed longitudinally from presentation, found a highly significant association between genotype at the tau locus and the cumulative risk of dementia.[66] Over three and a half years of follow-up only individuals homozygous for the H1 allele reached criteria for dementia. The H1 haplotype has previously been shown to be associated with both progressive supranuclear palsy (PSP)[67] and corticobasal degeneration (CBD),[68] but these are diseases, unlike PD, characterized histologically by the presence of tau aggregates.

The potential contribution of tau protein to the pathophysiology of PDD has been illuminated by a number of recent studies. Apaydin et al, in a post-mortem series of patients with PD dementia, found that in addition to limbic and neocortical Lewy bodies, neurofibrillary tangles, principally composed of aggregates of tau and more typically associated with AD, were also present in these regions, their concentration correlating significantly with Lewy body load.[49] This effect was not seen in non-demented PD and could not be attributed to age-related changes. Thus, although AD did not appear to be the primary substrate for dementia, tau-containing neuropathological markers were found associated with Lewy bodies. Recent work has also demonstrated protein-protein interactions between tau and α-synuclein,[69] although whether such interactions are pathological in vivo remains unclear. One intriguing hypothesis, however, is that the combination of tau genotype with Lewy body pathology creates the substrate for PDD. α-Synuclein pathology might "seed" the aggregation of tau in a process dependent upon tau genotype. The relative expression of different isoforms of tau, which has been shown to change with tau genotype in PD,[70] could thus mediate the rate of development of this superadded pathology.

The Role of Dopamine in Cognition

The contribution of dopaminergic deficiency to the cognitive profile of PD remains controversial. The functional neuroanatomy of subcortical circuits incorporating the striatum and substantia nigra is complex and incompletely understood, but one such circuit (the so-called dorsolateral prefrontal loop) which reciprocally connects the dorsolateral prefrontal cortex with the caudate nucleus, and thence the pallidum and thalamus, is considered to be intimately involved in executive behavior.[71] A number of functional imaging studies in PD provide evidence that executive dysfunction in PD is mediated at least in part by dysregulation at the level of the caudate nucleus as a consequence of nigrostriatal dopaminergic depletion.[72,73] However, it has also been suggested that dysfunction in the prefrontal cortex, which is in receipt of striatal afferents, may ultimately mediate the executive deficit.[74]

Executive function in PD is modulated by dopamine replacement therapy, with reports of both positive and deleterious effects.[75] This apparent paradox has been attributed to the non-uniform loss of striatal dopamine, with lesser-depleted areas, the ventral striatum in particular, potentially subject to supra-optimal dopamine levels with L-dopa therapy.[76] We have previously shown that these differential effects may also be explicable in terms of a common genetic polymorphism which influences the breakdown of synaptic dopamine, providing evidence that the locus of the deficit is indeed in the prefrontal cortex, not the striatum.[77]

The importance of dopamine in mediating executive function is further illustrated by patients with parkinsonism secondary to MPTP consumption who, in the context of relatively pure dopaminergic deficiency, show deficits in verbal fluency and other measures of executive dysfunction in the absence of impairment in other neuropsychological domains.[78]

Whilst executive impairment is common in PD, even at presentation,[8] when present in isolation it does not appear to confer any increased risk of later occurring dementia.[9]

Acetylcholine and PDD

It is well established that cholinergic systems are instrumental for cognition in humans and animals.[79] Dysfunction of these cholinergic systems in PD and PDD has been demonstrated in histopathological, neuropsychological, and molecular biological studies.[80]

Activity of the enzyme choline acetyltransferase (ChAT), responsible for the presynaptic synthesis of acetylcholine (ACh), is reduced not only in the neocortex, but also in basal ganglia and brainstem nuclei in PDD.[81–83] This reduction occurs earlier and is more extensive in Lewy body disorders than in AD.[84] Cortical levels of both acetyl- and butyryl-cholinesterase are reduced in PDD and DLB, but not in non-demented PD.[85] Loss of nicotinic receptors has been shown to occur in both cortical and subcortical regions, including the substantia nigra itself.[86,87] Other investigators have provided some evidence that this loss of receptors is subtype specific, with deficiency of the high-affinity $\alpha4\beta2$ occurring most widely in the cortex.[88] Muscarinic ACh receptors, by contrast, may be preserved or even upregulated in the temporal cortex,[89–91] which may be the neuropharmacological basis of the particularly beneficial clinical response of both PDD and DLB to acetylcholinesterase inhibitors, which we shall come to discuss in more detail below.

Reduction in markers of cholinergic transmission has been demonstrated in a number of clinicopathological series to correlate with the extent of cognitive impairment in PD.[92-94] Both cortical and subcortical regions are affected, and it is logical to ask which neuroanatomical loci, and by extension which cholinergic systems, are most relevant to the pathophysiology of cognitive impairment. Technically this is a difficult question to answer. A number of investigators have pointed out that cholinergic modulation of activity in the thalamo-cortical networks may be the main site for the expression of both up- and down-stream central cholinergic deficiencies.[95] Nevertheless, two subcortical loci have been implicated in the pathogenesis of PDD: the nucleus basalis of Meynert (NBM) and the pedunculopontine nucleus (PPN) (Figure 11-3).

The NBM is located in the substantia innominata of the basal forebrain, in the lateral part of the tuber cinereurm. It is composed almost exclusively

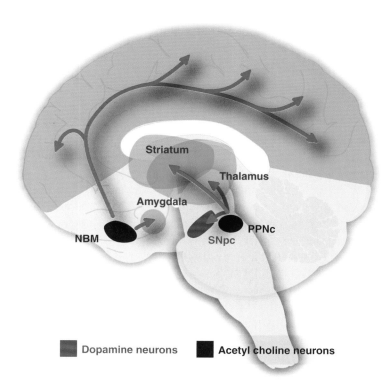

Figure 11-3. Representation of the main cholinergic regions in the brain and their projections. NBM=nucleus basalis, PPNc=pedunculopontine tegmental nucleus pars compacta, SNc=substantia nigra pars compacta.

of cholinergic neurons and projects widely to the neocortex and the amygdalae and pathology within this system is well recognized and has been identified in AD.[96] Independent involvement of the NBM in Lewy-body associated neurodegeneration has also been demonstrated,[97] and in both conditions a correlation between neuronal loss at this locus and dementia has been demonstrated.[98,99]

Recognition of the involvement of the PPN in PD has come more recently. Initial interest focused on a potential role for this nucleus as a pathological substrate of the gait and postural disturbances, features of PD known to respond poorly to dopamine replacement therapy. Subsequently, a number of other functions have been suggested, spanning both motor and non-motor domains.[100]

The PPN is located in the brainstem at the junction of the pons and cerebral peduncle, caudal to the substantia nigra, and adjacent to the superior cerebellar peduncle. Although the PPN has numerous interconnections with the basal ganglia, it is in fact part of the ascending reticular formation.[101] The PPN is not homogeneous. Architecturally, in fact, it shows striking analogy with the substantia nigra.[102] Two subdivisions of the PPN are recognized, one of which, the pars compacta of the PPN (PPNc), consists predominantly of neurons utilizing a single neurotransmitter, ACh (these neurons are designated the Ch5 subgroup).[101] These neurons project to the thalamus, striatum, substantia nigra pars compacta, and subthalamic nucleus. By contrast, the pars dissipatus (PPNd) harbors a largely non-cholinergic neuronal population, and receives efferents from corticostriatal regions as well as from the subthalamic nucleus and substantia nigra pars reticularis. This pattern of reciprocal connectivity illustrates that the PPN is well situated to exert a putative modulating effect upon corticostriatal loops. Furthermore, the cholinergic output of the PPN forms ascending connections with the thalamus,[103] which have been shown in experimental systems to influence thalamic firing patterns[104] and thus may have a potential effect upon cognitive processes.

Loss of cholinergic neurons from the PPN in PD has been well described.[105, 106] Whilst there is some experimental evidence supporting a role for the PPN in locomotion, there is also emerging evidence that it may also play a role in cognition. PPN lesion studies in rodents suggest reaction times and performance of stereotypic behaviors are impaired along with interference with the operant response to learned rewards, a phenomenon which suggests involvement of the nucleus in reinforcement and learning.[107,108] This hypothesis is neuroanatomically plausible, as the PPN projects to midbrain dopaminergic neurons known to be involved in the formation of causal associations,[109] but whether this is functionally important in PDD is unclear. Therapeutic stimulation of the PPN has been attempted in non-demented PD with beneficial motor effects ostensibly without neuropsychological sequelae, at least in the short term.[110]

Pharmacological manipulation of the cholinergic system in PD with anti-cholinergic agents consistently exacerbates cognitive dysfunction, particularly in the elderly.[111] This effect is not seen in age-matched controls, implying that even in non-demented PD a subthreshold cholinergic deficit may already be in existence. In these experiments prominent deficits in memory retrieval have been observed, with performance on tests of attention and visuospatial ability unchanged.[111] Conversely, the beneficial effects of acetylcholinesterase inhibitors in patients with established PDD and DLB have been conclusively demonstrated.[112] Improvements in both cognitive function and psychiatric symptoms are described with performance in memory and attentional domains improving the most.[113]

Noradrenaline and PDD

The locus coeruleus (LC) contains the cell bodies of noradrenergic neurons which project widely throughout the cerebral cortex, diencephalon, and brainstem (Figure 11-2). The presence of Lewy bodies and loss of these noradrenergic neurons are pathologic features of idiopathic PD.[114] Neuronal loss is more extensive than that observed in AD, and the degree of cell loss has been shown to correlate with dementia risk in clinicopathological series.[115] This is associated as one would expect with reductions in the levels of noradrenaline in both the neocortex and the hippocampus of patients with PD,[116] and indeed the relative degree of LC neuron loss in PD is greater than that seen in the NBM for cholinergic neurons.[117]

Pharmacological antagonism of NA in non-demented PD has been shown to increase distractibility and impair performance on tests of attention.[118,119] Conversely, the administration of a selective NA agonist in a similar patient group improves attentional processing and set-shifting.[119] Levels of the noradrenaline metabolite MPHG in the CSF of non-demented patients with PD have been shown to correlate with improved performance on tests of attention and reaction time.[120] On the basis of such results it has been suggested that the physiological function of the noradrenergic system is to enhance the signal:noise ratio in frontal processing areas.[121] Disruption of this process in PDD might therefore heighten distractibility, contributing to the fluctuation of attention considered a hallmark of the Lewy body-associated dementias. However, given the close association of the noradrenergic system to depression it is difficult to know ultimately what underlies the basis of any cognitive changes.[122]

Serotonin and PDD

The raphe nuclei are a group of serotonergic (5 hydroxy-tryptophan; 5-HT) nuclei located medially in the brainstem and forming part of the reticular formation. Their arborizations are widespread throughout the brain with those situated in the midbrain and pons (i.e. the linear, dorsal and median raphe nuclei) projecting to the neocortex and striatum. The theory that dysfunction of serotonergic neurons might underlie clinically significant symptoms in PD, in particular non-motor symptoms, has generated much interest.[123] 5-HT deficiency has been heavily implicated in the neuropsychiatric and behavioral symptoms of PD,[124] and the possibility of a wider role in PD cognitive dysfunction is a theory which is gaining experimental support.

In PDD and DLB, Lewy bodies are seen in these raphe nuclei and both 5-HT levels and binding-sites are markedly reduced in the neocortex and throughout the striatum.[125–127] 5-HT metabolites are also reduced in the CSF in PD.[128] The extent of the deficit has been correlated with disease progression as evidenced by increasing Hoehn-Yahr stage, the implication being that this is likely to reflect degeneration of serotonergic neurons.[129] However, there is a considerable amount of heterogeneity in the pattern and extent of striatal 5-HT deficiency between patients, and some individuals have normal or near normal levels.[129] Similarly, the loss of serotonergic markers within the striatum is not uniform, with the caudate nucleus being affected to a greater extent than the putamen.[129] The caudate nucleus is believed to have a role in higher order cognitive processing (as opposed to the predominantly motor role of the putamen) through participation in cortico-subcortical association loops[130] and so the differential loss of the serotonergic input to the caudate nucleus might, therefore, contribute to the cognitive deficits seen in PDD.

Interactions between the neurochemistry of 5-HT and dopamine in the PD brain may, however, render such straightforward explanations inaccurate, as has become an issue of late in the genesis of levodopa-induced dyskinesias (LID) and graft-induced dyskinesias (GID). Exogenously administered dopamine appears to compete with 5-HT for striatal decarboxylase sites and may also displace endogenous 5-HT from its neuronal storage sites.[131] It follows that dopamine replacement therapy may be reducing the availability of striatal 5-HT independently of any losses occurring secondary to degeneration of serotonergic neurons as part of the intrinsic disease process. Thus, although the availability of 5-HT is clearly decreased in the PD brain, we must be circumspect in our interpretation of this and it should be reiterated that a correlation between serotonergic deficiency and cognitive dysfunction in PD has yet to be shown. Consistent with this, studies which have demonstrated the clinical efficacy of the 5-HT reuptake inhibitors (SSRIs) in the treatment of depression in PD do not report any coincident effects upon cognition.[132]

Glutamate and PDD

The role of glutamatergic dysfunction in PD cognitive dysfunction, and in PD in general, has been little studied. One study reported reduced expression of hippocampal glutamate receptors in DLB,[133] but others have found no change in glutamatergic markers.[134] From a clinical perspective amantadine, a glutamate antagonist, has been used in PD therapy for some years, principally for the amelioration of treatment-induced dyskinesias.[135] Amantadine not infrequently causes cognitive side-effects, particularly in the elderly, but as its pharmacological spectrum of action is wide (including antagonism at nicotinic ACh receptors) it is relatively unlikely that this is a direct effect of glutamatergic blockade. Furthermore, the more selective NMDA antagonist memantine is currently undergoing trials as a treatment for the cognitive impairment of PDD and DLB, based on its reported efficacy in AD.[136]

Conclusion

On the basis of the available evidence, dopamine deficiency alone is insufficient to account for the cognitive dysfunction seen in PD and PDD. Involvement of other neurotransmitter systems, including cholinergic and noradrenergic systems, and possibly serotonergic and glutamatergic, is likely to contribute to the development of the syndrome. Assessing the significance and relative contribution of each is difficult as for many of the brainstem nuclei implicated in the process the relationship between structure and function has yet to be established. Thus when dealing with distributed Lewy body pathology simultaneously involving numerous cortical and subcortical structures, it is difficult to know which of the observed lesions are relevant to the clinical presentation. In the case of PDD it has not yet even been possible to establish definitively whether cortico-limbic or subcortical involvement is most relevant. The balance of evidence would seem to suggest limbic and neocortical Lewy body pathology as the most likely substrate of dementia, probably synergizing with the effects of disease in other subcortical and brainstem areas. A role for tau and/or amyloid at some stage in this process would also appear plausible, but many questions remain unanswered. Furthermore, there is likely to be interaction between the neurotransmitter systems involved, both with each other and with dopamine, as suggested in the case of 5-HT. Any such putative interactions, which might be synergistic or antagonistic in nature, add a further layer of complexity to any pathophysiological model of PDD.

This seeming complexity should, perhaps, be anticipated given the clinical heterogeneity of PD and the neuropsychological heterogeneity of PDD. Some patterns do, however, emerge. The noradrenergic system appears to have a prominent role in mediating attentional processing, with cholinergic deficiencies probably impacting more upon memory functions. Alteration in dopamine levels more obviously results in impairment of executive function. Serotonergic dysfunction may have a direct role upon cognition in PD, but alternatively may exert an indirect effect, either neurochemically through modulating dopaminergic neurotransmission, or neuropsychiatrically by influencing mood and consequently attentional function. This model is illustrated in Figure 11-4.

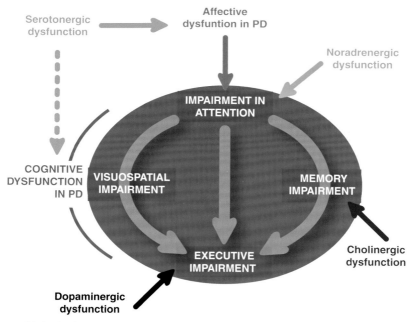

Figure 11-4. An integrated model of the contribution of different neurotransmitter systems to the cognitive dysfunction of PD. The core cognitive deficits in PD are represented in the central oval. As previously discussed, the operation of higher executive functions requires other lower domains to be intact. It is unclear if serotonergic dysfunction affects cognition directly or indirectly, either through influencing mood or through interactions with exogenously-delivered dopamine (not shown).

The pharmacological correction of these neurochemical imbalances offers an attractive therapeutic target. However, in vivo neuronal loss per se may prove less important than, for example, the necessary reorganization of subcortical circuits occurring as a consequence of neurodegeneration. The clinical effect of the anti-cholinesterase inhibitors, for example, is comparatively modest.[112] A better understanding of the pathophysiology of the dementing process in PDD may suggest new targets for treatment.

In summary, the existing evidence suggests not only that non-dopaminergic systems are involved in PDD, but that their involvement is at the core of the syndrome. Neuropathology at sites outside of the substantia nigra, including the neocortex and subcortical and limbic regions, are etiologically important. Whilst Lewy body-associated neurodegeneration appears to be the most likely pathogenic mechanism, an emerging role for tau is an area of considerable interest and one which, ultimately, may re-define our understanding of extra-nigral pathology in PD. Future studies combining detailed neuropsychological data with post-mortem information are needed to further our understanding of clinico-pathological correlations in PDD, improving our models of the condition and suggesting new, possibly individualized symptomatic treatments depending upon the pattern of cognitive deficits shown by a particular patient.

Acknowledgments
JE is supported by the Van Geest Foundation and holds a Raymond and Beverley Sackler studentship.

References

1. Schrag A, Hovris A, Morley d, Quinn N, Jahanshahi M. Caregiver-burden in Parkinson'd isease is closely associated with pschiatric symptoms, falls and disability. *Parkinsinism Relat Disord*. Jan 2006;12(1):35–41.
2. Brundin P, Li JY, Holton JL, Lindvall O, Revesz T. Research in motion: the enigma of Parkinson's disease pathology spread. *Nat Rev Neurosci*. Oct 2008;9(10):741–745.
3. Braak H, Del Tredici K, Rub U, de Vos RA, Jansen Steur EN, Braak E. Staging of brain pathology related to sporadic Parkinson's disease. *Neurobiol Aging*. Mar-Apr 2003;24(2):197–211.
4. Aarsland, D., K., Andersen, et al. (2001). " K, Larsen JP, Lolk A, Nielsen H, Kragh-Sorensen P. Risk of dementia in Parkinson's disease: a community-based, prospective study." *Neurology*. Mar 27 2001;56(6): 730–736.
5. Hobson P, Gallacher J, Meara J. Cross-sectional survey of Parkinson's disease and parkinsonism in a rural area of the United Kingdom. *Mov Disord*. Aug 2005;20(8): 995–998.

6. Marder K, Tang MX, Cote L, Stern Y, Mayeux R. The frequency and associated risk factors for dementia in patients with Parkinson's disease. *Arch Neurol.* Jul 1995;52(7):695–701.

7. Hely MA, Reid WG, Adena MA, Halliday GM, Morris JG. The Sydney multicenter study of Parkinson's disease: the inevitability of dementia at 20 years. *Mov Disord.* Apr 30 2008;23(6):837–844.

8. Foltynie T, Brayne CE, Robbins TW, Barker RA. The cognitive ability of an incident cohort of Parkinson's patients in the UK. The CamPaIGN study. *Brain.* Mar 2004;127(Pt 3):550–560.

9. Williams-Gray CH, Foltynie T, Brayne CE, Robbins TW, Barker RA. Evolution of cognitive dysfunction in an incident Parkinson's disease cohort. *Brain.* Jul 2007;130 (Pt 7):1787–1798.

10. Richard IH, Papka M, Rubio A, Kurlan R. Parkinson's disease and dementia with Lewy bodies: one disease or two? *Mov Disord.* Nov 2002;17(6):1161–1165.

11. Ballard C, Ziabreva I, Perry R, et al. Differences in neuropathologic characteristics across the Lewy body dementia spectrum. *Neurology.* Dec 12 2006;67(11): 1931–1934.

12. Polymeropoulos MH, Lavedan C, Leroy E, et al. Mutation in the alpha-synuclein gene identified in families with Parkinson's disease. *Science.* Jun 27 1997;276(5321):2045–2047.

13. Zarranz JJ, Alegre J, Gomez-Esteban JC, et al. The new mutation, E46K, of alpha-synuclein causes Parkinson and Lewy body dementia. *Ann Neurol.* Feb 2004;55(2): 164–173.

14. Emre M, Aarsland D, Brown R, et al. Clinical diagnostic criteria for dementia associated with Parkinson's disease. *Mov Disord.* Sep 15 2007;22(12):1689–1707; quiz 1837.

15. Aarsland D, Litvan I, Salmon D, Galasko D, Wentzel-Larsen T, Larsen JP. Performance on the dementia rating scale in Parkinson's disease with dementia and dementia with Lewy bodies: comparison with progressive supranuclear palsy and Alzheimer's disease. *J Neurol Neurosurg Psychiatry.* Sep 2003;74(9):1215–1220.

16. Litvan I, Mohr E, Williams J, Gomez C, Chase TN. Differential memory and executive functions in demented patients with Parkinson's and Alzheimer's disease. *J Neurol Neurosurg Psychiatry.* Jan 1991;54(1):25–29.

17. Cahn-Weiner DA, Grace J, Ott BR, Fernandez HH, Friedman JH. Cognitive and behavioral features discriminate between Alzheimer's and Parkinson's disease. *Neuropsychiatry Neuropsychol Behav Neurol.* Jun 2002;15(2):79–87.

18. McKeith IG, Dickson DW, Lowe J, et al. Diagnosis and management of dementia with Lewy bodies: third report of the DLB Consortium. *Neurology.* Dec 27 2005;65(12):1863–1872.

19. Ballard CG, Aarsland D, McKeith I, et al. Fluctuations in attention: PD dementia vs DLB with parkinsonism. *Neurology.* Dec 10 2002;59(11):1714–1720.

20. Noe E, Marder K, Bell KL, Jacobs DM, Manly JJ, Stern Y. Comparison of dementia with Lewy bodies to Alzheimer's disease and Parkinson's disease with dementia. *Mov Disord.* Jan 2004;19(1):60–67.

21. Pillon B, Boller F, Levy R, Dubois B. Cognitive deficits and dementia in Parkinson's disease. In: Boller F, Cappa S, eds. *Handbook of Neuropsychology*. 2nd ed. Amsterdam: Elsevier; 2001:311–371.

22. Higginson CI, Wheelock VL, Carroll KE, Sigvardt KA. Recognition memory in Parkinson's disease with and without dementia: evidence inconsistent with the retrieval deficit hypothesis. *J Clin Exp Neuropsychol*. May 2005;27(4):516–528.

23. Cummings JL, Darkins A, Mendez M, Hill MA, Benson DF. Alzheimer's disease and Parkinson's disease: comparison of speech and language alterations. *Neurology*. May 1988;38(5):680–684.

24. Cahn-Weiner DA, Williams K, Grace J, Tremont G, Westervelt H, Stern RA. Discrimination of dementia with lewy bodies from Alzheimer disease and Parkinson disease using the clock drawing test. *Cogn Behav Neurol*. Jun 2003;16(2):85–92.

25. Mosimann UP, Mather G, Wesnes KA, O'Brien JT, Burn DJ, McKeith IG. Visual perception in Parkinson disease dementia and dementia with Lewy bodies. *Neurology*. Dec 14 2004;63(11):2091–2096.

26. Janvin CC, Larsen JP, Salmon DP, Galasko D, Hugdahl K, Aarsland D. Cognitive profiles of individual patients with Parkinson's disease and dementia: comparison with dementia with lewy bodies and Alzheimer's disease. *Mov Disord*. Mar 2006;21(3): 337–342.

27. Dubois B, Pillon B. Cognitive deficits in Parkinson's disease. *J Neurol*. Jan 1997;244(1):2–8.

28. Obeso JA, Rodriguez-Oroz MC, Benitez-Temino B, et al. Functional organization of the basal ganglia: therapeutic implications for Parkinson's disease. *Mov Disord*. 2008;23 Suppl 3:S548–559.

29. Lewis SJ, Foltynie T, Blackwell AD, Robbins TW, Owen AM, Barker RA. Heterogeneity of Parkinson's disease in the early clinical stages using a data driven approach. *J Neurol Neurosurg Psychiatry*. Mar 2005;76(3):343–348.

30. Levy G, Tang MX, Cote LJ, et al. Motor impairment in PD: relationship to incident dementia and age. *Neurology*. Aug 22 2000;55(4):539–544.

31. Aarsland D, Andersen K, Larsen JP, Lolk A, Kragh-Sorensen P. Prevalence and characteristics of dementia in Parkinson disease: an 8-year prospective study. *Arch Neurol*. Mar 2003;60(3):387–392.

32. Zetusky WJ, Jankovic J, Pirozzolo FJ. The heterogeneity of Parkinson's disease: clinical and prognostic implications. *Neurology*. Apr 1985;35(4):522–526.

33. Burn DJ, Rowan EN, Allan LM, Molloy S, O'Brien JT, McKeith IG. Motor subtype and cognitive decline in Parkinson's disease, Parkinson's disease with dementia, and dementia with Lewy bodies. *J Neurol Neurosurg Psychiatry*. May 2006;77(5): 585–589.

34. Burn DJ, Rowan EN, Minett T, et al. Extrapyramidal features in Parkinson's disease with and without dementia and dementia with Lewy bodies: A cross-sectional comparative study. *Mov Disord*. Aug 2003;18(8):884–889.

35. Francis PT, Palmer AM, Snape M, Wilcock GK. The cholinergic hypothesis of Alzheimer's disease: a review of progress. *J Neurol Neurosurg Psychiatry*. Feb 1999; 66(2):137–147.

36. Francis PT. Glutamatergic systems in Alzheimer's disease. *Int J Geriatr Psychiatry*. Sep 2003;18(Suppl 1):S15–21.

37. Aarsland D, Ballard CG, Halliday G. Are Parkinson's disease with dementia and dementia with Lewy bodies the same entity? *J Geriatr Psychiatry Neurol.* Sep 2004;17(3):137–145.
38. Double KL, Halliday GM, McRitchie DA, Reid WG, Hely MA, Morris JG. Regional brain atrophy in idiopathic Parkinson's disease and diffuse Lewy body disease. *Dementia.* Nov-Dec 1996;7(6):304–313.
39. Cordato NJ, Halliday GM, Harding AJ, Hely MA, Morris JG. Regional brain atrophy in progressive supranuclear palsy and Lewy body disease. *Ann Neurol.* Jun 2000;47(6):718–728.
40. Ince PG, Clark B, Holton JL, Revesz T, Wharton S. Disorders of movement and system degenerations. In: Ellison DW, Louis DN, Love S, eds. *Greenfield's Neuropathology.* Vol 1. London: Arnold; 2008:889–1030.
41. Halliday G, Hely M, Reid W, Morris J. The progression of pathology in longitudinally followed patients with Parkinson's disease. *Acta Neuropathol.* Apr 2008;115(4): 409–415.
42. Parkkinen L, Kauppinen T, Pirttila T, Autere JM, Alafuzoff I. Alpha-synuclein pathology does not predict extrapyramidal symptoms or dementia. *Ann Neurol.* Jan 2005;57(1):82–91.
43. Parkkinen L, Pirttila T, Alafuzoff I. Applicability of current staging/categorization of alpha-synuclein pathology and their clinical relevance. *Acta Neuropathol.* Apr 2008;115(4):399–407.
44. Kalaitzakis ME, Graeber MB, Gentleman SM, Pearce RK. The dorsal motor nucleus of the vagus is not an obligatory trigger site of Parkinson's disease: a critical analysis of alpha-synuclein staging. *Neuropathol Appl Neurobiol.* Jun 2008;34(3): 284–295.
45. Jellinger KA. A critical evaluation of current staging of alpha-synuclein pathology in Lewy body disorders. *Biochim Biophys Acta.* Aug 5 2008.
46. Tsuboi Y, Dickson DW. Dementia with Lewy bodies and Parkinson's disease with dementia: are they different? *Parkinsonism Relat Disord.* Jun 2005;11 Suppl 1:S47–51.
47. Harding AJ, Halliday GM. Cortical Lewy body pathology in the diagnosis of dementia. *Acta Neuropathol.* Oct 2001;102(4):355–363.
48. Harding AJ, Broe GA, Halliday GM. Visual hallucinations in Lewy body disease relate to Lewy bodies in the temporal lobe. *Brain.* Feb 2002;125(Pt 2):391–403.
49. Apaydin H, Ahlskog JE, Parisi JE, Boeve BF, Dickson DW. Parkinson disease neuropathology: later-developing dementia and loss of the levodopa response. *Arch Neurol.* Jan 2002;59(1):102–112.
50. Hurtig HI, Trojanowski JQ, Galvin J, et al. Alpha-synuclein cortical Lewy bodies correlate with dementia in Parkinson's disease. *Neurology.* May 23 2000;54(10): 1916–1921.
51. Aarsland D, Perry R, Brown A, Larsen JP, Ballard C. Neuropathology of dementia in Parkinson's disease: a prospective, community-based study. *Ann Neurol.* Nov 2005;58(5):773–776.
52. Mattila PM, Roytta M, Torikka H, Dickson DW, Rinne JO. Cortical Lewy bodies and Alzheimer-type changes in patients with Parkinson's disease. *Acta Neuropathol.* Jun 1998;95(6):576–582.

53. Schneider JA, Arvanitakis Z, Bang W, Bennett DA. Mixed brain pathologies account for most dementia cases in community-dwelling older persons. *Neurology*. Dec 11 2007;69(24):2197–2204.

54. Fujishiro H, Ferman TJ, Boeve BF, et al. Validation of the neuropathologic criteria of the third consortium for dementia with Lewy bodies for prospectively diagnosed cases. *J Neuropathol Exp Neurol*. Jul 2008;67(7):649–656.

55. Braak H, Rub U, Jansen Steur EN, Del Tredici K, de Vos RA. Cognitive status correlates with neuropathologic stage in Parkinson disease. *Neurology*. Apr 26 2005;64(8):1404–1410.

56. Colosimo C, Hughes AJ, Kilford L, Lees AJ. Lewy body cortical involvement may not always predict dementia in Parkinson's disease. *J Neurol Neurosurg Psychiatry*. Jul 2003;74(7):852–856.

57. Hyman BT, Trojanowski JQ. Consensus recommendations for the postmortem diagnosis of Alzheimer disease from the National Institute on Aging and the Reagan Institute Working Group on diagnostic criteria for the neuropathological assessment of Alzheimer disease. *J Neuropathol Exp Neurol*. Oct 1997;56(10):1095–1097.

58. Jellinger KA, Attems J. Prevalence and impact of vascular and Alzheimer pathologies in Lewy body disease. *Acta Neuropathol*. Apr 2008;115(4):427–436.

59. Kraybill ML, Larson EB, Tsuang DW, et al. Cognitive differences in dementia patients with autopsy-verified AD, Lewy body pathology, or both. *Neurology*. Jun 28 2005;64(12):2069–2073.

60. Mattila PM, Rinne JO, Helenius H, Dickson DW, Roytta M. Alpha-synuclein-immunoreactive cortical Lewy bodies are associated with cognitive impairment in Parkinson's disease. *Acta Neuropathol*. Sep 2000;100(3):285–290.

61. Pletnikova O, West N, Lee MK, et al. Abeta deposition is associated with enhanced cortical alpha-synuclein lesions in Lewy body diseases. *Neurobiol Aging*. Aug-Sep 2005;26(8):1183–1192.

62. Masliah E, Rockenstein E, Veinbergs I, et al. beta-amyloid peptides enhance alpha-synuclein accumulation and neuronal deficits in a transgenic mouse model linking Alzheimer's disease and Parkinson's disease. *Proc Natl Acad Sci U S A*. Oct 9 2001;98(21):12245–12250.

63. Lashley T, Holton JL, Gray E, et al. Cortical alpha-synuclein load is associated with amyloid-beta plaque burden in a subset of Parkinson's disease patients. *Acta Neuropathol*. Apr 2008;115(4):417–425.

64. Kalaitzakis ME, Graeber MB, Gentleman SM, Pearce RK. Striatal beta-amyloid deposition in Parkinson disease with dementia. *J Neuropathol Exp Neurol*. Feb 2008;67(2):155–161.

65. Jellinger KA. Striatal beta-amyloid deposition in Parkinson disease with dementia. *J Neuropathol Exp Neurol*. May 2008;67(5):484; author reply 484–485.

66. Goris A, Williams-Gray CH, Clark GR, et al. Tau and alpha-synuclein in susceptibility to, and dementia in, Parkinson's disease. *Ann Neurol*. Aug 2007;62(2):145–153.

67. Baker M, Litvan I, Houlden H, et al. Association of an extended haplotype in the tau gene with progressive supranuclear palsy. *Hum Mol Genet*. Apr 1999;8(4):711–715.

68. Houlden H, Baker M, Morris HR, et al. Corticobasal degeneration and progressive supranuclear palsy share a common tau haplotype. *Neurology*. Jun 26 2001;56(12):1702–1706.

69. Giasson BI, Lee VM, Trojanowski JQ. Interactions of amyloidogenic proteins. *Neuromolecular Med.* 2003;4(1-2):49–58.

70. Williams-Gray CH, Evans JR, Goris A, et al. The distinct cognitive syndromes of Parkinson's disease: 5 year follow-up of the CamPaIGN cohort. *Brain.* Nov 2009;132(11):2958–69

71. Cummings JL. Frontal-subcortical circuits and human behavior. *Arch Neurol.* Aug 1993;50(8):873–880.

72. Owen AM, Doyon J, Dagher A, Sadikot A, Evans AC. Abnormal basal ganglia outflow in Parkinson's disease identified with PET. Implications for higher cortical functions. *Brain.* May 1998;121 (Pt 5):949–965.

73. Lewis SJ, Dove A, Robbins TW, Barker RA, Owen AM. Striatal contributions to working memory: a functional magnetic resonance imaging study in humans. *Eur J Neurosci.* Feb 2004;19(3):755–760.

74. Williams-Gray CH, Hampshire A, Robbins TW, Owen AM, Barker RA. Catechol O-methyltransferase Val158Met genotype influences frontoparietal activity during planning in patients with Parkinson's disease. *J Neurosci.* May 2 2007;27(18): 4832–4838.

75. Cools R, Barker RA, Sahakian BJ, Robbins TW. Enhanced or impaired cognitive function in Parkinson's disease as a function of dopaminergic medication and task demands. *Cereb Cortex.* Dec 2001;11(12):1136–1143.

76. Lewis SJ, Dove A, Robbins TW, Barker RA, Owen AM. Cognitive impairments in early Parkinson's disease are accompanied by reductions in activity in frontostriatal neural circuitry. *J Neurosci.* Jul 16 2003;23(15):6351–6356.

77. Foltynie T, Goldberg TE, Lewis SG, et al. Planning ability in Parkinson's disease is influenced by the COMT val158met polymorphism. *Mov Disord.* Aug 2004;19(8):885–891.

78. Stern Y, Tetrud JW, Martin WR, Kutner SJ, Langston JW. Cognitive change following MPTP exposure. *Neurology.* Feb 1990;40(2):261–264.

79. Everitt BJ, Robbins TW. Central cholinergic systems and cognition. *Annu Rev Psychol.* 1997;48:649–684.

80. Francis PT, Perry EK. Cholinergic and other neurotransmitter mechanisms in Parkinson's disease, Parkinson's disease dementia, and dementia with Lewy bodies. *Mov Disord.* Aug 13 2007;22(S17):S351-S357.

81. Perry EK, Marshall E, Kerwin J, et al. Evidence of a monoaminergic-cholinergic imbalance related to visual hallucinations in Lewy body dementia. *J Neurochem.* Oct 1990;55(4):1454–1456.

82. Perry EK, Marshall E, Perry RH, et al. Cholinergic and dopaminergic activities in senile dementia of Lewy body type. *Alzheimer Dis Assoc Disord.* Summer 1990;4(2): 87–95.

83. Tiraboschi P, Hansen LA, Alford M, et al. Cholinergic dysfunction in diseases with Lewy bodies. *Neurology.* Jan 25 2000;54(2):407–411.

84. Tiraboschi P, Hansen LA, Alford M, et al. Early and widespread cholinergic losses differentiate dementia with Lewy bodies from Alzheimer disease. *Arch Gen Psychiatry.* Oct 2002;59(10):946–951.

85. Piggott MA, Owens J, O'Brien J, et al. Muscarinic receptors in basal ganglia in dementia with Lewy bodies, Parkinson's disease and Alzheimer's disease. *J Chem Neuroanat.* Mar 2003;25(3):161–173.

86. Perry EK, Morris CM, Court JA, et al. Alteration in nicotine binding sites in Parkinson's disease, Lewy body dementia and Alzheimer's disease: possible index of early neuropathology. *Neuroscience.* Jan 1995;64(2):385–395.

87. Martin-Ruiz C, Court J, Lee M, et al. Nicotinic receptors in dementia of Alzheimer, Lewy body and vascular types. *Acta Neurol Scand Suppl.* 2000;176:34–41.

88. Rei RT, Sabbagh MN, Corey-Bloom J, Tiraboschi P, Thal LJ. Nicotinic receptor losses in dementia with Lewy bodies: comparisons with Alzheimer's disease. *Neurobiol Aging.* Sep-Oct 2000;21(5):741–746.

89. Ballard C, Piggott M, Johnson M, et al. Delusions associated with elevated muscarinic binding in dementia with Lewy bodies. *Ann Neurol.* Dec 2000;48(6):868–876.

90. Shiozaki K, Iseki E, Hino H, Kosaka K. Distribution of m1 muscarinic acetylcholine receptors in the hippocampus of patients with Alzheimer's disease and dementia with Lewy bodies-an immunohistochemical study. *J Neurol Sci.* Dec 15 2001;193(1):23–28.

91. Shiozaki K, Iseki E, Uchiyama H, et al. Alterations of muscarinic acetylcholine receptor subtypes in diffuse Lewy body disease: relation to Alzheimer's disease. *J Neurol Neurosurg Psychiatry.* Aug 1999;67(2):209–213.

92. Rinne JO, Myllykyla T, Lonnberg P, Marjamaki P. A postmortem study of brain nicotinic receptors in Parkinson's and Alzheimer's disease. *Brain Res.* Apr 26 1991;547(1): 167–170.

93. Perry EK, Curtis M, Dick DJ, et al. Cholinergic correlates of cognitive impairment in Parkinson's disease: comparisons with Alzheimer's disease. *J Neurol Neurosurg Psychiatry.* May 1985;48(5):413–421.

94. Bohnen NI, Kaufer DI, Hendrickson R, et al. Cognitive correlates of cortical cholinergic denervation in Parkinson's disease and parkinsonian dementia. *J Neurol.* Feb 2006;253(2):242–247.

95. Ziabreva I, Ballard CG, Aarsland D, et al. Lewy body disease: thalamic cholinergic activity related to dementia and parkinsonism. *Neurobiol Aging.* Mar 2006;27(3): 433–438.

96. Whitehouse PJ, Price DL, Clark AW, Coyle JT, DeLong MR. Alzheimer disease: evidence for selective loss of cholinergic neurons in the nucleus basalis. *Ann Neurol.* Aug 1981;10(2):122–126.

97. Nakano I, Hirano A. Parkinson's disease: neuron loss in the nucleus basalis without concomitant Alzheimer's disease. *Ann Neurol.* May 1984;15(5):415–418.

98. Dubois B, Ruberg M, Javoy-Agid F, Ploska A, Agid Y. A subcortico-cortical cholinergic system is affected in Parkinson's disease. *Brain Res.* Dec 12 1983;288(1-2): 213–218.

99. Perry RH, Perry EK, Smith CJ, et al. Cortical neuropathological and neurochemical substrates of Alzheimer's and Parkinson's diseases. *J Neural Transm Suppl.* 1987;24: 131–136.

100. Pahapill PA, Lozano AM. The pedunculopontine nucleus and Parkinson's disease. *Brain.* Sep 2000;123 (Pt 9):1767–1783.

101. Mesulam MM, Geula C, Bothwell MA, Hersh LB. Human reticular formation: cholinergic neurons of the pedunculopontine and laterodorsal tegmental nuclei and some cytochemical comparisons to forebrain cholinergic neurons. *J Comp Neurol.* May 22 1989;283(4):611–633.

102. Winn P. How best to consider the structure and function of the pedunculopontine tegmental nucleus: evidence from animal studies. *J Neurol Sci.* Oct 25 2006;248 (1-2):234–250.

103. Usunoff KG, Kharazia VN, Valtschanoff JG, Schmidt HH, Weinberg RJ. Nitric oxide synthase-containing projections to the ventrobasal thalamus in the rat. *Anat Embryol (Berl).* Sep 1999;200(3):265–281.

104. McCormick DA, Prince DA. Acetylcholine induces burst firing in thalamic reticular neurones by activating a potassium conductance. *Nature.* Jan 30-Feb 5 1986; 319(6052):402–405.

105. Jellinger K. The pedunculopontine nucleus in Parkinson's disease, progressive supranuclear palsy and Alzheimer's disease. *J Neurol Neurosurg Psychiatry.* Apr 1988;51(4):540–543.

106. Hirsch EC, Graybiel AM, Duyckaerts C, Javoy-Agid F. Neuronal loss in the pedunculopontine tegmental nucleus in Parkinson disease and in progressive supranuclear palsy. *Proc Natl Acad Sci U S A.* Aug 1987;84(16):5976–5980.

107. Alderson HL, Brown VJ, Latimer MP, Brasted PJ, Robertson AH, Winn P. The effect of excitotoxic lesions of the pedunculopontine tegmental nucleus on performance of a progressive ratio schedule of reinforcement. *Neuroscience.* 2002;112(2): 417–425.

108. Alderson HL, Latimer MP, Blaha CD, Phillips AG, Winn P. An examination of d-amphetamine self-administration in pedunculopontine tegmental nucleus-lesioned rats. *Neuroscience.* 2004;125(2):349–358.

109. Fiorillo CD, Tobler PN, Schultz W. Discrete coding of reward probability and uncertainty by dopamine neurons. *Science.* Mar 21 2003;299(5614):1898–1902.

110. Stefani A, Lozano AM, Peppe A, et al. Bilateral deep brain stimulation of the pedunculopontine and subthalamic nuclei in severe Parkinson's disease. *Brain.* Jun 2007;130(Pt 6):1596–1607.

111. Bedard MA, Pillon B, Dubois B, Duchesne N, Masson H, Agid Y. Acute and long-term administration of anticholinergics in Parkinson's disease: specific effects on the subcortico-frontal syndrome. *Brain Cogn.* Jul 1999;40(2):289–313.

112. Emre M, Aarsland D, Albanese A, et al. Rivastigmine for dementia associated with Parkinson's disease. *N Engl J Med.* Dec 9 2004;351(24):2509–2518.

113. Poewe W, Wolters E, Emre M, et al. Long-term benefits of rivastigmine in dementia associated with Parkinson's disease: an active treatment extension study. *Mov Disord.* Apr 2006;21(4):456–461.

114. Gaspar P, Gray F. Dementia in idiopathic Parkinson's disease. A neuropathological study of 32 cases. *Acta Neuropathol.* 1984;64(1):43–52.

115. Zweig RM, Cardillo JE, Cohen M, Giere S, Hedreen JC. The locus ceruleus and dementia in Parkinson's disease. *Neurology.* May 1993;43(5):986–991.

116. Scatton B, Javoy-Agid F, Rouquier L, Dubois B, Agid Y. Reduction of cortical dopamine, noradrenaline, serotonin and their metabolites in Parkinson's disease. *Brain Res.* Sep 26 1983;275(2):321–328.

117. Zarow C, Lyness SA, Mortimer JA, Chui HC. Neuronal loss is greater in the locus coeruleus than nucleus basalis and substantia nigra in Alzheimer and Parkinson diseases. *Arch Neurol.* Mar 2003;60(3):337–341.

118. Sharpe MH. Auditory attention in early Parkinson's disease: an impairment in focused attention. *Neuropsychologia*. Jan 1992;30(1):101–106.
119. Bedard MA, el Massioui F, Malapani C, et al. Attentional deficits in Parkinson's disease: partial reversibility with naphtoxazine (SDZ NVI-085), a selective noradrenergic alpha 1 agonist. *Clin Neuropharmacol*. Mar-Apr 1998;21(2):108–117.
120. Cash R, Dennis T, L'Heureux R, Raisman R, Javoy-Agid F, Scatton B. Parkinson's disease and dementia: norepinephrine and dopamine in locus ceruleus. *Neurology*. Jan 1987;37(1):42–46.
121. Everitt BJ, Robbins TW, Selden SRW. Functions of the locus coeruleus noradrenergic system: a neurobiological and behavioural synthesis. In: Heal DJ, Marsden CD, eds. *The Pharmacology of Noradrenaline in the Central Nervous System*. New York: Oxford University Press; 1990:349–378.
122. Nutt DJ. Relationship of neurotransmitters to the symptoms of major depressive disorder. *J Clin Psychiatry*. 2008;69 Suppl E1:4–7.
123. Kish SJ. Biochemistry of Parkinson's disease: is a brain serotonergic deficiency a characteristic of idiopathic Parkinson's disease? *Adv Neurol*. 2003;91:39–49.
124. Lemke MR. Depressive symptoms in Parkinson's disease. *Eur J Neurol*. Apr 2008;15 Suppl 1:21–25.
125. Chinaglia G, Landwehrmeyer B, Probst A, Palacios JM. Serotoninergic terminal transporters are differentially affected in Parkinson's disease and progressive supranuclear palsy: an autoradiographic study with [3H]citalopram. *Neuroscience*. Jun 1993;54(3):691–699.
126. Halliday GM, Blumbergs PC, Cotton RG, Blessing WW, Geffen LB. Loss of brainstem serotonin- and substance P-containing neurons in Parkinson's disease. *Brain Res*. Feb 26 1990;510(1):104–107.
127. Ballard C, Johnson M, Piggott M, et al. A positive association between 5HT reuptake binding sites and depression in dementia with Lewy bodies. *J Affect Disord*. May 2002;69(1-3):219–223.
128. Mayeux R, Stern Y, Sano M, Williams JB, Cote LJ. The relationship of serotonin to depression in Parkinson's disease. *Mov Disord*. 1988;3(3):237–244.
129. Kish SJ, Tong J, Hornykiewicz O, et al. Preferential loss of serotonin markers in caudate versus putamen in Parkinson's disease. *Brain*. Jan 2008;131(Pt 1):120–131.
130. Alexander GE, DeLong MR, Strick PL. Parallel organization of functionally segregated circuits linking basal ganglia and cortex. *Annu Rev Neurosci*. 1986;9:357–381.
131. Carta M, Carlsson T, Kirik D, Bjorklund A. Dopamine released from 5-HT terminals is the cause of L-DOPA-induced dyskinesia in parkinsonian rats. *Brain*. Jul 2007;130(Pt 7):1819–1833.
132. Lemke MR, Fuchs G, Gemende I, et al. Depression and Parkinson's disease. *J Neurol*. Sep 2004;251 Suppl 6:VI/24–27.
133. Thorns V, Mallory M, Hansen L, Masliah E. Alterations in glutamate receptor 2/3 subunits and amyloid precursor protein expression during the course of Alzheimer's disease and Lewy body variant. *Acta Neuropathol*. Dec 1997;94(6):539–548.
134. Scott HL, Pow DV, Tannenberg AE, Dodd PR. Aberrant expression of the glutamate transporter excitatory amino acid transporter 1 (EAAT1) in Alzheimer's disease. *J Neurosci*. Feb 1 2002;22(3):RC206.

135. Danysz W, Parsons CG, Kornhuber J, Schmidt WJ, Quack G. Aminoadamantanes as NMDA receptor antagonists and antiparkinsonian agents–preclinical studies. *Neurosci Biobehav Rev.* Jul 1997;21(4):455–468.
136. Reisberg B, Doody R, Stoffler A, Schmitt F, Ferris S, Mobius HJ. Memantine in moderate-to-severe Alzheimer's disease. *N Engl J Med.* Apr 3 2003;348(14): 1333–1341.

Chapter 12

Systemic Manifestations of Parkinson's Disease

Dominic B. Rowe

Introduction

Parkinson's disease (PD) is a systemic disease with involvement of the central and peripheral nervous system, with effects on many organ systems. Although abnormalities of dopaminergic transmission are responsible for many of the major motor abnormalities in PD, many other non-dopaminergic aspects of neurotransmission are involved. This chapter attempts to summarize the literature of some of the other aspects of PD that are not already covered. Of necessity, the chapter will attempt to highlight some of the interesting observations of the systemic manifestations of PD. Because of the wide scope of this chapter, the references are eclectic rather than comprehensive.

This chapter begins with a discussion on the considerable literature on changes in the immune system in PD, as well as infection and cancer in PD, either as a consequence or a manifestation of PD. The respiratory system is affected in PD, which is commonly a source of symptoms in patients with advanced PD. In addition, dopamine replacement therapies can sometimes produce respiratory disturbances, either via direct toxicity or as a manifestation of motor fluctuation. Although Chapter 5 dealt in detail with the disturbances that occur in the gastrointestinal tract in PD patients, it is worth considering the effect of PD on nitrogen balance, weight loss, and overall nutrition. The largest organ of the human body, the skin, is also involved in PD, and this will be reviewed. Finally, the ocular manifestations of PD will be discussed.

The Immune System, Infections and Parkinson's Disease

For many years, researchers have failed to identify the events that precipitate and propagate the relentless neuronal destruction that occurs in sporadic PD. Apart from the relatively small percentage of patients with monogenic forms of PD, no mechanisms have been proven in sporadic PD. Because of the history of post-encephalitic parkinsonism, it was plausible to study possible infectious and immunological mechanisms in sporadic PD. As a result, multiple changes have been identified in the immune systems of PD patients, by many different investigators. Numerous studies have documented changes in lymphocyte, monocyte, natural killer cell, and cytokine levels in blood, cerebrospinal fluid, and CNS tissue from patients with PD (Table 12-1).[1] In general, there is a T-lymphocyte reduction in PD, with activation of some lymphocyte populations towards a T_H1-type immune response. Some studies have identified an increase in T_{REG} lymphocyte populations (CD4+CD25+),[2] and others an increase of gamma delta+ T-cells.[3] Some of these changes occur prior to the commencement of dopamine replacement therapy. What is still not known is whether these changes are part of the pathogenesis of PD, or whether they represent changes that occur in the immune system as a result of PD.[1]

It does not appear that auto-immune disease is more prevalent in PD subjects.[34] A recent large population-based case control study from Denmark of 13,695 patients with PD could not demonstrate any association between autoimmune disease and the subsequent risk of developing PD (odds ratio 0.96; 95% confidence interval 0.85-1.08). Intriguingly, in a subgroup of patients with rheumatoid arthritis, there was a decrease in risk for PD of 30%.[34] This might be due to an under-diagnosis of PD in patients with this inflammatory arthropathy, or might be a real protective effect.

Despite multiple studies over decades, there are no data thus far to support the hypothesis that PD is triggered by any specific infection, whether bacterial, viral or from any other organism.

Cancer and PD

There is substantial evidence based from epidemiologic studies for atypical cancer rates in patients with PD.[35] There is a risk reduction for

Table 12-1. Immune and Inflammatory Changes in Parkinson Disease

Central Nervous System

Microglial Proliferation and Activation[4-8]
β2 microglobulin elevation[9]
Complement activated oligodendroglia[10]
Lymphocyte infiltration[6,8]
Lewy Body immunohistochemistry
   Complement deposition[10]
   Other relevant molecules[11]
Cytokine and growth factor elevation
   Tumour Necrosis Factor-α[12,13]
   Interferon-γ[5]
   Interleukin-1β[14]
   Interleukin-6[14]
Apoptosis markers[15-18]
Immunoglobulin deposition[8]

Blood and Cerebrospinal Fluid

$\gamma\delta$ lymphocytes[3]
Lymphocyte - population changes[2,19]
Lymphocyte - impaired responses[20-22]
Monocyte activation[23]
Natural Killer cell - impaired function[24]
Neutrophil - impaired phagocytosis[25]
Immunoglobulin - level changes[26]
Immunoglobulin - impaired production[20]
Circulating Antibodies to dopaminergic tissue[27-31]
Elevated CSF cytokines and growth factors[14,32,33]

malignancy that cannot be attributed to the recognized low life-long incidence of smoking in patients with PD, as not only smoking-related cancers but also non-smoking-related ones are less common in PD. Whereas the risk for most cancers appears to be relatively low in patients with PD, breast cancer, melanomas, and non-melanotic skin cancer occur more frequently in the PD population as compared with controls.[36] The relationship between this peculiar pattern of cancer rates and PD might be related to the involvement of common genes in both diseases, but at present the mechanisms involved in this phenomenon are unknown.

Hoehn and Yahr were among the first to report the reduced mortality from cancer in PD.[37] Most of the studies of cancer in PD are case-control studies that assess the incidence of cancer after the diagnosis of PD.

However, there are 4 studies that determined the frequency of cancer prior to the onset of PD.[38–41] The first study of 59 PD patients from the Mayo Clinic identified an overall lower frequency of cancer in PD patients than controls (19.4% v 23.5%).[39] A larger study of 222 PD patients from Italy confirmed the inverse association between cancer and PD.[41] The frequency of cancer was 6.8% for PD cases, 12.6% for controls. Patients with PD had an overall decreased risk for neoplasms (adjusted OR, 0.4; 95% confidence interval [CI], 0.2-0.7). Interestingly, the risk was reduced only for women (adjusted OR, 0.3; 95% CI, 0.1-0.7), even though breast cancer was twice as common among PD cases as in controls. A large study in Denmark of 8090 PD patients showed a two-fold higher incidence of malignant melanoma in patients with PD than in the general population.[38] This study showed increased prevalence of malignant melanoma (OR 1.44; 95% CI, 1.03-2.01) and skin carcinoma (OR 1.26; 95% CI, 1.11-1.43) prior to the first hospital contact for PD. It also demonstrated a reduced prevalence of cancers at smoking-related sites in patients before their first hospital contact for PD. Lastly, in a very large study using a matched cohort analysis of the 22,071 males in the Physician's Health Study, a total of 487 incident cases of PD without preceding cancer were identified, and matched to appropriate controls.[42] Those with PD developed less cancer (11.0% versus 14.0%), with a reduced adjusted relative risk (RR, 0.85; 95% CI, 0.59-1.22). Reduced risk was present for smoking-related cancers such as lung (RR, 0.32), colorectal (RR, 0.54), and bladder (RR, 0.68), as well as for most non-smoking-related cancers such as prostate cancer (RR, 0.74). In contrast, PD patients were at significantly increased risk (RR, 6.15; 95% CI, 1.77-21.37) for melanoma. PD patients who smoked were at reduced risk for smoking-related cancer (RR, 0.33; 95% CI, 0.12-0.92), whereas nonsmokers with PD were at increased risk (RR, 1.80; 95% CI, 0.60-5.39), which was statistically significant (p = 0.02).

Studies of cancer following the diagnosis of PD are more common. The first, in 1985, used data from 2 separate surveys and calculated the expected incidence rates for malignancies in a sample of 406 PD patients.[43] Cancer incidence was about one-third that of the general population. Relative risk of cancer increased after the onset of PD and after the treatment was started, but it was still half that of the general population. In a large Danish cohort of 7046 patients with PD which were matched to the Danish cancer registry and the Danish registry of deaths,[44] cancer incidence in PD patients (observed number of cases) was compared to the expected number of cancer cases. A significantly lower risk of cancer was observed for PD patients (RR 0.88). In particular, PD patients had a lower risk of smoking-related cancer (lung and bladder), while they showed a two-fold increased risk of malignant melanoma.

Two recent studies have reproduced the increased risk of breast cancer in PD.[36,45] In the first of these studies of 246 PD patients, although the overall rate of cancer was not significantly reduced, the risk of breast cancer was 5.5 fold higher.[45] In the second much larger study of 14,088 PD patients from Denmark, there was an increased incidence of breast cancer and melanomas, and a slight increased incidence of non-melanocytic skin cancers.[36] In the latest study, 487 incident cases of PD without cancer preceding PD onset were identified and matched to PD-free individuals.[40] PD patients had a lower cancer risk. PD patients had in particular less lung (RR 0.3), colorectal (RR 0.54), and bladder (RR 0.68) malignancies. The risk for melanoma skin cancer was very high (RR 6.15). As in other studies, smoking status significantly modified the relationship between PD and smoking-related cancers, suggesting a gene–environment interaction. PD patients who smoked were in fact at a reduced risk for smoking-related cancers (RR 0.33), whereas nonsmoker PD patients were at increased risk (RR 1.8).

The mechanisms underlying this inverse relationship between PD and most forms of cancer, and a positive relationship with melanoma, non-melanotic skin cancer, and breast cancer are unknown. The discovery of gene mutations associated with familial parkinsonian disorders and understanding their role in cell survival and cell death may unravel the relationship between cancer and PD. However, the field is largely unexplored, especially in sporadic PD.

The Respiratory System in PD

While it is commonly observed in the PD clinic that patients with PD are less likely to develop viral respiratory tract infections, there are only a few studies to support this observation.[46,47] There is a complex and underestimated involvement of the respiratory system in PD. Patients with PD often have restrictive deficits later in the disease course and upper airway obstructive abnormalities on objective testing of respiratory function are most commonly asymptomatic. In addition, there are several effects of medical therapies relevant to respiration in PD. Motor fluctuations due to dopamine replacement therapy can produce 'off' dyspnea that is poorly understood and can be severely disabling. Even though this 'off' dyspnea is frequently observed in advanced PD, there is little published on this disabling phenomenon. Dopamine agonists derived from ergot alkaloids have pulmonary toxicity including serositis, pleural effusion, and interstitial lung disease that requires monitoring. Silent aspiration from dysphagia and sialorrhea is observed in the later stages of PD, which can produce aspiration pneumonia as a terminal event in end-stage patients. Lastly, pulmonary embolism can also occur co-incidentally rather than as a consequence of PD, and together with pneumonia, are two of the most common causes of death in advanced PD patients at post mortem.

Parkinson himself noted a patient that 'fetched the breath rather hard,' and as early as 1957 10% of patients with PD were recognized to have significant respiratory involvement.[48] Patients with PD in both ON and OFF states have significant impairments on respiratory function testing, which is most often asymptomatic.[49–51] The pattern of respiratory abnormality is usually that of a restrictive lung deficit, with reductions in forced vital capacity, FEV1, peak expiratory flow rate, maximum inspiratory and expiratory pressures.[50,52] Abnormal flow-volume loop contour is also found in PD that reflects involvement of the upper airway musculature.[53] In some patients this can produce upper airway obstruction; however, generalized airflow limitation is not an important characteristic of PD (as is the case often in multiple systems atrophy). Most reports suggest that these spirometric abnormalities improve to a limited extent with levodopa therapy.[49,50,54,55] The restrictive spirometric defect is probably due to an incoordinated expiratory effort or abnormally low chest wall compliance, although the underlying pathophysiology for this is unknown.[56] There is objective evidence of a physiological reduction of muscle function in the chest wall of patients with PD.[57] There are no systematic research articles on the involvement of the respiratory centers in the brainstem in PD, nor of the efferent neural pathways from the cervical cord to the diaphragm. To my knowledge, there are no original research articles on the pathogenesis and pathology of the pulmonary abnormalities in PD, apart from post mortem ascertainment of pneumonia and pulmonary embolism as the commonest causes of death.[58]

Several patterns of respiration have been identified in advanced PD, but there is usually no disturbance of nocturnal oxygenation early in the course of PD.[59] Sleep apnea syndrome may occur in PD.[60] In a retrospective study of PD patients referred for polysomnography, sleep apnea was identified in 21of 49 PD patients. Of these patients, the sleep apnea was classified as severe in 7 patients of this very selected cohort. There are as yet no systematic studies on the frequency of sleep apnea in PD, but given the paucity of other reports,[61] it seems unlikely to be a common disturbance. Levodopa-induced respiratory dysfunction has been described,[62, 63] which may be a heterogeneous disorder of choreiform movements of the respiratory muscles, rigidity-akinesis of the respiratory muscles, and abnormal central control with hyperventilation.[63] In addition, the ergot-derived dopamine agonists such as bromocriptine, cabergoline, and pergolide can cause pleural and pulmonary inflammation even in low doses.[64–67] Although the risk of these side effects is probably quite low,[68, 69] they should still be considered with patients on these therapies. These complications generally resolve with early recognition and discontinuation of the medication.

Pneumonia is the one of the commonest causes of death in PD.[70] The incidence of pneumonia as the cause of death ranges between 20% and 75%.[58,71,72] There are only a few detailed reports on the cause of death in patients with PD, and most reports lack postmortem verification. In one large series, 60 complete autopsies were performed on patients with a parkinsonian syndrome, all from one institution. Pulmonary embolism was second only to pneumonia as the most common cause of death overall.[58] Pulmonary embolism has been reported as an infrequent terminal event, but may be an important cause of respiratory dysfunction in PD.[73] While immobility and respiratory dysfunction clearly contribute to the development of pneumonia, impaired swallowing may also be a factor. In the early stages of PD the motor component of cough can be impaired.[74] In advanced stages of the disease, both the motor and sensory components of cough can be impaired, which may play an important role in the development of aspiration pneumonia in PD.

The assessment of patients with PD regarding respiratory function begins with a history and examination for intercurrent pulmonary disease. Medications are critical in the history, as past ergot exposure may well be relevant. Simple tests such as a chest x-ray may be informative regarding intercurrent diseases such as asbestos exposure, although most respiratory physicians would now require a high resolution CT scan of the chest in the initial investigations of a patient with a significant history of respiratory disease. CT pulmonary angiography is an accurate method for the diagnosis of significant pulmonary emboli, which may also require a ventilation perfusion scan. A discourse on the relative merits of these investigations regarding sensitivity and specificity is beyond the scope of this chapter, but the importance regarding the suspicion of pulmonary embolism as a cause of dyspnea in the PD patient deserves highlighting. Respiratory function testing including forced vital capacity, flow loops, and diffusion of carbon monoxide (DLCO or Kco – transfer factor) are routinely available and should be performed. Oximetry, blood gases, and capnography are sometimes required, but the assistance of a respiratory physician should be employed in this detailed assessment. If ergot-derived dopamine agonists are to be considered, then the patient should be counseled about the relatively small risk this conveys to their respiratory system. Baseline spirometry including a DLCO is often performed and specific investigations undertaken in the patient who develops new onset dyspnea, chest pain, or cough.

Regarding therapy of dyspnea in PD there are several small trials assessing the value of respiratory muscle training to alleviate the perception of dyspnea in PD. As most patients with PD do not have subjective dyspnea, there are as yet no trials to suggest that respiratory muscle training is of significance in preventing respiratory symptomatology.[75-77] It is intuitive that PD patients should have adequate dopaminergic replacement, and while this partially improves some of the objective respiratory measurements in PD, whether this helps the symptomatic respiratory involvement in PD is as yet unknown. The use of ergot derivatives (pergolide, cabergoline) in the therapy of PD requires adequate assessment of respiratory function, including DLCO before initiation of therapy and consideration of significant intercurrent disease. There is no literature to suggest that pre-existing lung disease either predisposes a PD patient to ergot-related lung disease, or that exposure to ergot drugs exacerbates existing pulmonary pathology, although it has been suggested in the literature that asbestos exposure may contribute to the pulmonary toxicity of ergot dopamine agonists.[65] The dyspnea that occurs as a consequence of dyskinesia from dopamine replacement therapy is very difficult to treat, and standard approaches to motor fluctuations should be adopted. Systemic anticoagulation is recommended in patients with proven pulmonary embolism, but this decision becomes more difficult in the presence of falls and the risk of subdural hematomas and so has to be made in the context of the individual patient.

The Skin in PD

Although symptoms concerning skin are very common in PD, there is only a small literature regarding the involvement of skin. Abnormalities of the skin were described more than fifty years ago,[78] although authors of the 19th century had already commented on this, particularly with reference to seborrheic dermatitis, abnormalities of sweating[79] and the autonomic innervation of the skin, and skin malignancies. There are uncommon skin manifestations of therapy that deserve brief mention in passing, such as cutaneous allergic reactions to levodopa preparations, livedo reticularis as a consequence of amantadine, and apomorphine-associated panniculitis and pigmentation.

Despite its name, seborrheic dermatitis is not associated with excessive secretion of sebum,[80] nor does it primarily involve the sebaceous glands. Fungi of the genus *Malassezia* are thought to be pathogenic in seborrheic dermatitis, since they are present on affected skin and antifungal agents are useful in treatment.[80] There are multiple references in the literature to seborrheic dermatitis in PD,[81-84] and conflicting results regarding the secretion of sebum in PD,[81,85-87] although recent well conducted studies show no increase in the amount of sebum secretion in PD.[85] Although seborrheic dermatitis is a very common observation in PD, even recent reviews on this condition are unable to agree on whether there is an association with PD.[86] In the clinic, a pragmatic approach should be adopted towards seborrheic dermatitis and patients advised to use topical antifungal agents such as ketoconazole daily for a month, as well as shampoo once a week.[80] Maintenance therapy is effective at maintaining remission, as there have been at least 10 randomized controlled trials on the use of ketoconazole for the treatment of seborrheic dermatitis.[80]

There is considerable evidence of skin sympathetic abnormalities in PD. Abnormalities of sweating with both dry skin and hyperhidrosis indicate vasomotor instability. For many years, neurophysiological measures of sympathetic skin responses (SSR) have identified abnormalities in the autonomic function of the skin in PD.[88-93] In general, there is a significant association between altered SSR and PD and an inverse correlation in this group of patients between SSR values and older age, greater severity, and later onset of disease. Therefore, the study of SSR may provide valuable information on cholinergic sympathetic function in patients with PD.[94] Several investigators have commented on the inconsistent association of abnormal SSR with other features of autonomic dysfunction such as orthostatic hypotension and R-R interval variation,[95, 96] arguing for the pleiotropic nature of involvement of the autonomic nervous system in PD.

Over recent years, pathological examination of biopsy material has confirmed abnormalities of sympathetic innervation that do correlate with clinical and neurophysiological abnormalities in PD. α-Synuclein was first identified semi-quantitatively in skin biopsies by Barker and colleagues,[97] although there is as yet no evidence that skin deposition of α-synuclein will be a sensitive biomarker or an indicator of the pre-motor phase of PD. Even though Kawada was able to identify quantitative abnormalities with reduction of the sudomotor axon reflex test in PD subjects, there was no detectable α-synuclein deposition in the sweat glands of patients with PD.[98]

More recently, peripheral nervous system de-afferentation in PD was identified, suggesting a major role for this in the pathogenesis of the sudomotor and sensory dysfunction.[99] Nolano and coworkers demonstrated that PD patients showed a significant increase in tactile and thermal thresholds (P <0.01), a significant reduction in mechanical pain perception (P <0.01), and significant loss of epidermal nerve fibers and Meissner's corpuscles (P <0.01). In patients with bilateral biopsies, loss of pain perception and epidermal nerve fibers was higher on the more affected side (P <0.01). There was also evidence of increased branching, sprouting of nerves, and enlargement of the vascular bed to suggest compensatory re-innervation.

Age and disease duration did not correlate with morphological and functional findings, but did correlate with the degree of loss of Meissner's corpuscles and reduction in cold and pain perception. In summary, the
denervation of skin that occurs in PD is variable, just as the motor manifestations of PD vary between patients. There are abnormalities of small nerve
fibers that produce changes in tactile and sudomotor function, and the skin
has much more to reveal in the systematic study of PD.

The possible association of melanoma and PD was first noted in 1972.[100]
There are many small series and case reports, as well as case-control studies with much larger cohorts. It does appear that there is an increased risk
of melanoma in PD, with a relative risk approximately 50% higher than
controls.[101] The risk is there before diagnosis and before the initiation of
levodopa therapy and in fact does not appear to be an increased risk of
developing melanoma from levodopa use.[102] As such, the ubiquitous warning that there is an increased risk of melanoma and that levodopa use is
contraindicated with a past or intercurrent melanoma appears to be without substance.[101] This quite common misconception should be discussed
with all PD patients and ideally patients should be surveyed for melanoma
as PD patients have a nearly two fold incidence of it.[103] The reasons for
this are not yet understood.

The incidence of skin allergy to the yellow dye in C/L 25/100 is rare.
Several large multicenter randomized controlled trials did not identify
allergic skin rash as more common than placebo.[104] Nevertheless, neurolo-
gists should be aware that a skin rash associated with Sinemet™ may be
due to the D&C Yellow 10 and FD&C Yellow 6 dye in the 100/25 formulation, and a different preparation of Sinemet™ or Madopar™ should be tried
before concluding that the patient has a levodopa or carbidopa allergy.[104]
Amantadine can cause livedo reticularis[105–107] and photosensitivity,[108] and
this is important to recognize given the increased use of this drug in patients
to treat L-dopa-induced dyskinesias. Subcutaneous apomorphine can produce panniculitis[109] as well as pigmentation due to oxidation of the apomorphine.[110] While both can be troublesome for the patient, the
panniculitis responds to local therapies.[111,112]

The Eye in PD

While dopamine is a neurotransmitter in the retina and plays an important
role in retinal function, most patients with PD do not have subjective visual
deficits, but rather may be troubled by positive visual illusions and hallucinations. There are only a few postmortem studies of the retina in PD,[113,114] and
while these studies identified a deficit of tyrosine hydroxylase neurons in the

retina and lower dopamine concentrations, there is caution as to whether these changes account for the clinical abnormalities identified in the eyes of patients with PD. As far as can be ascertained in the referenced literature, there are no studies suggesting α-synuclein deposition in the retina.

The retinal changes in PD patients have been the subject of recent reviews.[115,116] Although visual acuity is usually not affected in PD, the most common visual abnormalities identified on special testing in PD are loss of color discrimination, color contour perception, and contrast sensitivity.[117–119] However, these changes on testing do not appear to correlate with degeneration of the nigrostriatal system as measured by β-CIT imaging,[120] and therefore the basis for these visual disturbances has yet to be determined. More recently, optical coherence tomography has been used in several studies to demonstrate thinning of both the inferior and superior inner retinal layer (IRL) in the macular region in PD eyes.[121] In the largest study to date, retinal thickness was quantified in patients with PD. Forty-five eyes of 24 PD patients and 31 eyes of 17 control subjects underwent a comprehensive ophthalmologic examination. Optical coherence tomography was used to examine retinal thickness, separately quantifying the inner and outer retinal layers. No difference was found in either the superior or inferior outer retinal layer thickness of PD vs control eyes, but the inner retinal layer was significantly thinner in PD patients than in healthy subjects.[121] The clinical utility of these measures is as yet unclear, but this technique might prove to be useful in the early assessment of PD.

The size and reactivity of the pupils are controlled by the sympathetic and parasympathetic components of the autonomic nervous system. Constriction of the pupils is mediated via the parasympathetic fibers of the third cranial nerve that arise from the Edinger-Westphal nucleus of the midbrain, which is involved in PD.[122] Pupillary dilatation is mediated via the sympathetic pathways, which are also variably affected in PD. Abnormally slow pupillary responses to light and pain in PD patients were initially identified.[123] More recent studies of pupillary responses in PD have found that resting diameters are normal, but the response to changes in light is less than in matched controls.[124] Early studies using the application of pharmacological agents to stimulate pupillary reactions demonstrated the peripheral autonomic nervous system to be intact in PD patients, with pupillary abnormalities resulting from central autonomic dysfunction centered on the parasympathetic Edinger-Westphal nucleus of the midbrain.[122] There are several other studies of the pupil in PD to indicate both sympathetic[125] and parasympathetic deficits.[124] Indeed, there is a recent vogue for measuring the central cholinergic system via pupillometry of the pupillary light reflex (PLR) as a surrogate in PD.[126] Pupillary constriction to light is cholinergic, and several groups have identified that the peak amplitude of pupillary constriction, the maximum pupillary velocity and acceleration, are significantly lower in PD compared to controls, and are more impaired in patients with PD and cognitive impairment.[124,126] Parenthetically, pupillary diameter to dark adaption may be able to distinguish PD from other parkinsonian disorders such as PSP.[127] In summary, most of the detectable pupillary abnormalities that occur in PD are cholinergic and independent of any dopaminergic deficit—whether it is in the retina or in the CNS. These abnormalities, though, might give early insight into the central cholinergic deficits that underlie the cognitive abnormalities in early PD, in the dementia of PD, and in other Lewy body diseases.

There is scant literature on the ocular symptoms of PD, although in the clinic eye symptoms are one of the most common complaints. In one of the few systematic studies in early PD,[128] subjective complaints of surface irritation, including photophobia, tearing, crusting on lashes, eyes stuck in morning, dry eye, burning eye, gritty or sandy sensation, red eye, and eye pain were present in 19 of 30 PD subjects (compared with 9 of 31 controls (63.3% v 29.0% p=0.007). In a study of tear function tests, PD patients demonstrated abnormalities in several measures including blink rate and other objective measures of tear production including Schirmer's test.[129] These abnormalities correlated with PD severity as measured by the Hoehn–Yahr scale, similar to previous publications.[130,131] Although it is proposed that the ocular changes that occur in PD are related to underlying autonomic pathology, there are no data to support this assertion. Although these symptoms can be addressed with simple remedies such as ocular lubricants and punctual occlusion, there are no trial data to support these therapies.

Conclusion

This review of some of the systemic manifestations of PD demonstrates the protean nature of this common disease. Researchers are already moving away from the previous concepts of PD as a CNS-only disease, and one principally of the dopaminergic system. No doubt there are many clues to the pathogenesis and monitoring of PD, with a better understanding of these systemic abnormalities having the potential to lead to advances in the prevention and treatment of this condition.

References

1. Orr CF, Rowe DB, Halliday GM. An inflammatory review of Parkinson's disease. *Prog Neurobiol.* Dec 2002;68(5):325–340.

2. Bas J, Calopa M, Mestre M, et al. Lymphocyte populations in Parkinson's disease and in rat models of parkinsonism. *J Neuroimmunol*. Feb 1 2001;113(1):146–152.

3. Fiszer U, Mix E, Fredrikson S, Kostulas V, Olsson T, Link H. gamma delta+ T cells are increased in patients with Parkinson's disease. *J Neurol Sci*. Jan 1994;121(1):39–45.

4. Banati RB, Daniel SE, Blunt SB. Glial pathology but absence of apoptotic nigral neurons in long-standing Parkinson's disease. *Mov Disord*. Mar 1998;13(2):221–227.

5. Hunot S, Dugas N, Faucheux B, et al. FcepsilonRII/CD23 is expressed in Parkinson's disease and induces, in vitro, production of nitric oxide and tumor necrosis factor-alpha in glial cells. *J Neurosci*. May 1 1999;19(9):3440–3447.

6. McGeer PL, Itagaki S, Boyes BE, McGeer EG. Reactive microglia are positive for HLA-DR in the substantia nigra of Parkinson's and Alzheimer's disease brains. *Neurology*. Aug 1988;38(8):1285–1291.

7. Mirza B, Hadberg H, Thomsen P, Moos T. The absence of reactive astrocytosis is indicative of a unique inflammatory process in Parkinson's disease. *Neuroscience*. 2000;95(2):425–432.

8. Orr CF, Rowe DB, Mizuno Y, Mori H, Halliday GM. A possible role for humoral immunity in the pathogenesis of Parkinson's disease. *Brain*. Nov 2005;128(Pt 11): 2665–2674.

9. Mogi M, Harada M, Kondo T, Riederer P, Nagatsu T. Brain beta 2-microglobulin levels are elevated in the striatum in Parkinson's disease. *J Neural Transm Park Dis Dement Sect*. 1995;9(1):87–92.

10. Yamada T, Akiyama H, McGeer PL. Complement-activated oligodendroglia: a new pathogenic entity identified by immunostaining with antibodies to human complement proteins C3d and C4d. *Neurosci Lett*. May 4 1990;112(2–3):161–166.

11. Nakashima S, Ikuta F. Tyrosine hydroxylase protein in Lewy bodies of parkinsonian and senile brains. *J Neurol Sci*. Oct 1984;66(1):91–96.

12. Boka G, Anglade P, Wallach D, Javoy-Agid F, Agid Y, Hirsch EC. Immunocyto-chemical analysis of tumor necrosis factor and its receptors in Parkinson's disease. *Neurosci Lett*. May 19 1994;172(1–2):151–154.

13. Mogi M, Harada M, Riederer P, Narabayashi H, Fujita K, Nagatsu T. Tumor necrosis factor-alpha (TNF-alpha) increases both in the brain and in the cerebrospinal fluid from parkinsonian patients. *Neurosci Lett*. Jan 3 1994;165(1–2):208–210.

14. Mogi M, Harada M, Kondo T, et al. Interleukin-1 beta, interleukin-6, epidermal growth factor and transforming growth factor-alpha are elevated in the brain from parkinsonian patients. *Neurosci Lett*. Oct 24 1994;180(2):147–150.

15. Mogi M, Harada M, Kondo T, et al. The soluble form of Fas molecule is elevated in parkinsonian brain tissues. *Neurosci Lett*. Dec 20 1996;220(3):195–198.

16. Mogi M, Harada M, Kondo T, et al. bcl-2 protein is increased in the brain from parkinsonian patients. *Neurosci Lett*. Sep 6 1996;215(2):137–139.

17. Hirsch EC, Hunot S, Faucheux B, et al. Dopaminergic neurons degenerate by apoptosis in Parkinson's disease. *Mov Disord*. Mar 1999;14(2):383–385.

18. Marshall KA, Daniel SE, Cairns N, Jenner P, Halliwell B. Upregulation of the anti-apoptotic protein Bcl-2 may be an early event in neurodegeneration: studies on Parkinson's and incidental Lewy body disease. *Biochem Biophys Res Commun*. Nov 7 1997;240(1):84–87.

19. Chiba S, Matsumoto H, Saitoh M, Kasahara M, Matsuya M, Kashiwagi M. A correlation study between serum adenosine deaminase activities and peripheral lymphocyte subsets in Parkinson's disease. *J Neurol Sci.* Oct 1995;132(2):170–173.

20. Marttila RJ, Eskola J, Soppi E, Rinne UK. Immune functions in Parkinson's disease lymphocyte subsets, concanavalin A-induced suppressor cell activity and in vitro immunoglobulin production. *J Neurol Sci.* Jul 1985;69(3):121–131.

21. Bessler H, Djaldetti R, Salman H, Bergman M, Djaldetti M. IL-1 beta, IL-2, IL-6 and TNF-alpha production by peripheral blood mononuclear cells from patients with Parkinson's disease. *Biomed Pharmacother.* Apr 1999;53(3):141–145.

22. Kluter H, Vieregge P, Stolze H, Kirchner H. Defective production of interleukin-2 in patients with idiopathic Parkinson's disease. *J Neurol Sci.* Nov 1995;133(1–2):134–139.

23. Fiszer U, Mix E, Fredrikson S, Kostulas V, Link H. Parkinson's disease and immunological abnormalities: increase of HLA-DR expression on monocytes in cerebrospinal fluid and of CD45RO+ T cells in peripheral blood. *Acta Neurol Scand.* Sep 1994;90(3):160–166.

24. Bokor M, Farago A, Garam T, Malatinszky G, Schnabel R. Antibody-dependent cell-mediated cytotoxicity (ADCC) in Parkinson's disease. *J Neurol Sci.* Mar 1993;115(1):47–50.

25. Salman H, Bergman M, Djaldetti R, Bessler H, Djaldetti M. Decreased phagocytic function in patients with Parkinson's disease. *Biomed Pharmacother.* Apr 1999;53(3):146–148.

26. Fiszer U, Piotrowska K, Korlak J, Czlonkowska A. The immunological status in Parkinson's disease. *Med Lab Sci.* Jul 1991;48(3):196–200.

27. Emile J, Pouplard A, Bossu Van Nieuwenhuyse C, Bernat-Viallet C. Parkinson's disease, dysautonomy, and auto-antibodies directed against sympathetic neurones. *Rev Neurol (Paris).* 1980;136(3):221–233.

28. McRae Degueurce A, Gottfries CG, Karlsson I, Svennerholm L, Dahlstrom A. Antibodies in the CSF of a Parkinson patient recognizes neurons in rat mesencephalic regions. *Acta Physiol Scand.* Feb 1986;126(2):313–315.

29. Pouplard A, Emile J. Autoimmunity in Parkinson's disease. *Adv Neurol.* 1984;40:307–313.

30. Le W, Rowe D, Xie W, Ortiz I, He Y, Appel SH. Microglial activation and dopaminergic cell injury: an in vitro model relevant to Parkinson's disease. *J Neurosci.* Nov 1 2001;21(21):8447–8455.

31. Rowe DB, Le W, Smith RG, Appel SH. Antibodies from patients with Parkinson's disease react with protein modified by dopamine oxidation. *J Neurosci Res.* Sep 1 1998;53(5):551–558.

32. Le WD, Rowe DB, Jankovic J, Xie W, Appel SH. Effects of cerebrospinal fluid from patients with Parkinson disease on dopaminergic cells. *Arch Neurol.* Feb 1999;56(2):194–200.

33. Mogi M, Harada M, Narabayashi H, Inagaki H, Minami M, Nagatsu T. Interleukin (IL)-1 beta, IL-2, IL-4, IL-6 and transforming growth factor-alpha levels are elevated in ventricular cerebrospinal fluid in juvenile parkinsonism and Parkinson's disease. *Neurosci Lett.* Jun 14 1996;211(1):13–16.

34. Rugbjerg K, Friis S, Ritz B, Schernhammer ES, Korbo L, Olsen JH. Autoimmune disease and risk for Parkinson disease: a population-based case-control study. *Neurology.* Nov 3 2009;73(18):1462–1468.
35. D'Amelio M, Ragonese P, Sconzo G, Aridon P, Savettieri G. Parkinson's disease and cancer: insights for pathogenesis from epidemiology. *Ann N Y Acad Sci.* Feb 2009;1155:324–334.
36. Olsen JH, Friis S, Frederiksen K, McLaughlin JK, Mellemkjaer L, Moller H. Atypical cancer pattern in patients with Parkinson's disease. *Br J Cancer.* Jan 17 2005;92(1):201–205.
37. Hoehn MM, Yahr MD. Parkinsonism: onset, progression and mortality. *Neurology.* May 1967;17(5):427–442.
38. Olsen JH, Friis S, Frederiksen K. Malignant melanoma and other types of cancer preceding Parkinson disease. *Epidemiology.* Sep 2006;17(5):582–587.
39. Elbaz A, Peterson BJ, Yang P, et al. Nonfatal cancer preceding Parkinson's disease: a case-control study. *Epidemiology.* Mar 2002;13(2):157–164.
40. Driver JA, Kurth T, Buring JE, Gaziano JM, Logroscino G. Prospective case-control study of nonfatal cancer preceding the diagnosis of Parkinson's disease. *Cancer Causes Control.* Sep 2007;18(7):705–711.
41. D'Amelio M, Ragonese P, Morgante L, et al. Tumor diagnosis preceding Parkinson's disease: a case-control study. *Mov Disord.* Jul 2004;19(7):807–811.
42. Driver JA, Logroscino G, Buring JE, Gaziano JM, Kurth T. A prospective cohort study of cancer incidence following the diagnosis of Parkinson's disease. *Cancer Epidemiol Biomarkers Prev.* Jun 2007;16(6):1260–1265.
43. Jansson B, Jankovic J. Low cancer rates among patients with Parkinson's disease. *Ann Neurol.* May 1985;17(5):505–509.
44. Moller H, Mellemkjaer L, McLaughlin JK, Olsen JH. Occurrence of different cancers in patients with Parkinson's disease. *BMJ.* Jun 10 1995;310(6993):1500–1501.
45. Minami Y, Yamamoto R, Nishikouri M, Fukao A, Hisamichi S. Mortality and cancer incidence in patients with Parkinson's disease. *J Neurol.* Jun 2000;247(6):429–434.
46. Kawaguchi N, Yamada T, Hattori T. Rare tendency of catching cold in Parkinson's disease. *Parkinsonism Relat Disord.* Dec 1998;4(4):207–209.
47. Nomoto M, Igata A. Do parkinsonian patients have a greater resistance to the common cold? *J Neurol Neurosurg Psychiatry.* Dec 1983;46(12):1153–1154.
48. Woltman HW. Encephalitis: historical review and perspective. *Can Med Assoc J.* Dec 1 1957;77(11):995–1001.
49. Mehta AD, Wright WB, Kirby BJ. Ventilatory function in Parkinson's disease. *Br Med J.* Jun 3 1978;1(6125):1456–1457.
50. Pal PK, Sathyaprabha TN, Tuhina P, Thennarasu K. Pattern of subclinical pulmonary dysfunctions in Parkinson's disease and the effect of levodopa. *Mov Disord.* Feb 15 2007;22(3):420–424.
51. Sabate M, Gonzalez I, Ruperez F, Rodriguez M. Obstructive and restrictive pulmonary dysfunctions in Parkinson's disease. *J Neurol Sci.* Jun 1996;138(1–2):114–119.
52. De Pandis MF, Starace A, Stefanelli F, et al. Modification of respiratory function parameters in patients with severe Parkinson's disease. *Neurol Sci.* Sep 2002;23 Suppl 2:S69–70.

53. Hovestadt A, Bogaard JM, Meerwaldt JD, van der Meche FG, Stigt J. Pulmonary function in Parkinson's disease. *J Neurol Neurosurg Psychiatry*. Mar 1989;52(3):329–333.

54. Herer B, Arnulf I, Housset B. Effects of levodopa on pulmonary function in Parkinson's disease. *Chest*. Feb 2001;119(2):387–393.

55. Sathyaprabha TN, Kapavarapu PK, Pall PK, Thennarasu K, Raju TR. Pulmonary functions in Parkinson's disease. *Indian J Chest Dis Allied Sci*. Oct-Dec 2005;47(4): 251–257.

56. Izquierdo-Alonso JL, Jimenez-Jimenez FJ, Cabrera-Valdivia F, Mansilla-Lesmes M. Airway dysfunction in patients with Parkinson's disease. *Lung*. 1994;172(1):47–55.

57. Tzelepis GE, McCool FD, Friedman JH, Hoppin FG, Jr. Respiratory muscle dysfunction in Parkinson's disease. *Am Rev Respir Dis*. Aug 1988;138(2):266–271.

58. Mosewich RK, Rajput AH, Shuaib A, Rozdilsky B, Ang L. Pulmonary embolism: an under-recognized yet frequent cause of death in parkinsonism. *Mov Disord*. May 1994;9(3):350–352.

59. Apps MC, Sheaff PC, Ingram DA, Kennard C, Empey DW. Respiration and sleep in Parkinson's disease. *J Neurol Neurosurg Psychiatry*. Dec 1985;48(12):1240–1245.

60. Diederich NJ, Vaillant M, Leischen M, et al. Sleep apnea syndrome in Parkinson's disease. A case-control study in 49 patients. *Mov Disord*. Nov 2005;20(11):1413–1418.

61. Steffen A, Hagenah J, Graefe H, Mahlerwein M, Wollenberg B. [Obstructive sleep apnea in patients with Parkinson's disease–report of two cases and review]. *Laryngorhinootologie*. Feb 2008;87(2):107–111.

62. Jankovic J, Nour F. Respiratory dyskinesia in Parkinson's disease. *Neurology*. Feb 1986;36(2):303–304.

63. Rice JE, Antic R, Thompson PD. Disordered respiration as a levodopa-induced dyskinesia in Parkinson's disease. *Mov Disord*. May 2002;17(3):524–527.

64. Brown LK. Respiratory dysfunction in Parkinson's disease. *Clin Chest Med*. Dec 1994;15(4):715–727.

65. Frank W, Moritz R, Becke B, Pauli R. Low dose cabergoline induced interstitial pneumonitis. *Eur Respir J*. Oct 1999;14(4):968–970.

66. Tintner R, Manian P, Gauthier P, Jankovic J. Pleuropulmonary fibrosis after long-term treatment with the dopamine agonist pergolide for Parkinson Disease. *Arch Neurol*. Aug 2005;62(8):1290–1295.

67. Haro-Estarriol M, Sabater-Talaverano G, Rodriguez-Jerez F, Obrador-Lagares A, Genis-Batlle D, Sendra-Salillas S. Pleural effusion and pulmonary hypertension in a patient with Parkinson disease treated with cabergoline. *Arch Bronconeumol*. Feb 2009;45(2):100–102.

68. Agarwal P, Fahn S, Frucht SJ. Diagnosis and management of pergolide-induced fibrosis. *Mov Disord*. Jun 2004;19(6):699–704.

69. Dhawan V, Medcalf P, Stegie F, et al. Retrospective evaluation of cardio-pulmonary fibrotic side effects in symptomatic patients from a group of 234 Parkinson's disease patients treated with cabergoline. *J Neural Transm*. May 2005;112(5):661–668.

70. Wermuth L, Stenager EN, Stenager E, Boldsen J. Mortality in patients with Parkinson's disease. *Acta Neurol Scand*. Jul 1995;92(1):55–58.

71. Aboussouan LS. Respiratory disorders in neurologic diseases. *Cleve Clin J Med*. Jun 2005;72(6):511–520.

72. Wang X, You G, Chen H, Cai X. Clinical course and cause of death in elderly patients with idiopathic Parkinson's disease. *Chin Med J (Engl)*. Sep 2002;115(9): 1409–1411.

73. Hung SC, Tai CT. Parkinson's disease with recurrent pulmonary embolism. *Zhonghua Yi Xue Za Zhi (Taipei)*. Jun 2000;63(6):487–491.

74. Ebihara S, Saito H, Kanda A, et al. Impaired efficacy of cough in patients with Parkinson disease. *Chest*. Sep 2003;124(3):1009–1015.

75. Inzelberg R, Peleg N, Nisipeanu P, Magadle R, Carasso RL, Weiner P. Inspiratory muscle training and the perception of dyspnea in Parkinson's disease. *Can J Neurol Sci*. May 2005;32(2):213–217.

76. Saleem AF, Sapienza CM, Okun MS. Respiratory muscle strength training: treatment and response duration in a patient with early idiopathic Parkinson's disease. *NeuroRehabilitation*. 2005;20(4):323–333.

77. Silverman EP, Sapienza CM, Saleem A, et al. Tutorial on maximum inspiratory and expiratory mouth pressures in individuals with idiopathic Parkinson disease (IPD) and the preliminary results of an expiratory muscle strength training program. *NeuroRehabilitation*. 2006;21(1):71–79.

78. Kvorning SA. Excretion of skin lipids in patients with Parkinson's syndrome. *Acta Derm Venereol Suppl (Stockh)*. 1952;32(29):201–203.

79. Gower WR. *A Manual of Diseases of the Nervous System*. 2nd ed. London: Churchill; 1893.

80. Naldi L, Rebora A. Clinical practice. Seborrheic dermatitis. *N Engl J Med*. Jan 22 2009;360(4):387–396.

81. Burton JL, Cartlidge M, Cartlidge NE, Shuster S. Sebum excretion in Parkinsonism. *Br J Dermatol*. Mar 1973;88(3):263–266.

82. Burton JL, Shuster S. Effect of L-dopa on seborrhoea of Parkinsonism. *Lancet*. Aug 8 1970;2(7667):311.

83. Appenzeller O, Harville D. Effect of L-dopa on seborrhea of Parkinsonism. *Lancet*. Aug 8 1970;2(7667):311–312.

84. Pochi PE, Strauss JS, Mescon H. Sebum production and fractional 17-ketosteroid excretion in parkinsonism. *J Invest Dermatol*. Jan 1962;38:45–51.

85. Mastrolonardo M, Diaferio A, Logroscino G. Seborrheic dermatitis, increased sebum excretion, and Parkinson's disease: a survey of (im)possible links. *Med Hypotheses*. Jun 2003;60(6):907–911.

86. Fischer M, Gemende I, Marsch WC, Fischer PA. Skin function and skin disorders in Parkinson's disease. *J Neural Transm*. 2001;108(2):205–213.

87. Kohn SR, Pochi PE, Strauss JS, Sax DS, Feldman RG, Timberlake WH. Sebaceous gland secretion in Parkinson's disease during L-dopa treatment. *J Invest Dermatol*. Mar 1973;60(3):134–136.

88. Hirashima F, Yokota T, Miyatake T, Hayashi M, Tanabe H. Sudomotor dysfunction in Parkinson's disease. *Rinsho Shinkeigaku*. Jul 1993;33(7):709–714.

89. De Marinis M, Stocchi F, Testa SR, De Pandis F, Agnoli A. Alterations of thermoregulation in Parkinson's disease. *Funct Neurol*. Jul-Sep 1991;6(3):279–283.

90. Ishida G, Nakashima K, Takahashi K. Skin nerve sympathetic activity reflex latency in Parkinson's disease. *Acta Neurol Scand*. Feb 1990;81(2):121–124.

91. Turkka JT, Myllyla VV. Sweating dysfunction in Parkinson's disease. *Eur Neurol.* 1987;26(1):1–7.

92. Goetz CG, Lutge W, Tanner CM. Autonomic dysfunction in Parkinson's disease. *Neurology.* Jan 1986;36(1):73–75.

93. Jost WH, Kirchhofer U, Houy S, Schimrigk K. [Sympathetic skin response in Parkinson syndrome]. *Nervenarzt.* Oct 1995;66(10):777–780.

94. Schestatsky P, Ehlers JA, Rieder CR, Gomes I. Evaluation of sympathetic skin response in Parkinson's disease. *Parkinsonism Relat Disord.* Dec 2006;12(8): 486–491.

95. Wang SJ, Fuh JL, Shan DE, et al. Sympathetic skin response and R-R interval variation in Parkinson's disease. *Mov Disord.* Apr 1993;8(2):151–157.

96. Akaogi Y, Asahina M, Yamanaka Y, Koyama Y, Hattori T. Sudomotor, skin vasomotor, and cardiovascular reflexes in 3 clinical forms of Lewy body disease. *Neurology.* Jul 7 2009;73(1):59–65.

97. Michell AW, Luheshi LM, Barker RA. Skin and platelet alpha-synuclein as peripheral biomarkers of Parkinson's disease. *Neurosci Lett.* Jun 24 2005;381(3): 294–298.

98. Kawada M, Tamada Y, Simizu H, et al. Reduction in QSART and vasoactive intestinal polypeptide expression in the skin of Parkinson's disease patients and its relation to dyshidrosis. *J Cutan Pathol.* May 2009;36(5):517–521.

99. Nolano M, Provitera V, Estraneo A, et al. Sensory deficit in Parkinson's disease: evidence of a cutaneous denervation. *Brain.* Jul 2008;131(Pt 7):1903–1911.

100. Skibba JL, Pinckley J, Gilbert EF, Johnson RO. Multiple primary melanoma following administration of levodopa. *Arch Pathol.* Jun 1972;93(6):556–561.

101. Vermeij JD, Winogrodzka A, Trip J, Weber WE. Parkinson's disease, levodopa-use and the risk of melanoma. *Parkinsonism Relat Disord.* Sep 2009;15(8):551–553.

102. Zanetti R, Loria D, Rosso S. Melanoma, Parkinson's disease and levodopa: causal or spurious link? A review of the literature. *Melanoma Res.* Jun 2006;16(3):201–206.

103. Zanetti R, Rosso S. Levodopa and the risk of melanoma. *Lancet.* Jan 27 2007;369(9558):257–258.

104. Chou KL, Stacy MA. Skin rash associated with Sinemet does not equal levodopa allergy. *Neurology.* Mar 27 2007;68(13):1078–1079.

105. Loffler H, Habermann B, Effendy I. [Amantadine-induced livedo reticularis]. *Hautarzt.* Mar 1998;49(3):224–227.

106. Silver DE, Sahs AL. Livedo reticularis in Parkinson's disease patients treated with amantadine hydrochloride. *Neurology.* Jul 1972;22(7):665–669.

107. Parkes JD, Baxter RC, Curzon G, et al. Treatment of Parkinson's disease with amantadine and levodopa. A one-year study. *Lancet.* May 29 1971;1(7709):1083–1086.

108. van Ketel WG, Goedhart-van Dijk B. Fotosensitization by Amantadine (Symmetrel). *Dermatologica.* 1974;148(2):124–126.

109. Pot C, Oppliger R, Castillo V, Coeytaux A, Hauser C, Burkhard PR. Apomorphine-induced eosinophilic panniculitis and hypereosinophilia in Parkinson disease. *Neurology.* Jan 25 2005;64(2):392–393.

110. Loewe R, Puspok-Schwarz M, Petzelbauer P. [Apomorphine hyperpigmentation]. *Hautarzt.* Jan 2003;54(1):58–63.

111. Poltawski L, Edwards H, Todd A, Watson T, Lees A, James CA. Ultrasound treatment of cutaneous side-effects of infused apomorphine: a randomized controlled pilot study. *Mov Disord.* Jan 15 2009;24(1):115–118.
112. Todd A, James CA. Apomorphine nodules in Parkinson's disease: best practice considerations. *Br J Community Nurs.* Oct 2008;13(10):457–463.
113. Harnois C, Di Paolo T. Decreased dopamine in the retinas of patients with Parkinson's disease. *Invest Ophthalmol Vis Sci.* Nov 1990;31(11):2473–2475.
114. Nguyen-Legros J. Functional neuroarchitecture of the retina: hypothesis on the dysfunction of retinal dopaminergic circuitry in Parkinson's disease. *Surg Radiol Anat.* 1988;10(2):137–144.
115. Archibald NK, Clarke MP, Mosimann UP, Burn DJ. The retina in Parkinson's disease. *Brain.* May 2009;132(Pt 5):1128–1145.
116. Bodis-Wollner I. Retinopathy in Parkinson Disease. *Journal of neural transmission (Vienna, Austria : 1996).* Nov 1 2009;116(11):1493–1501.
117. Bodis-Wollner I. Visual electrophysiology in Parkinson's disease: PERG, VEP and visual P300. *Clin Electroencephalogr.* Jul 1997;28(3):143–147.
118. Buttner T, Kuhn W, Muller T, Patzold T, Heidbrink K, Przuntek H. Distorted color discrimination in 'de novo' parkinsonian patients. *Neurology.* Feb 1995;45(2):386–387.
119. Price MJ, Feldman RG, Adelberg D, Kayne H. Abnormalities in color vision and contrast sensitivity in Parkinson's disease. *Neurology.* Apr 1992;42(4):887–890.
120. Muller T, Kuhn W, Buttner T, et al. Colour vision abnormalities do not correlate with dopaminergic nigrostriatal degeneration in Parkinson's disease. *J Neurol.* Oct 1998;245(10):659–664.
121. Hajee ME, March WF, Lazzaro DR, et al. Inner retinal layer thinning in Parkinson disease. *Arch Ophthalmol.* Jun 2009;127(6):737–741.
122. Hunter S. The rostral mesencephalon in Parkinson's disease and Alzheimer's disease. *Acta Neuropathol.* 1985;68(1):53–58.
123. Micieli G, Tassorelli C, Martignoni E, et al. Disordered pupil reactivity in Parkinson's disease. *Clin Auton Res.* Mar 1991;1(1):55–58.
124. Stergiou V, Fotiou D, Tsiptsios D, et al. Pupillometric findings in patients with Parkinson's disease and cognitive disorder. *Int J Psychophysiol.* May 2009;72(2):97–101.
125. Sawada H, Yamakawa K, Yamakado H, et al. Cocaine and phenylephrine eye drop test for Parkinson disease. *JAMA.* Feb 23 2005;293(8):932–934.
126. Fotiou DF, Stergiou V, Tsiptsios D, Lithari C, Nakou M, Karlovasitou A. Cholinergic deficiency in Alzheimer's and Parkinson's disease: evaluation with pupillometry. *Int J Psychophysiol.* Aug 2009;73(2):143–149.
127. Schmidt C, Herting B, Prieur S, et al. Pupil diameter in darkness differentiates progressive supranuclear palsy (PSP) from other extrapyramidal syndromes. *Mov Disord.* Oct 31 2007;22(14):2123–2126.
128. Biousse V, Skibell BC, Watts RL, Loupe DN, Drews-Botsch C, Newman NJ. Ophthalmologic features of Parkinson's disease. *Neurology.* Jan 27 2004;62(2):177–180.

129. Tamer C, Melek IM, Duman T, Oksuz H. Tear film tests in Parkinson's disease patients. *Ophthalmology*. Oct 2005;112(10):1795.
130. Kwon OY, Kim SH, Kim JH, Kim MH, Ko MK. Schrimer test in Parkinson's disease. *J Korean Med Sci*. Jun 1994;9(3):239–242.
131. Bagheri H, Berlan M, Senard JM, Rascol O, Montastruc JL. Lacrimation in Parkinson's disease. *Clin Neuropharmacol*. Feb 1994;17(1):89–91.

Index

Note: Page numbers followed by "*f*" and "*t*" denote figures and tables, respectively.

312

Index